THE PARAI
REVIEW

•

BOB ELLING, MPA, REMT-P
KIRSTEN M. ELLING, BS, REMT-P

Technical Reviewer

TERRY DEVITO, RN, MEd, EMT-P, CEN

DELMAR

THOMSON LEARNING™

Albany Bonn Boston Cincinnati Detroit London Madrid Melbourne
Mexico City New York Pacific Grove Paris San Francisco
Singapore Tokyo Toronto Washington

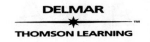

DELMAR
™
THOMSON LEARNING

The Paramedic Review
by Bob Elling and Kirsten M. Elling

Health Care Publishing Director:
William Brottmiller

Executive Editor:
Cathy L. Esperti

Development Editor:
Darcy M. Scelsi

Executive Marketing Manager:
Dawn F. Gerrain

Channel Manager:
Jennifer McAvey

Production Editor:
Mary Colleen Liburdi

For permission to use material from this text or product, contact us by
Tel   (800) 730-2214
Fax   (800) 730-2215
www.thomsonrights.com

Library of Congress Cataloging-in-Publication Data
Elling, Bob
    The paramedic review / Bob Elling, Kristen M. Elling ; technical
reviewer, Terry Devito.
        p. ; cm.
    Includes bibliographical references and index.
    ISBN 0-7668-3118-3
    1. Emergency medical technicians—Examinations, questions, etc.   I.
Elling, Kirsten M.   II. Title
    [DNLM: 1. Emergency Medical Services—Examination Questions. 2.
Emergency Medical Technicians—Examination Questions. WX 18.2
E46p 2002]
RC86.9 .E43 2002
616.02'5'076—dc21   2001054381

NOTICE TO THE READER

Contents

Dedication

This work is dedicated to Kirsten and my daughters Laura and Caitlin.
May you always maintain humility as your accomplishments meet the stars.

—BOB ELLING

In memory of my mother Inge Nicholson, 1940–2000, whose love and support I miss very much;
To my husband Bob, whose support and inspiration continue to drive me to
continuously improve patient care in the field.

—KIRSTEN M. ELLING

Special Thanks

Our deepest thanks to our close friend and colleague Mikel A. Rothenberg, MD
for all his hard work, insight, and guidance during the development of
the companion text, "Why-Driven EMS Enrichment" book.

About the Authors

Bob Elling, MPA, REMT-P

Bob has been involved in EMS since 1975 and is currently a faculty member for the Institute of Prehospital Emergency Medicine at Hudson Valley Community College in Troy, NY. Bob teaches in the EMT–Basic, Paramedic, and recertification courses. Bob has served as the Institute's Program Director and was responsible for providing leadership in the expansion of the Institute, accreditation of the paramedic program, as well as the development of the AAS: EMT–Paramedic degree.

Bob is an active paramedic with the Town of Colonie EMS Department. He is a member of the NYS Department of Health EMS Bureau's Regional Faculty as well as an American Heart Association National Faculty member.

Bob is also a Professor of management at the American College of Prehospital Medicine, Richardson University, which is a distance learning college in Florida. He is a member of the JEMS editorial review board, as well as the author of many articles, video scripts and books such as: *Essentials of Emergency Care, First Responder Exam Preparation and Review, Emergency Care Student Workbook, Pocket Reference For The EMT–Basic and First Responder, Essentials of Emergency Care Instructor's Resource Manual, MedReview For The EMT–Basic*, a co-author of *Why–Driven EMS Enrichment*, a contributing author for *Paramedic Care: Principles & Practice*, a co-author of the *National First Responder, Paramedic and EMT–Intermediate Curricula.*

Bob has served as a paramedic and lieutenant for NYC EMS, the Associate Director for NYS EMS, Education Coordinator for PULSE: Emergency Medical Update, Evaluation Coordinator for REMO, and a firefighter-paramedic in Colonie throughout his 26-year EMS career.

Kirsten M. Elling, BS, REMT-P

Kirsten (Kirt) Elling is a career paramedic who works in the Town of Colonie in upstate New York. She began work in EMS in 1988 as an EMT/firefighter and has been a National Registered paramedic since 1991. She has been an EMS educator since 1990 and teaches basic and advanced EMS programs at the Institute of Prehospital Emergency Medicine in Troy, New York. Kirt serves as Regional Faculty NYS DOH, Bureau of EMS and Regional Faculty American Heart Association, Northeast region. She has written numerous scripts for the EMS training video series *PULSE: Emergency Medical Update*, is a co-author of *Why–Driven EMS Enrichment,* contributing author of the *Paramedic Lab Manual* for the IPEM, and an adjunct writer for the 1998 revision of the National Highway Traffic Safety Administration, EMT–Paramedic and EMT–Intermediate: National Standard Curricula.

Preface

Paramedic training has evolved quite a bit since I first completed the program at the Institute of Albert Einstein Medical School in "da-Bronx" back in 1978. I remember the first day of class when Dr. J. and the instructor coordinator wheeled in a hand truck piled high with papers that we used as our textbook. Most of the materials consisted of the yet-unpublished draft of the Paramedic book that Nancy Caroline, MD had just completed for the U.S. DOT and lots of interesting articles from the medical journals.

These days, it is hard to find a 15-module trained medic still working in the field. Both Kirsten, my co-author and partner, and I have seen the curriculum become more enriched and sophisticated in 1985 with the six division program and then again in 1998 with the latest revision. Working as paramedics and EMS educators for the past 12 years and 26 years respectively, both Kirsten and I have seen medic training evolve firsthand.

Today there are many choices of books, magazines, video, workbooks, and websites for instructors to use to prepare their students for the streets. We sincerely hope you will agree that this book, *The Paramedic Review*, will be a valuable tool to help review and prepare for state and national examinations.

Earlier this year, together with our colleague Mikel Rothenberg, MD, we completed the companion text to the review book *Why-Driven EMS Enrichment*. That book as well as this review book are designed to follow the organizational chapter format of the DOT Paramedic curriculum (with the excepetion of the two resuscitation chapters 9 and 52).

The *Enrichment* book is designed for all levels of EMS providers, whereas the information tested in this book is specifically for paramedics. To save space in this book, so we could devote the majority of the book to review questions rather than the answer key, you will find the answer key at the end of the book listing just the letter of the correct answer. If you would like a more detailed explanation to the questions in this boook as well as enrichment of the parmedic objectives, we suggest you purchase the companion text, *Why-Driven EMS Enrichment*. Both books use the same chapter names and numbers to make it easy to refer back and forth.

Early in this project we made a decision that the questions would only be the multiple choice style with the standard format of three distractors and one correct answer to each question. Since this book will be used to prepare for both State and National paramedic examinations, it makes the most sense to use the format and style of questions used on these types of exams.

For each question there is one correct answer. When you have difficulty narrowing the choice down always read through all four choices and select the best choice. There are over 2,800 questions in this book. We suggest you tackle a chapter at a time and after taking each exam, check the answer key and mark the ones you need to review the material on.

We sincerely hope you will enjoy *The Paramedic Review* and benefit from the test-taking review to expand your knowledge base. After all, when the real test occurs, in the field, our patients rely on us to be prepared.

See you in the streets!

—*Bob & Kirsten Elling*

The Paramedic Review consists of multiple choice questions covering all topics in the 1999 DOT National Standard Curriculum. The chapter order follows that of the curriculum for ease of reference and use. *The Paramedic Review* is the perfect resource for preparing for the National Registry written exam. The CD that accompanies the text mimics typical state and national exam formats. A practice exam will be generated that will present the same number of questions from the same topic areas that are covered in the National Registry exam. This will allow you to time yourself and track your progress. The CD will summarize your results and show you the topic areas that you need to study in greater depth.

1

The Well-Being of the EMS Provider

1. _____ is defined as a state of complete physical, mental and social well being.

   a. Health
   b. Wellness
   c. Fitness
   d. Nutrition

2. The components of wellness include physical well-being, proper nutrition and:

   a. vaccinations.
   b. past medical history.
   c. mental and emotional health.
   d. compliance with prescribed medications.

3. Proper nutrition involves an understanding of nutrients the body needs, as well as the principles of:

   a. mental health.
   b. emotional well-being.
   c. exercise.
   d. weight control.

4. According to the Surgeon General's Report on Nutrition and Health, diet-related diseases account for over _____ of all deaths in the United States.

   a. one-quarter
   b. one-third
   c. one-half
   d. two-thirds

5. Poor diet and nutrition contribute to the development of degenerative diseases that include all the following major killers, *except*:

   a. heart disease.
   b. gout.
   c. diabetes.
   d. stroke.

6. The diets of EMS providers are often complicated by meals that are rushed, interrupted, and:

   a. limited access to choices of food types.
   b. increased susceptibility to lactose intolerance.
   c. low in cholesterol.
   d. high in vitamins and complex carbohydrates.

7. All the following are ways the EMS provider can eat better at work, *except*:

   a. prepare meals in advance.
   b. expand the range of foods from your normal choices.
   c. stop for fast food when you did not bring a meal.
   d. bring along a small cooler with fresh fruits or vegetables.

8. Reasonable changes in diet include all the following, *except*:

   a. watching only the calories, not the fat.
   b. making a slow transition.
   c. making small changes.
   d. drinking more fluids before and during meals.

9. Snacking will not make you fat unless you overdo it. All the following are accurate tips on snacking, *except*:

   a. high fiber snacks are better for dental health.
   b. eating a low calorie snack two hours before a meal will decrease your appetite for the meal.
   c. waiting until you are starving before you eat a snack will better satisfy your hunger.
   d. snacks can fill the voids in meals throughout the day and should be a part of your food plan.

10. Being physically fit involves a combination of all the following elements, *except*:

    a. aerobic conditioning.
    b. having a personal trainer.
    c. strength and endurance.
    d. attitude.

11. Before starting a fitness program, it is a good idea to get a physical examination by a physician because:

    a. a physician will identify any specific limitations to consider.
    b. most gyms require medical clearance before joining.
    c. athletic trainers require medical clearance before working with new clients.
    d. your physician will prescribe steroids to help you increase muscle mass.

12. All the following immunizations are required for paramedics, *except*:

    a. tetanus & diphtheria.
    b. rubella.
    c. Lyme disease.
    d. hepatitis B

13. All the following are benefits of being physically fit, *except*:

    a. improved personal appearance and self-image.
    b. increased resistance to injury.
    c. increased blood pressure and resting heart rate.
    d. increased muscle mass and metabolism.

14. Routine aerobic exercise lasting at least 20 minutes, three times a week improves the cardiac stroke volume of the heart while increasing:

    a. the resting heart rate.
    b. wear and tear on the heart.
    c. nutritional fortitude.
    d. physical endurance.

15. _____ are regular changes in mental and physical characteristics that occur in the course of a day.

    a. Anxieties
    b. Circadian rhythms
    c. Addictions
    d. Stimulants

16. Major industrial accidents, such as the Exxon Valdez oil spill, have been attributed partly to errors made by:

    a. fatigued night shift workers.
    b. smokers who suffered a stroke.
    c. stressed obese shift workers.
    d. overdose on No Doz®.

17. When considering the risk assessment for cardiovascular disease, the paramedic should take into account all the following, *except*:

    a. blood pressure.
    b. stress.
    c. exposure to the sun.
    d. triglycerides.

18. In relationship to cancer, the paramedic should consider all the following in the risk assessment, *except*:

    a. dietary changes.
    b. the need for regular examinations.
    c. exposure to the sun.
    d. personal hygiene.

19. Which of the following is not a recommended safety tip for proper lifting techniques?

    a. Use caution and know your limits.
    b. Avoid bending at the hips and knees.
    c. Do not twist when lifting.
    d. Keep the load close to your body.

20. All the following are recommended tips for managing a hostile scene situation, *except*:

    a. stand your ground while waiting for the police.
    b. always leave yourself an exit.
    c. always bring the radio.
    d. retreat when danger is imminent.

21. The typical profile of an ambulance collision is one that occurs in the:

    a. winter while driving on snow and ice.
    b. daytime on clear, dry roads.
    c. fall when the roads are covered with wet leaves.
    d. night involving intoxicated drivers.

22. Knowledge of the proper use of lights and sirens as well as the public's typical reactions includes the understanding that:

    a. these devices guarantee you the right of way.
    b. there are limitations with these device.
    c. the public has to yield the right of way.
    d. driving an emergency vehicle requires a special course.

23. All the following can reduce the risks associated with driving an emergency vehicle, *except*:

    a. using a police escort whenever possible.
    b. using due regard for the safety of all others.
    c. always driving with the headlights on to be more easily seen.
    d. use proper child restraints when transporting children.

24. When developing strategies to help eliminate ambulance collisions, you should consider all the following areas, *except*:

    a. hands-on-training.
    b. knowledge of standard operating procedures (SOPs).
    c. familiarity with the ambulance size and weight.
    d. knowledge of the use of global position systems (GPS).

25. EMS agencies should have an SOP for their drivers consisting of all the following, *except*:

    a. how to qualify drivers.
    b. the proper way to change a tire.
    c. what to do when a collision occurs.
    d. a policy on prudent speed.

26. Safety equipment that EMS personnel use at the scene of a crash includes:

    a. head protection, such as a helmet.
    b. eye protection, such as safety goggles or shields.
    c. a turnout coat to protect from sharp objects.
    d. all of the above.

27. Twenty minutes after the cessation of smoking cigarettes all the following physical changes occur, *except* the:

    a. blood pressure decreases.
    b. blood pressure increases.
    c. pulse rate drops.
    d. body temperature of the hands and feet increases.

28. At one year after the cessation of cigarette smoking the excess risk of coronary heart diseases is decreased to _____ of a smoker.

    a. one-fourth
    b. one-third
    c. one-half
    d. two-thirds

29. Which of the following is not accurate about the cessation of cigarette smoking?

    a. Even heavy smokers can benefit significantly by stopping.
    b. For long-time smokers stopping is not of any benefit.
    c. At 5–10 years after quitting the stroke risk is reduced to that of non-smokers.
    d. Nicotine is a drug that causes addiction.

30. All the following are accurate about the effects of nicotine, *except*:

    a. nicotine has no effect on nerve cells.
    b. withdrawal is difficult with nicotine.
    c. nicotine can act as a stimulant.
    d. nicotine can act as a sedative.

31. A/an _____ is a compulsive need for and use of a habit-forming substance.

    a. anxiety
    b. addiction
    c. biorhythm
    d. stimulant

32. Stress is defined as a factor that induces bodily or mental tension. Which of the following is not correct in reference to stress?

    a. Stress is a natural and necessary emotion.
    b. Stress is a harmful emotion that should be avoided.
    c. Stress is experienced with positive events.
    d. Stress is experienced with negative events.

33. There are three distinct phases in a stress response which include all the following, *except* the:

    a. alarm reaction.
    b. resistance phase.
    c. denial phase.
    d. exhaustion phase.

34. The physiologic response of the alarm reaction includes all the following, *except*:

    a. increased pulse and B/P.
    b. decreased blood sugar.
    c. dilation of the pupils.
    d. slowed digestion.

35. A person can become desensitized or adapted to extreme stressors. This is a result of an increase in the:

    a. level of resistance in the resistance phase.
    b. production of epinephrine in the alarm reaction phase.
    c. norepinephrine released during the denial phase.
    d. glucose production from a pituitary response.

36. As stress continues, and coping mechanisms are exhausted, the body will have an increased:

    a. release of adrenocorticotrophic hormones.
    b. pulse rate and blood pressure.
    c. resistance to stressors.
    d. susceptibility to physical and psychological ailments.

37. Factors that can trigger a stress response include all the following, *except*:

   a. glucose production.
   b. poor health or nutrition.
   c. injury to the body.
   d. ineffective coping.

38. Which of the following is not usually considered a physical sign or symptom of stress?

   a. Chest tightness or pain.
   b. Flushed skin.
   c. Aching muscles and joints.
   d. Dry skin.

39. The emotional signs and symptoms of stress include all the following, *except*:

   a. panic reactions.
   b. poor concentration.
   c. feeling overwhelmed.
   d. anger.

40. All the following are cognitive signs and symptoms of stress, *except*:

   a. fear.
   b. disorientation.
   c. memory problems.
   d. distressing dreams.

41. Which of the following is not usually considered a behavioral sign or symptom of stress?

   a. Hyperactivity
   b. Increased smoking
   c. Withdrawal
   d. Heart palpitations

42. _____ is an example of an environmental stress trigger.

   a. Siren noise
   b. Inclement weather
   c. Confined workspace
   d. All of the above.

43. An example of a psychosocial stress trigger is:

   a. a conflict with a supervisor or coworker.
   b. a rapid scene response.
   c. life and death decision making.
   d. hyperventilation syndrome.

44. Personality or emotional stress are often triggered by any of the following, *except*:

   a. personal expectations.
   b. feelings of guilt.
   c. feelings of incompetence.
   d. nausea or vomiting.

45. _____ is an active process of confronting the stress or cause of the stress.

   a. Putting up defenses
   b. Coping
   c. Exposure
   d. Gaining experience

46. Examples of techniques used to manage stress include all the following, *except*:

   a. reframing.
   b. controlled breathing.
   c. progressive relaxation.
   d. guided hyperactivity.

47. _____ is an organized process that enables emergency personnel to vent feelings and facilitates understanding of stressful situations.

   a. Coping for EMS providers (CEMSP)
   b. EMS problem solving (EMSPS)
   c. Emergency EMS distress (EEMSD)
   d. Critical incident stress management (CISM)

48. The components of the organized process described in question 47 include all the following, *except*:

   a. a defusing after a large scale event.
   b. on-scene support of distressed personnel at a major incident.
   c. financial support of post-traumatic stress syndrome.
   d. follow-up mental health services.

49. Examples of common situations that the services provided by the process described in question 48 include all the following, *except*:

   a. disaster situations.
   b. reversal of a cardiac arrest.
   c. emergency worker suicide.
   d. an extreme threat to emergency workers.

50. The key techniques for reducing crisis-induced stress include all the following, *except*:

   a. getting plenty of rest.
   b. replacing food and fluids.
   c. increased cigarette smoking.
   d. limiting exposure to the incident.

51. During the grieving process it is not unusual for families to vent their anger on the paramedic. As long as there is no perceived physical harm to you it is best to:

   a. allow them to express their feelings as best as you can.
   b. walk away as it could get personal.
   c. give them your opinion based on your experience.
   d. let them argue with the police instead.

52. In which developmental age group do children begin to understand the finality of death?

    a. 3 to 6 years old
    b. 6 to 9 years old
    c. 9 to 12 years old
    d. Adolescents

53. Which of the following statements about helping children deal with grief is most accurate?

    a. It is less distressing for the child to see that "everything is normal."
    b. Tell the truth and be straightforward when talking about the death of a loved one.
    c. Shielding a child from grief may protect them in the long run.
    d. A child seeing his father cry over mom's death is an unnecessary burden on a child.

54. The stages of the grieving process include all the following, *except*:

    a. shock.
    b. withdrawal.
    c. denial.
    d. bargaining.

55. Prevention of disease transmission by the EMS provider includes all the following, *except*:

    a. protection against airborne pathogens.
    b. protection against blood-borne pathogens.
    c. following recommended guidelines for proper cleaning and disinfection.
    d. sterilizing all ambulance equipment on a regular basis.

56. A/an _____ is contact with a potentially infectious body fluid substance that may be carrying a pathogen.

    a. exposure
    b. removal
    c. body substance isolation
    d. preventive measure

57. All the following are included as part of the procedure for managing an exposure, *except*:

    a. documenting the situation in which the exposure occurred.
    b. safeguarding against disciplinary action.
    c. cooperating with incident investigation.
    d. completing the required medical follow-up.

58. When documenting an exposure the paramedic should include:

    a. periodic risk assessment.
    b. ongoing exposure control training.
    c. actions taken to reduce chances of infection.
    d. obtaining proper immunization boosters.

59. _____ is cleaning the surface of objects with a specific agent designed to kill pathogens that may have come in contact with the object.

    a. Cleaning
    b. Disinfection
    c. Sterilization
    d Isolation precaution

60. BSI is an acronym for body substance isolation procedures, which are a series of practices designed to:

    a. prevent lapses in immunizations.
    b. improve screening for exposures.
    c. improve personal hygiene habits.
    d. prevent contact with body substances such as blood and urine.

61. There are a number of ways to positively deal with excessive stress, such as:

    a. alcohol.
    b. biofeedback.
    c. decreasing exercise.
    d. overeating.

62. All the following are used to treat stress, *except*:

    a. vaccination.
    b. patient education.
    c. medication.
    d. psychotherapy.

Test #1 Answer Form

	A	B	C	D			A	B	C	D
1.	❏	❏	❏	❏		26.	❏	❏	❏	❏
2.	❏	❏	❏	❏		27.	❏	❏	❏	❏
3.	❏	❏	❏	❏		28.	❏	❏	❏	❏
4.	❏	❏	❏	❏		29.	❏	❏	❏	❏
5.	❏	❏	❏	❏		30.	❏	❏	❏	❏
6.	❏	❏	❏	❏		31.	❏	❏	❏	❏
7.	❏	❏	❏	❏		32.	❏	❏	❏	❏
8.	❏	❏	❏	❏		33.	❏	❏	❏	❏
9.	❏	❏	❏	❏		34.	❏	❏	❏	❏
10.	❏	❏	❏	❏		35.	❏	❏	❏	❏
11.	❏	❏	❏	❏		36.	❏	❏	❏	❏
12.	❏	❏	❏	❏		37.	❏	❏	❏	❏
13.	❏	❏	❏	❏		38.	❏	❏	❏	❏
14.	❏	❏	❏	❏		39.	❏	❏	❏	❏
15.	❏	❏	❏	❏		40.	❏	❏	❏	❏
16.	❏	❏	❏	❏		41.	❏	❏	❏	❏
17.	❏	❏	❏	❏		42.	❏	❏	❏	❏
18.	❏	❏	❏	❏		43.	❏	❏	❏	❏
19.	❏	❏	❏	❏		44.	❏	❏	❏	❏
20.	❏	❏	❏	❏		45.	❏	❏	❏	❏
21.	❏	❏	❏	❏		46.	❏	❏	❏	❏
22.	❏	❏	❏	❏		47.	❏	❏	❏	❏
23.	❏	❏	❏	❏		48.	❏	❏	❏	❏
24.	❏	❏	❏	❏		49.	❏	❏	❏	❏
25.	❏	❏	❏	❏		50.	❏	❏	❏	❏

	A	B	C	D			A	B	C	D
51.	❏	❏	❏	❏		57.	❏	❏	❏	❏
52.	❏	❏	❏	❏		58.	❏	❏	❏	❏
53.	❏	❏	❏	❏		59.	❏	❏	❏	❏
54.	❏	❏	❏	❏		60.	❏	❏	❏	❏
55.	❏	❏	❏	❏		61.	❏	❏	❏	❏
56.	❏	❏	❏	❏		62.	❏	❏	❏	❏

2

Roles and Responsibilities
of the EMS Provider

1. The first civilian ambulance service was started in _____ in 1865.

    a. New York City
    b. Cincinnati
    c. Philadelphia
    d. Chicago

2. In _____ the first known air medical transport occurred during the retreat of the Serbian army from Albania.

    a. 1915
    b. 1930
    c. 1955
    d. 1962

3. In the _____ many of the first volunteer rescue squads were organized in Roanoke, Virginia and along the New Jersey coast.

    a. 1920s
    b. 1930s
    c. 1940s
    d. 1950s

4. In 1960 _____ was first shown to be an effective treatment method for cardiac arrest.

    a. intubation
    b. epinephrine administration
    c. sodium bicarbonate
    d. CPR

5. In 1966 landmark legislation called the _____ created the U.S. Department of Transportation (DOT) as a cabinet level department and required the Secretary of DOT to develop EMS training programs.

    a. White Paper
    b. Highway Safety Act
    c. Committee on Traffic Safety report
    d. EMT–Ambulance curriculum

6. In 1970 the _____ was established with DOT to provide leadership to the EMS community and states as well as federal agencies involved in EMS.

    a. television show EMERGENCY
    b. Board of Directors of the National Registry of EMTs
    c. Emergency Medical Services Systems Act
    d. National Highway Traffic Safety Administration

7. In 1974 DOT published the "KKK-A-1822" Federal:

    a. educational standards.
    b. Emergency Medical Dispatch system.
    c. Ambulance Specifications.
    d. Standards for CPR.

8. In 1983 the American College of Surgeons identified the:

    a. standard equipment to be carried on BLS ambulances.
    b. standard equipment to be carried on ALS ambulances.
    c. first trauma training program.
    d. first trauma care system.

9. The _____ EMT–Basic curriculum included the use of the automated external defibrillator as a skill taught to the EMT, rather than reserved for only the advanced levels of EMTs.

    a. 1985
    b. 1990
    c. 1995
    d. 1998

10. A/an _____ is a coordinated effort to bring together at least ten key components to reduce out-of-hospital morbidity and mortality.

    a. EMS curriculum
    b. NHTSA Act
    c. EMS system
    d. emergency medical dispatch flow chart

11. Permission that is granted by a government authority to practice in a profession, business or activity is called:

    a. certification.
    b. licensure.
    c. public access.
    d. registration.

12. A _____ is a document testifying to the fulfillment of the requirements for practice in the field.

    a. certification
    b. licensure
    c. public access
    d. registration

13. Which of the following is not one of the four national levels of out-of-hospital training that is recognized by the National Registry of Emergency Medical Technicians?

    a. First Responder
    b. EMT–Basic
    c. Critical Care Technician
    d. EMT–Paramedic

14. The level of provider that is not intended to be utilized as the minimum staffing for an ambulance is the:

    a. First responder.
    b. Critical Care Technician.
    c. EMT–A.
    d. EMT–B.

15. The roles and responsibilities of the _____ include: providing safety, initial assessment and treatment, including immediate resuscitative measures, and portraying a professional and positive appearance.

    a. First Responder
    b. EMT–Intermediate
    c. EMT–Paramedic
    d. All the above

16. All the following are roles of the National Registry, *except*:

    a. contributing to the development of professional standards.
    b. verifying competency of EMS providers.
    c. simplifying the process of state-to-state reciprocity or credentialing.
    d. licensing the EMS provider once competency has been verified.

17. The recertification of EMS providers varies from state to state and includes all the following methods, *except*:

    a. taking a recertification course.
    b. "challenging" by demonstrating competency through testing.
    c. giving credit through reciprocity with another state.
    d. utilizing continuing medical education.

18. _____ is the legal recognition of training obtained in another state.

    a. Recertification
    b. Challenging
    c. Reciprocity
    d. National Registration

19. The benefits of continuing education for the EMS provider include all the following, *except*:

    a. it is better than taking a refresher course.
    b. increasing the EMS provider's knowledge base.
    c. increasing the EMS provider's understanding of relevant EMS issues.
    d. refreshing skills.

20. In EMS, examples of professionalism include all the following, *except*:

    a. indifference.
    b. a good practice ethic.
    c. good personal hygiene.
    d. good time management.

21. All the following are accurate statements about health care professionals, *except*:

    a. health care providers work to instill pride in their profession.
    b. health care providers conform to the standards of health care by providing quality patient care.
    c. there are high expectations by society of health care professionals on duty.
    d. the expectations by society of health care professionals is lower when off duty.

22. _____ are moral principles of one's practice in his or her profession.

    a. Standards of care
    b. Ethics
    c. Peer review
    d. Professional conduct

23. Constructive feedback by other EMS providers in a genuine effort to improve future performance is called:

    a. quality control.
    b. quality improvement.
    c. peer review.
    d. the standard of care.

24. One of the most important attributes of an EMS provider is integrity. All the following are examples of this attribute, *except*:

    a. showing a coworker how to lift a patient.
    b. always telling the truth.
    c. never stealing.
    d. providing complete and accurate documentation.

25. Examples of behavior demonstrating empathy include all the following, *except*:

    a. showing caring and compassion for others.
    b. being supportive and reassuring to others.
    c. demonstrating an understanding of the patients feelings.
    d. suppressing your own feelings when you are overwhelmed.

26. _____ acknowledges the patient's circumstances and how serious they must be without the provider becoming emotionally involved.

    a. Empathy
    b. Sympathy
    c. Pity
    d. Kindness

27. Examples of demonstrating self-confidence include:

    a. consulting with Medical Direction after the patient's condition deteriorates.
    b. having a good understanding of your limitations.
    c. calling for backup after realizing the patient you are lifting is too heavy.
    d. being able to call for help once you are overwhelmed.

28. A neat and professional appearance, well groomed and clean, are important and:

    a. very subjective qualities of an EMT–B.
    b. an indication of your competency and skills.
    c. show respect to the patient and their family.
    d. help to instill confidence in the patient and their families.

29. Good time management skills involve all the following, *except*:

    a. prioritizing tasks during patient care.
    b. being punctual for meetings.
    c. attending a required continuing education class.
    d. being prepared to work when the shift begins.

30. In order for a patient to have a positive outcome, the paramedic must:

    a. work well as a member of a team.
    b. be punctual for all training classes.
    c. show up on time for work.
    d. be prepared to work alone.

31. _____ is defined as tact and skill in dealing with people.

    a. Respect
    b. Diplomacy
    c. Team work
    d. Communication

32. All the following are examples of behavior demonstrating teamwork, *except*:

    a. disagreeing with each other in private.
    b. disagreeing with each other in public.
    c. remaining flexible and open to change.
    d. communicating in an effort to solve problems.

33. Patients are at a disadvantage when thrust into the health care system because of a sudden illness or injury; this is why part of the responsibility of the paramedic is to:

    a. let their neighbors know which hospital you took them to.
    b. let them use your cell phone to call a friend.
    c. take their wallet or purse for safe keeping.
    d. be an advocate for your patient.

34. Patient advocate activities include all the following, *except*:

    a. being involved in EMS education.
    b. teaching the community about safety and prevention methods.
    c. being involved in your Regional EMS Council.
    d. telling the patient he made a stupid error when he did not buckle up.

35. Examples of behavior demonstrating patient advocacy include:

    a. placing the patient's safety above your own.
    b. protecting the patient's confidentiality.
    c. rushing a patient report to get out of work on time.
    d. allowing personal bias to influence patient care.

36. All the following are examples of behavior demonstrating a careful delivery of service, *except*:

    a. mastering and refreshing skills.
    b. following a good nutritional diet.
    c. performing complete equipment checks each shift.
    d. following medical protocols.

37. The primary role of the Medical Director of an EMS agency is to:

    a. ensure quality patient care.
    b. oversee all continuing education.
    c. delineate the quality control process.
    d. evaluate and revise patient access to definitive care.

38. _____ are guidelines for the management of specific patient presenting problems.

    a. Diagnosis
    b. Algorithms
    c. Protocols
    d. Definitive care standards

39. Typical roles of the EMS physician include all the following, *except*:

    a. education and training of personnel.
    b. participation in equipment selection.
    c. providing interface between EMS systems and the families of patients.
    d. serving as the medical conscience of the EMS organization.

40. Potential benefits of on-line (direct) medical control include:

    a. the ability to obtain real time direction and orders.
    b. interfacing with a physician for more effective treatment.
    c. treatment orders that are more efficient.
    d. quicker access to definitive care.

41. Off-line (indirect) medical control primarily relies on:

    a. stop lines.
    b. protocols.
    c. ACLS algorithms.
    d. advanced directives.

42. If a physician stops at the scene of your call and offers assistance, which of the following should you do before consenting to allow his/her assistance?

    a. Confirm that person is actually a medical doctor and not a Ph.D.
    b. Confirm that the physician is willing to come to the hospital with you and the patient.
    c. Let the physician speak to your medical control so they can work together.
    d. All of the above.

43. EMS providers are responsible for being prepared in which of the following ways?

    a. By getting a college education.
    b. By having a lawyer on retainer for potential law suits.
    c. By knowing as many residents personally in the area where you work.
    d. None of the above.

44. When determining the appropriate disposition for your patient you should consider all the following about the hospitals in your area, *except* their:

    a. resource capabilities.
    b. discharge facilities.
    c. clinical capabilities.
    d. levels of care.

45. Primary responsibilities for returning to service after a call includes all the following, *except*:

    a. disinfecting.
    b. restocking.
    c. regenerating.
    d. debriefing.

46. Which of the following is the most accurate benefit of having paramedics teach in the community?

    a. It enhances visibility and positive image of paramedics and their agencies.
    b. It ensures the safety of all the children in the community.
    c. It ensures proper utilization of the use of safety helmets.
    d. It helps to get the elderly compliant with medication use.

47. Examples of citizen involvement in EMS systems include all the following, *except*:

    a. learning how to access EMS.
    b. training and being willing to do bystander CPR.
    c. training to be a career paramedic/ firefighter.
    d. fundraising and lobbying for EMS improvements.

48. As the "scope of practice" evolves, the paramedic may be utilized in non-traditional activities such as:

a. patient checkup visits.
b. assisting with daily living activities.
c. assisting with physical therapy.
d. minor surgical procedures.

49. The expanded scope pilots have been utilized to bring medically trained health care professionals to the patients when they are underserved or:

a. the patient is in a Hospice program.
b. the transportation alternatives are very costly.
c. dental or chiropractic services are not affordable.
d. when a patient can not prepare his or her own meals.

50. In the document the *EMS Agenda for the Future*, integration of Health Services refers to:

a. EMS being aware of the special needs of the entire population.
b. allocating funding for HMOs.
c. developing paramedic jobs in private home care.
d. none of the above.

51. For the future, EMS research is developing strategies to:

a. develop information systems that provide linage between various health care services.
b. interpret informed consent rules to allow for clinical circumstances inherent to credible EMS research.
c. designate EMS as a physician subspecialty.
d. all of the above.

52. Legislation and regulation plans for the future in EMS are focused on all the following, *except*:

a. authorizing and funding a lead federal EMS agency.
b. establishing and funding the position of State EMS Medical Director in each state.
c. implementing laws that provide protection from liability for EMS providers when dealing with unusual situations.
d. implementing laws and funding that provide for liability insurance for all paid and volunteer providers.

53. System Finance in EMS is striving for which of the following?

a. To commission the development of government funded health care.
b. Collaboration with other health care providers and insurers to enhance patient care efficiency.
c. To compensate EMS on the basis of volume.
d. To provide immediate access to the Medicare approval process.

54. Strategies for the future in respect to Human Resources are working for all the following, *except* to:

a. develop a system for reciprocity of EMS provider credentials.
b. formalize paramedicine as a subspecialty of home health care.
c. develop collaborative relationships between EMS system and academic institutions.
d. conduct EMS occupations health research.

55. A key proposal for Medical Direction in the future is to:

a. require appropriate credentials for all those who provide on-line medical direction.
b. develop a system for reciprocity of EMS physician credentials.
c. ensure that Medical Directors are allocated federal funding for participating in an EMS system.
d. appoint national EMS Medical Directors.

56. Education Systems in EMS are striving to develop which of the following?

a. Accreditation for EMS education programs.
b. Bridging and transitioning EMS programs with all health professions' education.
c. National core contents to replace EMS program curricula.
d. All of the above.

57. Goals for EMS public education for the future include:

a. relying on HMOs to get the message out.
b. collaborating efforts with federally funded programs.
c. exploring and evaluating public education alternatives.
d. none of the above.

58. Goals for the future of EMS communications systems include all the following, *except* to:

    a. promulgate and update standards for EMS dispatching.
    b. provide the 9-1-1 emergency telephone service to GPS monitors.
    c. assess the effectiveness of resource attributes for EMS dispatching.
    d. update geographically integrated and functionally-based EMS communications networks.

59. One of the major goals in the clinical care aspect of EMS is to:

    a. commit to a common definition of what constitutes base line community EMS care.
    b. subject EMS clinical care to ongoing evaluation to determine its impact on patient outcomes.
    c. establish proactive relationships between EMS and other health care providers.
    d. all the above are major goals.

60. EMS information systems are working toward all the following goals, *except*:

    a. incorporating task analyses to configure staffing of patient transfers.
    b. developing a mechanism to generate and transmit data that are valid, reliable and accurate.
    c. developing integrated information systems with other health care providers.
    d. adopting uniform data elements and definitions.

61. In the document the *EMS Agenda for the Future*, elements of the evaluation component include all the following, *except*:

    a. developing valid models for EMS evaluations which incorporate consumer input.
    b. evaluating EMS standards for high earning potentials.
    c. evaluating EMS effects for various medical conditions.
    d. determining EMS effects for multiple outcome categories and cost-effectiveness.

62. Continuous quality improvement (CQI) is a process that is designed to:

    a. focus on specific problem individuals within an organization.
    b. uncover problems and provide solutions.
    c. correct life-threatening patient conditions.
    d. monitor the work performance of field paramedics.

63. Research in EMS is important for all the following reasons, *except*:

    a. research helps to enhance recognition and respect for EMS professionals.
    b. outcome studies are needed to assure the continued funding for EMS system grants.
    c. changes in professional standards, training and equipment need to be based on empirical data.
    d. research can be influenced by biases.

64. The role of EMS providers in data collection is to enthusiastically participate and honestly comply with the study requirements without:

    a. changing the sample size.
    b. obtaining informed consent.
    c. changing the initial hypothesis.
    d. negatively affecting patient care.

65. All the following are basic concepts of performing research, *except*:

    a. valuing peer review and publishing research.
    b. randomized and controlled groups.
    c. changing patient care standards.
    d. blinding the study.

66. Which of the following is not one of the typical steps in the procedure for conducting research in EMS?

    a. Collect the funding needs for the hypothesis development.
    b. Preparation of the question to be studied.
    c. Describe who the populations to be studied will be.
    d. Obtain legal advice on how to obtain informed consent.

67. Which of the following is not one of the three general areas of prehospital research?

    a. Arriving at conclusions based on scientifically sound procedures.
    b. Arriving at conclusions based on unethical procedures.
    c. Answering a clinically important question.
    d. Providing results that lead to system improvements.

68. When assessing the validity of research findings, all the following questions should be critically considered, *except*:

    a. was the research peer reviewed?
    b. who developed the hypothesis?
    c. what types of data were collected?
    d. was the data properly analyzed?

69. Which of the following is not an EMS provider level that is described in the DOT curriculum?

   a. EMT–B
   b. Cardiac rescue technician (CRT)
   c. EMT–Intermediate
   d. Paramedic

70. A _____ is a "calling" requiring specialized preparation and specific academic preparation.

   a. validation
   b. credential
   c. profession
   d. business

71. Which of the following is not accurate about the public image of health care workers?

   a. Your image and behavior in the public's eye are not significant.
   b. EMS providers are very visible role models whose behaviors are closely observed.
   c. Your actions in public represent the image of your peers as well as your own.
   d. If people see you not wearing your seat belt, they may think that seatbelts are really unnecessary.

72. Empathy should be demonstrated by the paramedic to all the following people, *except* to:

   a. patients.
   b. the families of patients.
   c. yourself.
   d. other health care providers.

73. Which of the following is an example of behavior that demonstrates self-motivation by the paramedic?

   a. Not accepting constructive feedback, because there is no such thing.
   b. Taking advantage of all learning opportunities.
   c. Taking on selective tasks as recommended by supervision.
   d. Making corrections to improve work performance when advised.

74. For the paramedic these days, being a diplomat also involves saying and doing things that are considered:

   a. status quo.
   b. newsworthy.
   c. "political suicide."
   d. "politically correct."

75. For the paramedic, examples of behavior demonstrating good communication includes all the following, *except*:

   a. speaking clearly over the radio.
   b. writing legibly on PCRs.
   c. using sign language.
   d. adjusting communications strategies to various situations.

Test #2 Answer Form

	A	B	C	D			A	B	C	D
1.	❑	❑	❑	❑		26.	❑	❑	❑	❑
2.	❑	❑	❑	❑		27.	❑	❑	❑	❑
3.	❑	❑	❑	❑		28.	❑	❑	❑	❑
4.	❑	❑	❑	❑		29.	❑	❑	❑	❑
5.	❑	❑	❑	❑		30.	❑	❑	❑	❑
6.	❑	❑	❑	❑		31.	❑	❑	❑	❑
7.	❑	❑	❑	❑		32.	❑	❑	❑	❑
8.	❑	❑	❑	❑		33.	❑	❑	❑	❑
9.	❑	❑	❑	❑		34.	❑	❑	❑	❑
10.	❑	❑	❑	❑		35.	❑	❑	❑	❑
11.	❑	❑	❑	❑		36.	❑	❑	❑	❑
12.	❑	❑	❑	❑		37.	❑	❑	❑	❑
13.	❑	❑	❑	❑		38.	❑	❑	❑	❑
14.	❑	❑	❑	❑		39.	❑	❑	❑	❑
15.	❑	❑	❑	❑		40.	❑	❑	❑	❑
16.	❑	❑	❑	❑		41.	❑	❑	❑	❑
17.	❑	❑	❑	❑		42.	❑	❑	❑	❑
18.	❑	❑	❑	❑		43.	❑	❑	❑	❑
19.	❑	❑	❑	❑		44.	❑	❑	❑	❑
20.	❑	❑	❑	❑		45.	❑	❑	❑	❑
21.	❑	❑	❑	❑		46.	❑	❑	❑	❑
22.	❑	❑	❑	❑		47.	❑	❑	❑	❑
23.	❑	❑	❑	❑		48.	❑	❑	❑	❑
24.	❑	❑	❑	❑		49.	❑	❑	❑	❑
25.	❑	❑	❑	❑		50.	❑	❑	❑	❑

	A	B	C	D			A	B	C	D
51.	❏	❏	❏	❏		64.	❏	❏	❏	❏
52.	❏	❏	❏	❏		65.	❏	❏	❏	❏
53.	❏	❏	❏	❏		66.	❏	❏	❏	❏
54.	❏	❏	❏	❏		67.	❏	❏	❏	❏
55.	❏	❏	❏	❏		68.	❏	❏	❏	❏
56.	❏	❏	❏	❏		69.	❏	❏	❏	❏
57.	❏	❏	❏	❏		70.	❏	❏	❏	❏
58.	❏	❏	❏	❏		71.	❏	❏	❏	❏
59.	❏	❏	❏	❏		72.	❏	❏	❏	❏
60.	❏	❏	❏	❏		73.	❏	❏	❏	❏
61.	❏	❏	❏	❏		74.	❏	❏	❏	❏
62.	❏	❏	❏	❏		75.	❏	❏	❏	❏
63.	❏	❏	❏	❏						

3

Illness and Injury Prevention

1. _____ is the study of occurrence of disease.

   a. Morbidity
   b. Mortality
   c. Incidence
   d. Epidemiology

2. The extent of an injury or illness is called:

   a. morbidity.
   b. mortality.
   c. incidence.
   d. epidemiology.

3. What is the leading cause of overall deaths in the United States?

   a. Heart disease
   b. Malignant tumors
   c. Cerebrovascular diseases
   d. COPD

4. All the following are accurate about the causes of death when it is broken down by gender, age and race, *except*:

   a. for ages 1–44 accidents were the leading cause of death.
   b. those who had never married had a higher mortality than those who had married.
   c. life expectancy for males has just recently surpassed that of females.
   d. for ages 45–64 cancer is the leading cause of death.

5. Which of the following is an effect that has occurred as a result of early release/discharge of patients from the hospital?

   a. Home health care will reduce the overall lifetime cost of injuries.
   b. There are more expectations for EMS services to provide care of patients being managed in the home setting.
   c. This cost-cutting trend is going to decrease the reliance on EMS.
   d. More hospitals will rely on EMS to care for and transport patients that have had outpatient procedures.

6. The leading cause of death for white males age 15–24 is:

   a. accidents.
   b. homicide.
   c. HIV infection.
   d. suicide.

7. _____ is defined as a real or potential hazardous situation that puts individuals at risk for sustaining an injury.

   a. Harm's way
   b. Injury surveillance
   c. Injury prevention
   d. Injury risk

8. An important part of any injury surveillance program is the timely dissemination of the data to those who need to use it for:

   a. prevention and control efforts.
   b. obtaining funding through grants.
   c. treatment of patients.
   d. reversal of management plans.

9. _____ injury prevention are activities involved in the care of an injury that has already occurred to prevent it from getting worse.

   a. Primary
   b. Secondary
   c. Tertiary
   d. Productive

10. Activities that are involved in the rehabilitation of an injured person, such as preventing infections, are known as:

    a. a teachable moment.
    b. tertiary injury prevention.
    c. sensible ongoing care.
    d. productive quality care.

11. All the following are reasons why paramedics should be involved in prevention efforts in the community, *except* that they are:

    a. often thought of as the experts on injury and prevention.
    b. often high profile role models.
    c. in rural areas where the paramedics are too few to advocate for customers.
    d. welcome in schools, nursing homes, and other environments.

12. Which of the following statements about bicycle-related head injuries is not accurate?

    a. Over 95% of victims of bicycle-related head injuries were not wearing helmets when injured.
    b. Over half a million Americans who sustain a bicycle related injury require ED care annually.
    c. The solution to the problem is clearly lack of parental supervision.
    d. The solutions to the problem include education, legislation and distribution of helmets.

13. All the following are solutions to assist in the prevention of drowning, *except*:

    a. supervision of adults who drink while boating.
    b. mandating for four-sided isolation fencing around pools.
    c. requiring PFDs be worn whenever children or adults who cannot swim are on or near water.
    d. Public education on recommendations for prevention.

14. The key strategy for reducing deaths from motor vehicles is:

    a. reducing speed limits in school zones.
    b. mandating lower speed limits on the highways.
    c. advocating for more vehicles to include airbags.
    d. getting everyone in the vehicle to wear seat belts.

15. In 1970, the Poison Prevention Act required the U.S. Consumer Product Safety Commission to require the:

    a. use of residential smoke detectors.
    b. use of carbon monoxide detectors in commercial properties.
    c. instillation of locks for the storage of toxic substances in schools.
    d. use of child-resistant packaging of toxic substances for in home use.

16. According to the U.S. Poison Control Centers, more than 90% of poison exposures occur in:

    a. schools.
    b. hospitals.
    c. homes.
    d. work facilities.

17. Strategies for fire safety include all the following, *except*:

    a. practicing family fire escape plans every six months.
    b. changing the batteries on carbon monoxide and smoke alarms every five years.
    c. never smoking in bed.
    d. knowing what to do if your clothing catches fire.

18. Key strategies to reduce injury and death that occur from motorcycle collisions include:

    a. educating riders to always wear a helmet and protective gear.
    b. educating motor vehicle drivers to give way to riders.
    c. increasing insurance rates for riders who drink and drive.
    d. all of the above.

19. Statistics on playground safety reveal that a child is injured every _____ on a playground in the United States.

    a. two and a half minutes
    b. two and a half hours
    c. two and a half weeks
    d. none of the above

20. All the following are accurate statements about common injuries from falls, *except*:

    a. the most common cause of falls in the elderly is falling down stairs.
    b. the injuries affect the very young and very old to the greatest degree.
    c. childhood falls account for an estimated two million ED visits annually.
    d. one in every three adults 65 years or older falls each year.

21. Which of the following is not a recommended strategy for prevention of falls?

    a. Installing metal grates on windows in high rise buildings.
    b. Installing slip resistant carpets in kitchens and baths.
    c. Eliminating throw rugs and other trip hazards.
    d. Using shopping carts with straps for holding toddlers.

22. Causes of strangulation and suffocation among infants and children include all the following, *except*:

    a. drawstrings on curtains or blinds in the home.
    b. unattended child in a vehicle during hot weather.
    c. being trapped in an unsafe old crib.
    d. unattended child on a playground.

23. Key strategies for the prevention of firearm injuries and fatalities include all the following, *except*:

    a. disassembling the National Rifle Association.
    b. gun control and proper storage.
    c. training and licensing of handgun owners.
    d. mandates for trigger locks and loading indicators.

24. Of the approximately 82,000 auto–pedestrian injuries that occur annually, over _____ of those include children who often receive serious brain injury.

    a. 10,000
    b. 20,000
    c. 35,000
    d. 50,000

25. Key strategies for pedestrian safety include all the following, *except*:

    a. avoid drinking and walking.
    b. wear reflective clothing after dark.
    c. avoid crossing the road with small children.
    d. teach children to always look left-right-left before crossing the street.

26. One of the most effective ways EMS leaders can provide leadership in the area of illness and injury prevention is to:

    a. say they are in support of prevention programs.
    b. set examples in all activities of the organization.
    c. give an in-service training program on injury prevention.
    d. advocate for state laws requiring helmet use.

27. When an EMS leader has the goal of protecting individual EMS providers from injury, that leader should do all the following, *except*:

    a. develop sensible polices and procedures promoting safety in all work activities.
    b. provide all EMS providers with appropriate PPE.
    c. provide all necessary safety training as required by OSHA.
    d. establish a wellness program for EMS providers, with exemption for the management and office staff.

28. The paramedic needs to be able to recognize exposure to the following, as a potential for injury, *except* for:

    a. temperature extremes.
    b. structural risks.
    c. communicable diseases.
    d. daycare centers.

29. Examples of resources the paramedic should be aware of as part of a prevention program, include all the following, *except*:

    a. child protective services.
    b. grief support.
    c. mental health resources.
    d. utility reimbursement resources.

30. Concepts of effective communication which the paramedic can use as part of the on-scene educational strategy for prevention include all the following, *except*:

    a. avoid consideration of ethnic, religious, or social diversity.
    b. recognize the teachable moments.
    c. have a good sense of timing.
    d. inform the patient or family how they can prevent a recurrence.

31. When a paramedic documents a safety hazard, which of the following should be included?

    a. Primary care provided.
    b. Primary injury data.
    c. Information required by the EMS agency.
    d. All of the above.

32. Which of the following is not an example of primary injury data?

    a. Queue time
    b. Scene time
    c. Scene conditions
    d. Absence of protective devices

33. Which of the following is associated with an overall lower risk of death?

    a. Higher education attainment
    b. Residing in warm climates
    c. Residing in cold climates
    d. Occupation in health care

34. Paramedics are in an ideal position to be front-line advocates for injury and disease prevention because:

    a. of the support provided by private sector groups.
    b. of their perspective offered in out-of-hospital care.
    c. of their knowledge of communicable diseases.
    d. all EMS leaders are progressive with injury prevention.

35. _____ is an effort to keep an injury from ever occurring.

    a. Incidence prevention
    b. Injury surveillance
    c. Primary injury prevention
    d. Accident Watch®

Test #3 Answer Form

	A	B	C	D
1.	❏	❏	❏	❏
2.	❏	❏	❏	❏
3.	❏	❏	❏	❏
4.	❏	❏	❏	❏
5.	❏	❏	❏	❏
6.	❏	❏	❏	❏
7.	❏	❏	❏	❏
8.	❏	❏	❏	❏
9.	❏	❏	❏	❏
10.	❏	❏	❏	❏
11.	❏	❏	❏	❏
12.	❏	❏	❏	❏
13.	❏	❏	❏	❏
14.	❏	❏	❏	❏
15.	❏	❏	❏	❏
16.	❏	❏	❏	❏
17.	❏	❏	❏	❏
18.	❏	❏	❏	❏

	A	B	C	D
19.	❏	❏	❏	❏
20.	❏	❏	❏	❏
21.	❏	❏	❏	❏
22.	❏	❏	❏	❏
23.	❏	❏	❏	❏
24.	❏	❏	❏	❏
25.	❏	❏	❏	❏
26.	❏	❏	❏	❏
27.	❏	❏	❏	❏
28.	❏	❏	❏	❏
29.	❏	❏	❏	❏
30.	❏	❏	❏	❏
31.	❏	❏	❏	❏
32.	❏	❏	❏	❏
33.	❏	❏	❏	❏
34.	❏	❏	❏	❏
35.	❏	❏	❏	❏

4

Medical/Legal Issues

1. Which of the following is a general type of law?

   a. legislative
   b. administrative
   c. criminal
   d. all of the above

2. The statues that are voted on and passed by the city council, county board, state legislature or U.S. Congress are called _____ law.

   a. legislative
   b. civil
   c. tort
   d. common

3. A state EMS Act is an example of _____ law.

   a. administrative
   b. criminal
   c. legislative
   d. civil

4. The rules and regulations that outline the specifics of the enacting EMS law in each state are called the:

   a. SOP.
   b. EMS code.
   c. State protocols.
   d. Practice Act.

5. Precedents are often decided in a court of law based upon _____ law.

   a. criminal
   b. tort
   c. case
   d. administrative

6. A paramedic found to be purposely hurting patients by withholding essential medications would be charged in a(an) _____ court.

   a. small claims
   b. criminal
   c. civil
   d. administrative

7. When a plaintiff sues a paramedic for a breach of confidentiality in which he/she felt harm was caused to his/her reputation in the community, this action would take place in _____ court.

   a. criminal
   b. administrative
   c. civil
   d. case law

8. The person or institution (corporation) being sued is called the:

   a. plaintiff.
   b. responder.
   c. claimant.
   d. defendant.

9. A less formal legal process, which involves a judge and attorneys but no jury, is called a/an:

   a. civil trial.
   b. hearing.
   c. common law action.
   d. appellate court.

10. In a trial court, the _____ is responsible for deciding the facts of the case as presented by the competing attorneys.

    a. judge
    b. jury
    c. hearing officer
    d. respondent's attorney

11. An appellate court has the option to:

    a. agree with the decision of the previous court.
    b. remand the decision to the lowest court.
    c. overrule the lower courts decision.
    d. all of the above.

12. A/an _____ is convened to help decide if the district attorney or prosecutor has enough evidence to indict an individual to stand trial for a crime.

    a. appellate court
    b. civil court
    c. grand jury
    d. higher court

13. Deviation from the accepted standard of care is called:

    a. abandonment.
    b. negligence.
    c. confidentiality.
    d. a civil tort.

14. When a plaintiff's objective is to receive a financial award for damages that were allegedly caused by the paramedic, this is conducted in a:

    a. grand jury.
    b. criminal court.
    c. civil court.
    d. administrative hearing.

15. If the paramedic has an established duty, to act and does not comply with that duty this is referred to as a(an):

    a. error of commission.
    b. breach of duty.
    c. error of omission.
    d. infraction of decorum.

16. The failure to do a required act or duty, such as CPR on a patient who has been down for five minutes prior to your arrival, is called:

    a. nonfeasance.
    b. breach.
    c. malfeasance.
    d. non-reliance.

17. In a malpractice case it is necessary to prove the paramedic who provides care:

    a. had a duty to act.
    b. breached her/his duty.
    c. caused the patient's injury.
    d. all of the above.

18. When an expert witness is called to testify in a malpractice case it is usually to establish:

    a. proximate cause.
    b. a duty was present.
    c. there was a breach of duty.
    d. commission incurred.

19. If a paramedic was found to have administered an excessive dose of lasix to a drug addict in order to get "pleasure" out of watching the patient urinate all over himself, this is an example of:

    a. proximate cause.
    b. gross negligence.
    c. abandonment.
    d. commission of duty.

20. The termination of a paramedic/ patient care relationship before assuring that a health care provider of equal or higher training will continue care is called:

    a. false imprisonment.
    b. confidentiality.
    c. malpractice.
    d. abandonment.

21. Detaining a patient without their consent or legal authority is considered:

    a. abandonment.
    b. false imprisonment.
    c. slander.
    d. kidnapping.

22. A crime in which a patient, his/her character or reputation is injured by false statements of another person is called:

    a. false imprisonment.
    b. libel.
    c. slander.
    d. abandonment.

23. A crime in which a person, his/her character or reputation, is injured by the false written statements of another person is called:

    a. libel.
    b. slander.
    c. graffiti.
    d. confidentiality.

24. The granting of medical privileges by a physician either on-line or off-line is called:

    a. libel.
    b. delegation.
    c. confiscation.
    d. scope of practice.

25. The range of duties and skills a paramedic is expected to perform when necessary is called the:

    a. scope of practice.
    b. delegated authority.
    c. protocol.
    d. negligence per se.

26. The Latin term _____ means "the thing speaks for itself."

    a. vini veni vechi
    b. semper fi
    c. res ipsa loquitor
    d. negligence per se

27. Negligence shown because the law was violated and an injury occurred is called:

    a. res ipsa locquitor.
    b. causation implied.
    c. negligence per se.
    d. contributory negligence.

28. In a rear-end collision the driver sustained a neck injury. Despite wearing a seat belt, the headrest was improperly positioned, which most likely contributed to the injury. At sentencing, the judge reduces the award to the injured party; this may be because of:

    a. negligence per se.
    b. government immunity.
    c. abandonment.
    d. contributory negligence.

29. Of the following steps, which is not involved in a typical court case?

    a. Depositions
    b. Information assessment
    c. Sentencing
    d. Answering the complaint

30. The period during the pretrial phase when opposing sides get the opportunity to obtain the facts and information from the other side in preparation for the trial is called:

    a. interrogations.
    b. discovery.
    c. settlement.
    d. deposition.

31. The damages and award that are to be given to the plaintiff are called the:

    a. settlement.
    b. interrogatory.
    c. sentencing.
    d. deposition.

32. Written answers to a list of questions about charges is/are called:

    a. interrogatories.
    b. settlement.
    c. deposition.
    d. discovery.

33. The responsibility for one's own actions is also called:

    a. immunity.
    b. per se negligence.
    c. liability.
    d. malpractice.

34. The time limit within which a lawsuit may be filled is called the:

    a. penalty clause.
    b. statute of limitations.
    c. maximum penalty.
    d. government immunity option.

35. Generally _____ years is a good period to save records for interactions with adult patients.

    a. 3
    b. 5
    c. 7
    d. 9

36. When an adult patient agrees to your care, this is called _____ consent.

    a. expressed
    b. informed
    c. implied
    d. detailed

37. After full disclosure or explanation, the patient is said to have given _____ consent.

    a. expressed
    b. implied
    c. involuntary
    d. informed

38. Another name for implied consent is the:

    a. writ of Hypheas.
    b. emergency doctrine.
    c. mental health law.
    d. nolo de solvo.

39. Minors who can refuse treatment include:

    a. those who are married.
    b. those who are parents themselves.
    c. members of the armed services.
    d. all of the above.

40. When a minor can refuse care or give consent, this is officially called:

    a. naturalization.
    b. emancipation.
    c. regionalization.
    d. authorization.

41. The process of patient refusal should include all the following steps, *except*:

    a. having a credible disinterested witness sign the release.
    b. enlisting the assistance of a significant other to help persuade.
    c. trying to convince the patient to accept care and transport.
    d. advising the patient he/she may not call back today after refusing.

42. If the steps described in question 41 are taken and you still have not persuaded the patient to go to the hospital, it may be helpful to:

    a. have the police arrest him/her.
    b. just go ahead and get a signature of release.
    c. consult medical control.
    d. leave the scene.

43. Can an intoxicated patient refuse care?

    a. Yes, if they do not want transport just leave them.
    b. Yes, unless they are a minor.
    c. No, persons with an altered mental status are not usually able to make a competent decision.
    d. No, they can only make decisions of implied consent.

44. Can a paramedic determine that a patient is intoxicated?

    a. Not without additional training.
    b. Yes.
    c. Only if the medical director agrees.
    d. Yes, after ruling out medical causes of the behavior.

45. If a patient who is refusing care becomes unconscious, can the paramedic treat him?

    a. Yes, under the informed consent provision.
    b. Yes, under the emergency doctrine.
    c. Not without the police present.
    d. Not without permission of medical control.

46. Who can just take a patient away against his/her will for evaluation in a hospital?

    a. A spouse.
    b. A mental health officer.
    c. The paramedic.
    d. The medical control physician.

47. When a police officer agrees that a patient who is refusing your care may be harmful to himself he/she can order the patient to the hospital under:

    a. executive powers.
    b. protective custody.
    c. mental health laws.
    d. all of the above.

48. You are called to the scene of a private residence. The patient is an elderly man whose two daughters meet you at the door and proceed to tell you how he is acting crazy and is so much trouble to care for. They would like you to take him to the hospital. If the patient refuses to go and is alert with no life-threats, what should you do?

    a. Just take him in restraints.
    b. Involve the police for some assistance.
    c. Call medical control to get an order to take him in.
    d. All of the above.

49. The Federal rules on sexual harassment are found in the:

    a. state harassment code.
    b. Civil Rights Act.
    c. OSHA regulations.
    d. NFPA guidelines.

50. A living will is a document that states the type of life saving medical treatment a patient wants or does not want to be employed in case of:

    a. terminal illness.
    b. coma.
    c. persistent vegetative state.
    d. all of the above.

51. A _____ allows a person to designate an agent in cases where the person is unable to make decisions for himself.

    a. living will
    b. health care proxy
    c. patient self-determination act
    d. release

52. All of the following are cases in which a paramedic or the EMS agency can release confidential information to others, *except* when:

   a. in response to a subpoena.
   b. a law requires the release of information.
   c. a third party requires the information for billing.
   d. the receiving hospital requests the patient's name over the radio.

53. _____ is/are the use of sheets, tape or leather padded restraints to reduce the potential harm to a patient who is unruly or violent.

   a. Humane restraints
   b. Hog tying
   c. Prove binding
   d. Mummy wrapping

54. The paramedic has a/an _____ responsibility to resuscitate all potential organ donors so that others may benefit from the organs.

   a. legal
   b. ethical
   c. moral
   d. religious

55. It is important for the paramedic to write the PCR "in the course of business" for all of the following reasons, *except*:

   a. completing the paper work at a later time looks suspicious.
   b. while the information is fresh in the paramedic's mind.
   c. the information has to be quickly available for billing.
   d. a copy needs to go to the ED to be placed in the patient's record.

56. Punitive damages are designed to punish the defendant for:

   a. his/her harmful actions.
   b. the extended response time.
   c. the delay in responding to the patients needs.
   d. discourteous language used.

57. All the following are examples of compensable damages that the paramedic may be required to pay as a result of a malpractice suit, *except*:

   a. medical expenses.
   b. wrongful death.
   c. lost earnings.
   d. adoption services.

58. Who has the burden of proof in a lawsuit?

   a. Defendant
   b. Plaintiff
   c. Responder
   d. Hearing officer

59. _____ is the range of skills and knowledge the paramedic is trained in.

   a. Scope of practice
   b. Standard of care
   c. Protocol
   d. Code of ethics

60. The _____ makes certain types of information collected by public agencies available to the media, legal council or the public upon demand.

   a. "standards of care"
   b. burden of proof act
   c. freedom of information act
   d. innocent until proven guilty pretext

61. The paramedic is responsible for the actions of the intern under the _____ concept.

   a. "cloak of secrecy"
   b. medical extender
   c. Good Samaritan
   d. "borrowed servant"

62. Except for the unconscious patient, all EMS providers must get the patient's consent for treatment or they could be charged with:

   a. battery and assault.
   b. sexual harassment.
   c. false imprisonment.
   d. no charges can be filed in this case.

63. In determining whether or not an ambulance operator was exercising due regard in the use of signaling equipment, the courts will consider all the following, *except*:

   a. was it reasonably necessary to use the signaling equipment, under all the circumstances?
   b. was the signaling equipment actually used?
   c. whether the signal given was audible and/or visible to the motorist and pedestrians?
   d. does the insurance company require the use of lights and sirens for all calls?

64. According to the American Heart Association, successful completion of an AHA course:

    a. warrants acceptable quality of care delivered to patients by the provider.
    b. authorizes the provider to perform the procedures learned in the course.
    c. ensures that the performance of procedures learned in the course are of the highest standard.
    d. does not warrant performance or quality or authorize a person to perform any procedures on a patient.

65. A _____ is a document testifying that one has fulfilled certain requirements such as a course of instruction.

    a. certificate
    b. license
    c. permit
    d. regents insignia

66. Which of the following driving courses provide immunity from lawsuits?

    a. Emergency Vehicle Operator Course (EVOC).
    b. Certified Emergency Vehicle Operator (CEVO).
    c. Defensive Driving Course (DDC).
    d. None of the above.

67. Who has the authority to decide the appropriate response mode for which to transport a patient to the hospital?

    a. The emergency vehicle operator.
    b. The highest medical authority attending to the patient.
    c. The paramedic supervisor still on the scene.
    d. All of the above.

68. Which of the following conditions are covered under the Americans with Disabilities Act (ADA)?

    a. Fractured leg
    b. Drug abuse
    c. Hearing impairment.
    d. All of the above.

69. The _____ is the federal law that has an impact on issues such as on-call pay, comp time, long shift and overtime pay.

    a. FMLA
    b. FLSA
    c. FICA
    d. OSHA

70. All the following are rationale that are included in OSHA, *except* to:

    a. encourage self-employed persons to report workplace injuries biannually.
    b. develop standards and guidelines for employers and employees to reduce the incidence of deaths on the job.
    c. develop an enforcement procedure for safety and health standards for the work place.
    d. encourage the improvement of existing safety and health programs.

71. It is good practice to wear an ID tag and introduce yourself to your patient by name and level of training because:

    a. it is the polite thing to do.
    b. so he/she knows who to sue if they feel treatment was inappropriate.
    c. so he/she knows to send a tip and thank you letter.
    d. patients have a right to know who you are and your level of training.

72. The Medical Director's liability for prehospital care falls into the two categories of:

    a. training and continuing education.
    b. on-line and off-line supervision.
    c. quality improvement and quality assurance.
    d. omission and commission.

73. The best way for a paramedic to avoid a lawsuit is to:

    a. always be respectful and pleasant to patients, their families and their property.
    b. Practice good medicine and be a competent caregiver.
    c. Accurately document the assessment and management of the patient clearly on the PCR.
    d. All of the above.

74. The first responsibility the paramedic has at a crime scene is to:

    a. protect potential evidence.
    b. provide care for the patient.
    c. protect him/herself and the crew.
    d. notify law enforcement if not already done.

75. To maintain the paramedic–patient relationship, all the following information must be kept confidential, *except*:

    a. assessment findings.
    b. treatment rendered.
    c. observations of the inside of a residence.
    d. revealing signs of suspected abuse.

Test #4 Answer Form

	A	B	C	D
1.	❏	❏	❏	❏
2.	❏	❏	❏	❏
3.	❏	❏	❏	❏
4.	❏	❏	❏	❏
5.	❏	❏	❏	❏
6.	❏	❏	❏	❏
7.	❏	❏	❏	❏
8.	❏	❏	❏	❏
9.	❏	❏	❏	❏
10.	❏	❏	❏	❏
11.	❏	❏	❏	❏
12.	❏	❏	❏	❏
13.	❏	❏	❏	❏
14.	❏	❏	❏	❏
15.	❏	❏	❏	❏
16.	❏	❏	❏	❏
17.	❏	❏	❏	❏
18.	❏	❏	❏	❏
19.	❏	❏	❏	❏
20.	❏	❏	❏	❏
21.	❏	❏	❏	❏
22.	❏	❏	❏	❏
23.	❏	❏	❏	❏
24.	❏	❏	❏	❏
25.	❏	❏	❏	❏
26.	❏	❏	❏	❏

	A	B	C	D
27.	❏	❏	❏	❏
28.	❏	❏	❏	❏
29.	❏	❏	❏	❏
30.	❏	❏	❏	❏
31.	❏	❏	❏	❏
32.	❏	❏	❏	❏
33.	❏	❏	❏	❏
34.	❏	❏	❏	❏
35.	❏	❏	❏	❏
36.	❏	❏	❏	❏
37.	❏	❏	❏	❏
38.	❏	❏	❏	❏
39.	❏	❏	❏	❏
40.	❏	❏	❏	❏
41.	❏	❏	❏	❏
42.	❏	❏	❏	❏
43.	❏	❏	❏	❏
44.	❏	❏	❏	❏
45.	❏	❏	❏	❏
46.	❏	❏	❏	❏
47.	❏	❏	❏	❏
48.	❏	❏	❏	❏
49.	❏	❏	❏	❏
50.	❏	❏	❏	❏
51.	❏	❏	❏	❏
52.	❏	❏	❏	❏

	A	B	C	D		A	B	C	D
53.	❏	❏	❏	❏	65.	❏	❏	❏	❏
54.	❏	❏	❏	❏	66.	❏	❏	❏	❏
55.	❏	❏	❏	❏	67.	❏	❏	❏	❏
56.	❏	❏	❏	❏	68.	❏	❏	❏	❏
57.	❏	❏	❏	❏	69.	❏	❏	❏	❏
58.	❏	❏	❏	❏	70.	❏	❏	❏	❏
59.	❏	❏	❏	❏	71.	❏	❏	❏	❏
60.	❏	❏	❏	❏	72.	❏	❏	❏	❏
61.	❏	❏	❏	❏	73.	❏	❏	❏	❏
62.	❏	❏	❏	❏	74.	❏	❏	❏	❏
63.	❏	❏	❏	❏	75.	❏	❏	❏	❏
64.	❏	❏	❏	❏					

5

Ethical Issues for the EMS Provider

1. The best way for a paramedic to stay out of the middle of an ethical dilemma is to think scenarios through ahead of time, and:

   a. maintain a high degree of suspicion.
   b. maintain a high degree of integrity.
   c. always defer to the request of the patient.
   d. always be honest with your patients.

2. Ethics are defined as:

   a. a system of principles governing moral conduct.
   b. not acting in a rude or crude manner.
   c. never cheating on your taxes.
   d. a true measure of honesty.

3. Morals relate to _____ standards and ethics relate to _____ standards.

   a. high: objective
   b. subjective: high
   c. personal: societal
   d. societal: personal

4. Which of the following questions should the paramedic consider when confronted with an ethical dilemma?

   a. "What is in the EMS agency's best interest?"
   b. "How will I keep from getting sued?"
   c. "How can my interest best be preserved?"
   d. "What is in the patient's best interest?"

5. Global concepts for the paramedic to consider when making an ethical decision include all the following, *except* will the decision:

   a. keep the patient calm.
   b. provide a benefit to the patient.
   c. avoid harm to the patient.
   d. acknowledge the patient's autonomy.

6. Some states have laws to provide immunity from _____ for the paramedic who begins CPR on a patient with a DNAR order.

   a. liability
   b. willful disregard
   c. wonton disregard
   d. malicious disregard

7. For the patient to be able to be well informed in his/her decisions regarding care, the paramedic, as a rule, should be honest and:

   a. have a family member involved when possible.
   b. use language/terms the patient can understand.
   c. ask the patient to sign for consent for treatment.
   d avoid having family involved whenever possible.

8. When the paramedic is faced with a global ethical conflict, which of the following should he/she avoid using to help resolve the conflict?

   a. Standards of care
   b. Treatment protocols
   c. Retrospective reviews of medical decisions
   d. Preplanned wills

9. The American Medical Association's Code of Medical Ethics states that patients have the right to:

   a. refuse payment when they are dissatisfied with care rendered.
   b. name the physician who will not do their surgery.
   c. waive their ethical options.
   d. make decisions on health care.

10. In which of the following areas might a paramedic have to make an ethical decision?

    a. Implied consent
    b. Refusal of medical assistance
    c. Transportation
    d. All of the above

11. In EMS systems with multiple hospitals and ill-defined transport protocols, the paramedic should use which of the following to influence the patient's decision on where to be transported?

    a. Capabilities of the hospital.
    b. The closest hospital to the patient's residence.
    c. The fastest trip to the hospital.
    d. Hospital that accepts the patient's insurance.

12. All the following are examples of prehospital ethical decisions paramedics may be confronted with, *except*:

    a. Deciding to stop to render assistance when not "on-duty."
    b. Deciding to stay home from work when you are injured.
    c. Dealing with patients who have no ability to pay for services.
    d. Receiving a physician order which does not seem medically acceptable.

13. All the following are accurate statements about ethics, *except*:

    a. ethics come from the Greek work "ethos."
    b. Socrates defined ethics as "how one should live."
    c. ethics involve larger issues than a paramedic's practice.
    d. there is really no difference between ethics and morals.

14. Examples of criteria that are used for allocating EMS resources include which of the following?

    a. True parity
    b. Need
    c. Earned
    d. All of the above

15. _____ is an attempt to make a comparison of all variables in an effort to arrive at a similarity.

    a. True parity
    b. Objective standard
    c. Subjective parity
    d. True standard

16. The paramedic is ethically accountable to all the following, *except*:

    a. the patient.
    b. the patient's advanced directives.
    c. the medical director.
    d. fulfilling the standard of care.

17. When answering an ethical question which of the following should not be considered?

    a. Emotion
    b. Reason
    c. Morals
    d. Good faith

18. When the paramedic is making the determination of "what is in the patient's best interest," all the following should be considered, *except*:

    a. the patient's statements.
    b. family input.
    c. the patient's lawyer's input.
    d. preplanned directives.

19. A husband called 9-1-1 when he found his wife unresponsive. You arrived and began resuscitation efforts, but shortly after the patient's son arrives and tells you that the patient did not want any type of resuscitation. There is no DNAR for the patient. What should you do next?

    a. Stop CPR and call the coroner.
    b. Call the patient's physician for his/her advice.
    c. Ask the police to keep the son away.
    d. When in doubt, resuscitate.

20. _____ as we know it today, stands for soundness of moral principle and character, uprightness, and honesty.

    a. Ethics
    b. Integrity
    c. Candor
    d. Sincerity

21. Examples of unethical behavior include all the following, *except*:

    a. making a medication error and hiding it.
    b. transporting a patient to the farthest hospital because you do not like the physician on staff at the closest hospital.
    c. transporting a trauma arrest patient to the nearest hospital instead of a trauma center.
    d. witnessing a coworker do something unethical and saying nothing.

22. Society attempts to resolve global ethical conflicts by using preplans such as wills and advanced directives to make a patient's wishes known, and by:

    a. preprogramming the phone to dial 9-1-1.
    b. using enhanced 9-1-1 and emergency medical dispatch.
    c. creating laws protecting patient's rights.
    d. researching prospective medical decisions.

23. Which of the following is an example of an ethical dilemma the paramedic may experience as a physician extender?

    a. An indirect (off-line) protocol is not in the patient's best interest.
    b. An indirect (off-line) protocol is contraindicated, but morally right.
    c. Receiving a direct (on-line) order which is not part of standing orders.
    d. Receiving a direct (on-line) order that is medically acceptable, but morally wrong.

24. When a patient wants to refuse treatment or transport, but the paramedic believes the patient needs immediate care, the paramedic can avoid an ethical dilemma by:

    a. using value judgment.
    b. acting in the patient's best interest.
    c. letting the patient sign a waiver of care.
    d. pre-emptively calling a personal lawyer after the call.

25. When we study and discuss ethical principles, this practice serves to:

    a. strengthen and validate our own inner value system.
    b. give direction to our moral compass.
    c. becomes the foundations upon which we can commit.
    d. all of the above.

Test #5 Answer Form

	A	B	C	D		A	B	C	D
1.	❏	❏	❏	❏	14.	❏	❏	❏	❏
2.	❏	❏	❏	❏	15.	❏	❏	❏	❏
3.	❏	❏	❏	❏	16.	❏	❏	❏	❏
4.	❏	❏	❏	❏	17.	❏	❏	❏	❏
5.	❏	❏	❏	❏	18.	❏	❏	❏	❏
6.	❏	❏	❏	❏	19.	❏	❏	❏	❏
7.	❏	❏	❏	❏	20.	❏	❏	❏	❏
8.	❏	❏	❏	❏	21.	❏	❏	❏	❏
9.	❏	❏	❏	❏	22.	❏	❏	❏	❏
10.	❏	❏	❏	❏	23.	❏	❏	❏	❏
11.	❏	❏	❏	❏	24.	❏	❏	❏	❏
12.	❏	❏	❏	❏	25.	❏	❏	❏	❏
13.	❏	❏	❏	❏					

6

General Principles of Pathophysiology

1. The study of abnormal function of the body is called:

   a. physiology.
   b. anatomy.
   c. pathology.
   d. pathophysiology.

2. What is the cause of a disease, also referred to as the:

   a. pathogenesis.
   b. etiology.
   c. pathology.
   d. prognosis.

3. When the symptoms of a disease become rapidly worse this is referred to as:

   a. remission.
   b. iatrogenic.
   c. exacerbation.
   d. prognosis.

4. Causes of disease include any of the following, *except*:

   a. heredity.
   b. relocation.
   c. infection.
   d. abnormal tissue growth.

5. A group of symptoms or conditions that may be caused by a disease or various related medical problems is called a/an:

   a. toxidrome.
   b. infection.
   c. syndrome.
   d. malignancy.

6. A decreased size in the cell leading to a decrease in the size of the tissue and organ is called:

   a. atrophy.
   b. hypertrophy.
   c. acceleration.
   d. cellular adaptation.

7. Of the following, which is not a major tissue type?

   a. epithelial
   b. adipose
   c. muscle
   d. nervous

8. Atrophy, hyperphasia and neoplasia are forms of:

   a. muscular dysfunction.
   b. dysplasia.
   c. cellular adaptation.
   d. dysfunction syndrome.

9. An increase in the actual number of cells by hormonal stimulation is called:

   a. hypertrophy.
   b. dysplasia.
   c. metaplasia.
   d. hyperplasia.

10. An alteration in the size and shape of cells as in a developing tumor is called:

    a. dysplasia.
    b. hyperplasia.
    c. metaplasia.
    d. hypertrophy.

11. The development of a new type of cell with an uncontrolled growth pattern is called:

    a. neoplasia.
    b. hyperplasia.
    c. metaplasia.
    d. hypertrophy.

12. The ability of microorganisms to cause disease is called:

    a. toxicity.
    b. infectabilty.
    c. carcinogenesis.
    d. virulence.

13. Many bacteria have a capsule that is designed to:

    a. hide the microorganism from its host.
    b. make it easier to infect the organism.
    c. protect it from ingestion and destruction by phagocytes.
    d. prevent destruction by a virus.

14. When large amounts of endotoxins are present in the body the patient may develop:

    a. renal failure.
    b. septic shock.
    c. hypovolemic shock.
    d. liver dysfunction.

15. Exotoxins are secretions found in the:

    a. wall of the white blood cells.
    b. wall of a gram-negative bacteria.
    c. medium surrounding the cell.
    d. capsule of the virus.

16. When white blood cells release endogenous pyrogens, it causes:

    a. the production of additional while blood cells.
    b. septic shock.
    c. the body to lower its temperature.
    d. fever to develop.

17. Inflammation is a common response to each of the following stimuli, except:

    a. trauma.
    b. immune response.
    c. over hydration.
    d. infection.

18. Each of the following are examples of an injurious genetic factor affecting the cell, *except*:

    a. hepatitis C.
    b. Down syndrome.
    c. premature atherosclerosis.
    d. some cases of obesity.

19. Why is good nutrition required by the cells?

    a. It helps the nerve cells to rejuvenate.
    b. It helps the cells in fighting off diseases.
    c. It helps the muscle cells multiply.
    d. It decreases the production of energy in the cells.

20. Which of the following is not part of the cellular environment?

    a. Changes in cell distribution with aging.
    b. The movement of water in and out of cells.
    c. The acid-base balance in the cells.
    d. The ability of the bladder to store urine.

21. How much of the body's weight is fluid?

    a. 10–12%
    b. 30–40%
    c. 50–60%
    d. 70–90%

22. Where, in the body, can most of the fluid be found?

    a. in the fluid between the cells
    b. intracellular fluids
    c. extracellular fluids
    d. in the bladder

23. How much fluid does the average adult take in each day?

    a. 1,500 cc
    b. 2,500 cc
    c. 3,500 cc
    d. 4,500 cc

24. When a person loses large quantities of water he/she also loses the major extracellular cation:

    a. sodium.
    b. calcium.
    c. potassium.
    d. chloride

25. Transcellular fluid includes all the following, *except*:

    a. glandular secretions.
    b. blood.
    c. vitreous humor.
    d. CSF.

26. The movement of a substance from an area of higher concentration to an area of lower concentration is called:

    a. osmosis.
    b. filtration.
    c. active transport.
    d. diffusion.

27. When a cell membrane ingests a substance, this is called:

    a. exocytosis.
    b. pinocytosis.
    c. endocytosis.
    d. phagocytosis.

28. The engulfing of liquid droplets is called:

    a. endocytosis.
    b. phagocytosis.
    c. pinocytosis.
    d. exocytosis.

29. The pressure that develops when two solutions of different concentrations are separated by a semipermeable membrane is called _____ pressure.

    a. intracranial
    b. osmotic
    c. colloid
    d. oncotic

30. Of the following age groups, which males have the greatest total body water percentage?

    a. 10–18
    b. 18–40
    c. 40–60
    d. over 60

31. A solution with a lower solute concentration than the blood is referred to as a/an _____ solution.

    a. hypertonic
    b. hypotonic
    c. isotonic
    d. neotonic

32. When a helper molecule, found within the membrane, helps the movement of a substance from areas of higher concentration to areas of lower concentration this is called:

    a. facilitated diffusion.
    b. active transport.
    c. osmosis.
    d. filtration.

33. Of the following, which is not a plasma protein?

    a. albumin
    b. WBC
    c. globulin
    d. fibrinogen

34. The pressure generated by dissolved proteins in the plasma that are too large to penetrate the capillary membrane is called:

    a. tissue colloidal osmotic pressure.
    b. capillary hydrostatic pressure.
    c. tissue hydrostatic pressure.
    d. capillary colloidal osmotic pressure.

35. The pressure pushing water out of the capillary into the interstitial space is referred to as the:

    a. tissue colloidal osmotic pressure.
    b. capillary colloidal osmotic pressure.
    c. capillary hydrostatic pressure.
    d. tissue hydrostatic pressure.

36. An accumulation of excess fluids in the interstitial space is called:

    a. edema.
    b. lymph.
    c. cellular swelling.
    d. none of the above.

37. Fluid that accumulates in the peritoneal cavity is referred to as:

    a. ascites.
    b. sacral edema.
    c. intestinal swelling.
    d. pitting edema.

38. Edema can be caused by:

    a. increased capillary pressure.
    b. decreased colloidal osmotic pressure.
    c. lymphatic vessel obstruction.
    d. all of the above.

39. When a patient has an extensive burn injury, swelling is caused by:

    a. increased capillary pressure.
    b. decreased colloidal osmotic pressure.
    c. dehydration.
    d. lymphatic vessel obstruction.

40. When edematous tissue, such as in the ankles, is compressed with a finger the fluid is pushed aside causing a temporary impression. This is referred to as:

    a. lymphatic edema.
    b. pitting edema.
    c. ascites.
    d. APE.

41. What is the main function of the sodium/potassium pump?

    a. To pump sodium into the cells.
    b. To move potassium out of the cells.
    c. To exchange 3 sodium ions for every 2 potassium ions.
    d. To exchange 2 sodium ions for every 3 potassium ions.

42. The tension exerted on cell size caused by water movement across the cell membrane is referred to as:

    a. tonicity.
    b. oncotic pressure.
    c. osmotic pressure.
    d. colloid pressure.

43. Cells with an osmolarity of 280 mOsm/L will neither shrink nor swell. This is because they:

    a. are considered hypotonic solutions.
    b. are high in both sodium and potassium.
    c. have the same osmolarity as intracellular fluid.
    d. are considered hypertonic solutions.

44. When a cell is placed in a _____ solution, it will shrink as the water is ____ the cell.

    a. hypotonic: pushed into
    b. hypotonic: pulled out of
    c. hypertonic: pushed into
    d. hypertonic: pulled out of

45. When a cell is placed in a hypotonic solution that has a _____ osmolarity than ICF, it will _____.

    a. lower: shrink
    b. lower: swell
    c. higher: shrink
    d. higher: swell

46. The most common cation in the body is:

    a. calcium.
    b. potassium.
    c. sodium.
    d. chloride.

47. Although the average adult ingests between 6 and 15 grams of sodium per day, the required amount is:

    a. 100 mg.
    b. 500 mg.
    c. 1000 mg.
    d. 4 mg.

48. Angiotensin II is responsible for:

    a. dilating the renal blood vessels.
    b. increasing kidney blood flow.
    c. stimulating sodium reabsorption.
    d. increasing the glomerular filtration rate.

49. The protein enzyme that is released by the kidney into the blood stream in response to changes in blood pressure is called:

    a. renin.
    b. epinephrine.
    c. tensin
    d. aldosterone.

50. Angiotensin II can stimulate aldosterone. It can also be stimulated by all of the following, *except*:

    a. decreased extracellular potassium levels.
    b. release of ACTH from the pituitary gland.
    c. decreased extracellular sodium levels.
    d. increased extracellular potassium levels.

51. When a patient has excess body water loss without a proportionate sodium loss he/she is said to be:

    a. hyponatremic.
    b. hypernatremic.
    c. dehydrated.
    d. edematous.

52. The manifestations of hypernatremia include any of the following, *except*:

    a. oliguria or anuria.
    b. a rough and fissured tongue.
    c. increased tears and salivation.
    d. seizures and coma.

53. The manifestation of hyponatremia includes any of the following, *except*:

    a. anorexia, nausea or vomiting.
    b. depression and confusion.
    c. altered mental status.
    d. constipation.

54. An athlete who has had excessive sweating for a three-hour period and has only been drinking water to rehydrate, may suffer the symptoms of:

    a. hypovolemia.
    b. hypertension.
    c. hyponatremia.
    d. hypernatremia.

55. The major intracellular cation, which is critical to many of the functions of the cell, is:

    a. sodium.
    b. potassium.
    c. chloride.
    d. calcium.

56. A patient may become hypokalemic from:

    a. excessive vomiting or diarrhea.
    b. a diet deficient in sodium.
    c. excessive eating.
    d. decreased sweating.

57. The manifestations of a deficiency in potassium may include all of the following, *except*:

    a. muscle tenderness and cramps.
    b. cardiac dysrhythmias.
    c. hypertension.
    d. paralysis or paresthesia.

58. When a patient has an elevated serum potassium level, this can be caused by:

    a. decreased potassium intake.
    b. excess use of diuretics.
    c. renal failure.
    d. treatment with angiotensin.

59. The clinical manifestations of hyperkalemia include:

    a. paresthesia and intestinal colic.
    b. feeling of euphoria.
    c. excessive urination.
    d. muscle overactivity.

60. A hyperkalemic patient may exhibit ECG changes such as:

    a. peaked ST segments.
    b. depressed T waves.
    c. widened QRS.
    d. peaked P waves.

61. Where is the vast majority of the body's calcium found?

    a. kidneys
    b. teeth
    c. liver
    d. bones

62. The purpose of calcium is to provide:

    a. strength and stability.
    b. increase conduction through muscles.
    c. enhanced renal effectiveness.
    d. maintenance of the blood pressure.

63. How does calcium enter the body?

    a. through the lungs
    b. by way of the bones
    c. through the GI tract
    d. through the skin

64. The causes of hypocalcemia include all the following, *except*:

    a. hyperparathyroidism.
    b. increased fatty acids.
    c. acute pancreatitis.
    d. renal failure.

65. Other causes of hypocalcemia include:

    a. hypermagnesemia.
    b. rapid transfusion of citrated blood.
    c. decreased pH.
    d. excess vitamin D.

66. A patient with hypocalcemia often presents with:

    a. skeletal muscle cramps.
    b. absence of tetany.
    c. hypertension.
    d. hypoactive reflexes.

67. A patient who has frequent skeletal muscle cramps, abdominal spasms and cramps, as well as frequent fractures, may benefit by supplementing his diet intake of:

    a. sodium.
    b. calcium.
    c. zinc.
    d. potassium.

68. Osteomalacia and carpopedal spasms have been found to be manifestations of:

    a. hyponatremia.
    b. hyperkalemia.
    c. hypophosphatemia.
    d. hypocalcemia.

69. Causes of hypercalcemia include any of the following, *except*:

    a. decreased vitamin D.
    b. lithium therapy.
    c. malignant neoplasms.
    d. Milk-alkali syndrome.

70. Kidney stones, constipation and polyuria are sometimes a manifestation of:

    a. hypocalcemia.
    b. hyponatremia.
    c. hypercalcemia.
    d. hypokalemia.

71. A shortening QT interval and A-V block on the ECG sometimes is found with which condition?

    a. hypercalcemia
    b. hyponatremia
    c. hypokalemia
    d. hyperkalemia

72. Alterations in the phosphate level are usually caused by any of the following, *except*:

    a. severe diarrhea.
    b. hypoglycemia.
    c. hyperparathyroidism.
    d. alkalosis.

73. The clinical manifestation of hypophosphatemia includes:

    a. impaired red blood cell function.
    b. hyperflexia.
    c. hemolytic anemia.
    d. excessive hunger.

74. Often patients who experience trauma and have kidney failure may develop:

    a. hypokalemia.
    b. hyperphosphatemia.
    c. hypocalcemia.
    d. hyponatremia.

75. Malnutrition or starvation can be caused by which of the following conditions?

    a. Hypocalcemia
    b. Hypomagnesemia
    c. Hypercalcemia
    d. Hyponatremia

76. Positive Babinski, positive Chvostek's sign and positive Trousseaus's sign may be found in the patient who has:

    a. hypomagnesemia.
    b. hypercalcemia.
    c. hypernatremia.
    d. hyponatremia.

77. A muscular spasm resulting from pressure applied to nerves and vessels of the upper arm is called _____ sign.

    a. Babinski's
    b. Chvostek's
    c. Trousseau's
    d. Cushing's

78. What is the normal pH range of the body?

    a. 7.15–7.25
    b. 7.25–7.35
    c. 7.35–7.45
    d. 7.45–7.55

79. A blood pH _____ than 7.45 is called _____.

    a. greater: acidosis
    b. greater: alkalosis
    c. greater: neutral
    d. lesser: alkalosis

80. Sepsis, diabetic ketoacidosis and salicylate poisoning may cause:

    a. respiratory acidosis.
    b. metabolic acidosis.
    c. metabolic alkalosis.
    d. respiratory alkalosis.

81. When CO_2 retention leads to increased levels of pCO_2, the patient develops:

    a. respiratory acidosis.
    b. respiratory alkalosis.
    c. metabolic acidosis.
    d. metabolic alkalosis.

82. Patients who experience a medical condition causing hypoventilation may develop:

    a. metabolic acidosis.
    b. metabolic alkalosis.
    c. respiratory acidosis.
    d. respiratory alkalosis.

83. When a patient has been hyperventilating from an anxiety attack, the patient may ultimately develop:

    a. metabolic acidosis.
    b. metabolic alkalosis.
    c. respiratory acidosis.
    d. respiratory alkalosis.

84. Analyzing disease risk involves reviewing all the following, *except*:

    a. genetic histories of population.
    b. rates of incidence.
    c. prevalence.
    d. mortality.

85. Examples of disease that are more prevalent in males include:

    a. osteoporosis.
    b. Parkinson's disease.
    c. breast cancer.
    d. rheumatoid arthritis.

86. Acquired hypersensitivity is called a/an:

    a. rheumatic fever.
    b. cancer.
    c. asthma.
    d. allergy.

87. You are treating a patient who tells you he had a recent strep throat, and he has a history of myocarditis and arthritis. Which of the following conditions could he most likely have?

    a. Parkinson's disease
    b. Rheumatic fever
    c. Lung cancer
    d. Diabetes

88. The signs of cancer include all the following, *except*:

    a. change in bowel or bladder habits.
    b. nagging cough or hoarseness.
    c. recent weight gain.
    d. difficulty swallowing.

89. A hypersensitivity reaction causing constriction of the bronchi, wheezing and dyspnea is a chronic illness called:

    a. diabetes.
    b. anemia.
    c. asthma.
    d. cardiomyopathy.

90. The leading cause of chronic illness in children is caused by:

    a. diabetes.
    b. chickenpox.
    c. cancer.
    d. asthma.

91. The leading cause of cancer deaths in both males and females combined is from _____ cancer.

    a. rectal
    b. brain
    c. lung
    d. breast

92. The difference between Type I and Type II diabetes is:

    a. Type I develops the disease as adults.
    b. Type II does not become hypoglycemic.
    c. Type I requires exogenous insulin.
    d. Type II requires injected insulin.

93. Why do diabetic patients need to *inject* insulin?

    a. So they can take an entire day's dose at once.
    b. Their digestive juices would destroy oral forms.
    c. Pills do not counteract low blood pressure.
    d. It is cheapest in this form.

94. Symptoms of diabetes include all the following, *except*:

    a. polydipsia.
    b. anorexia.
    c. glycosuria.
    d. polyuria.

95. What organ is responsible for the production of insulin?

    a. kidney
    b. liver
    c. spleen
    d. pancreas

96. Exposure to benzene and bacterial toxins can cause the patient to develop:

    a. hemophilia.
    b. hematochromatosis.
    c. drug-induced anemia.
    d. septal hypertrophy.

97. Typical symptoms experienced by the patient who tells you he is being treated for a mitral valve include all the following, *except*:

    a. dyspnea.
    b. prolonged chest pain.
    c. hallucinations.
    d. palpitations.

98. Risk factors for CAD include:

    a. hypercholesteremia.
    b. family history of CHD.
    c. cigarette smoking.
    d. all of the above.

99. A sex-linked hereditary disorder most commonly passed on from an asymptomatic mother to a male child is:

    a. anemia.
    b. hemophilia.
    c. ALS.
    d. hematochromatosis.

100. Incurable diseases of the heart, which ultimately lead to congestive heart failure or AMI, include:

    a. stroke.
    b. cardiomyopathies.
    c. mitral valve prolapse.
    d. hematochromatosis.

101. Of the following risk factors, which are considered "soft risk" factors?

    a. age
    b. hypertension
    c. diabetes
    d. high cholesterol

102. What is the leading cause of stroke in the prehospital setting?

    a. brain aneurysm
    b. diabetes
    c. cigarette smoking
    d. hypertension

103. A disorder of protein metabolism that primarily affects males leading to inflammation of the joints is called:

    a. arthritis.
    b. lactose intolerance.
    c. gout.
    d. ulcerative colitis.

104. All of the following are risk factors for essential hypertension, *except*:

    a. diet low in salt and fat.
    b. obesity.
    c. smoking.
    d. stress.

105. Why is smoking a risk factor for stroke?

    a. the carbon dioxide levels run higher.
    b. it damages the lung cells.
    c. nicotine causes vasoconstriction.
    d. it paralyzes the brain tissues.

106. The medical term for kidney stones is:

    a. uric acid crystals.
    b. renal calculi.
    c. hematuria.
    d. renal calcium.

107. Kidney stones are most common in _____ between the ages of _____

    a. males: 50–70
    b. females: 30–70
    c. males: 30–50
    d. females: 50–70

108. A disorder effecting the rectum and colon, causing inflammation, lesions and ulcerations of the musocal layer is called:

    a. lactose intolerance.
    b. irritable bowel syndrome.
    c. ulcerative colitis.
    d. Crohn's disease.

109. Patient's who are unable to break down the complex carbohydrates found in ice cream have:

    a. renal calculi.
    b. lactose intolerance.
    c. ulcerative colitis.
    d. irritable bowel syndrome.

110. A group of disorders that occurs in areas of the upper GI tract that are normally exposed to acid pepsin secretions is referred to as:

    a. peptic ulcers.
    b. muscular dystrophy.
    c. Crohn's disease.
    d. Huntington's disease.

111. Cholelithiasis is the medical term for:

    a. kidney stones.
    b. peptic ulcers.
    c. gallstones.
    d. Crohn's disease.

112. When the flow of bile is obstructed, the patient may be suffering from:

    a. renal calculi.
    b. lactose intolerance.
    c. gallstones.
    d. Huntington's disease.

113. Each of the following is considered a health risk associated with obesity, *except*:

    a. hyperlipidemia.
    b. hypotension.
    c. gallbladder disease.
    d. insulin resistance.

114. Morbidly obese patients often have sleep apnea and:

    a. lactose intolerance.
    b. hypolipidemia.
    c. multiple sclerosis.
    d. respiratory function impairment.

115. A rare hereditary disorder involving chronic progressive chorea, psychologic changes and dementia is called:

    a. Crohn's disease.
    b. Huntington's disease.
    c. multiple sclerosis.
    d. muscular dystrophy.

116. You are treating a patient who has a disease that manifests itself with acute episodes of paresthesia, optic neuritis, diplopia or gaze paralysis. You suspect he may have a history of:

    a. multiple sclerosis.
    b. Huntington's disease.
    c. muscular dystrophy.
    d. Alzheimer's.

117. A patient who has stage 2 Alzheimer's disease may exhibit:

    a. indifference to food and inability to communicate.
    b. memory loss and lack of spontaneity.
    c. impaired cognition and abstract thinking.
    d. inability to taste spicy food and disorientation to time and date.

118. Of the following, which is not a cause of cardiogenic shock?

    a. AMI
    b. heart failure
    c. envenomation
    d. ventricle septal defect

119. Of the following, which is *not* an example of obstructive shock?

    a. pericardial tamponade
    b. dissecting aortic aneurysm
    c. anaphylaxis
    d. all of the above

120. Causes of hypovolemic shock include:

    a. heart failure.
    b. ventricular septal defect.
    c. electrolyte loss from dehydration.
    d. pericardial tamponade.

121. What is MODS?

    a. a disease of the brain
    b. advice for managing shock
    c. multiple organ dysfunction syndrome
    d. none of the above

122. All of the following are autoimmune diseases, *except*:

    a. Graves' disease.
    b. lupus.
    c. myasthenia gravis.
    d. AIDS.

123. The body's first response to begin adapting to the new onset of circumstances is referred to as the:

    a. stage of exhaustion.
    b. alarm reaction.
    c. stage of resistance.
    d. final reaction.

124. The effect of catacholamines on the liver includes:

    a. hypersensitivity.
    b. autoimmunity.
    c. allergy.
    d. isoimmunity.

125. When a person's T cells or antibodies attack, causing tissue damage and organ dysfunction, this is called:

    a. allergy.
    b. autoimmunity.
    c. hypersensitivity.
    d. isoimmunity

126. The system that plays a vital role in attracting white blood cells to the site of the infection is called:

    a. bradykinin.
    b. imunocascade.
    c. complement.
    d. macrophage.

127. The cellular components of inflammation include all of the following, *except*:

    a. monocytes.
    b. phagocytes.
    c. erythrocytes.
    d. macrophages.

128. A bodily response to any substance that a patient is abnormally sensitive to is called a/an:

    a. contraction.
    b. allergy.
    c. increased renin secretion.
    d. lipolysis.

129. Natural immunity is acquired from:

    a. an injection of a vaccine.
    b. an anamnestic response.
    c. getting a childhood disease.
    d. none of the above.

130. When the body forms a "memory" for certain antigens this is referred to as a/an:

    a. native immunity.
    b. anamnestic response.
    c. nonspecific immunity.
    d. acquired immunity.

131. During an inflammation response the cells released by mast cells include:

    a. steroids.
    b. cortisol.
    c. histamine.
    d. lymphocytes.

Test #6 Answer Form

	A	B	C	D		A	B	C	D
1.	❏	❏	❏	❏	27.	❏	❏	❏	❏
2.	❏	❏	❏	❏	28.	❏	❏	❏	❏
3.	❏	❏	❏	❏	29.	❏	❏	❏	❏
4.	❏	❏	❏	❏	30.	❏	❏	❏	❏
5.	❏	❏	❏	❏	31.	❏	❏	❏	❏
6.	❏	❏	❏	❏	32.	❏	❏	❏	❏
7.	❏	❏	❏	❏	33.	❏	❏	❏	❏
8.	❏	❏	❏	❏	34.	❏	❏	❏	❏
9.	❏	❏	❏	❏	35.	❏	❏	❏	❏
10.	❏	❏	❏	❏	36.	❏	❏	❏	❏
11.	❏	❏	❏	❏	37.	❏	❏	❏	❏
12.	❏	❏	❏	❏	38.	❏	❏	❏	❏
13.	❏	❏	❏	❏	39.	❏	❏	❏	❏
14.	❏	❏	❏	❏	40.	❏	❏	❏	❏
15.	❏	❏	❏	❏	41.	❏	❏	❏	❏
16.	❏	❏	❏	❏	42.	❏	❏	❏	❏
17.	❏	❏	❏	❏	43.	❏	❏	❏	❏
18.	❏	❏	❏	❏	44.	❏	❏	❏	❏
19.	❏	❏	❏	❏	45.	❏	❏	❏	❏
20.	❏	❏	❏	❏	46.	❏	❏	❏	❏
21.	❏	❏	❏	❏	47.	❏	❏	❏	❏
22.	❏	❏	❏	❏	48.	❏	❏	❏	❏
23.	❏	❏	❏	❏	49.	❏	❏	❏	❏
24.	❏	❏	❏	❏	50.	❏	❏	❏	❏
25.	❏	❏	❏	❏	51.	❏	❏	❏	❏
26.	❏	❏	❏	❏	52.	❏	❏	❏	❏

	A	B	C	D
53.	❏	❏	❏	❏
54.	❏	❏	❏	❏
55.	❏	❏	❏	❏
56.	❏	❏	❏	❏
57.	❏	❏	❏	❏
58.	❏	❏	❏	❏
59.	❏	❏	❏	❏
60.	❏	❏	❏	❏
61.	❏	❏	❏	❏
62.	❏	❏	❏	❏
63.	❏	❏	❏	❏
64.	❏	❏	❏	❏
65.	❏	❏	❏	❏
66.	❏	❏	❏	❏
67.	❏	❏	❏	❏
68.	❏	❏	❏	❏
69.	❏	❏	❏	❏
70.	❏	❏	❏	❏
71.	❏	❏	❏	❏
72.	❏	❏	❏	❏
73.	❏	❏	❏	❏
74.	❏	❏	❏	❏
75.	❏	❏	❏	❏
76.	❏	❏	❏	❏
77.	❏	❏	❏	❏
78.	❏	❏	❏	❏
79.	❏	❏	❏	❏
80.	❏	❏	❏	❏
81.	❏	❏	❏	❏

	A	B	C	D
82.	❏	❏	❏	❏
83.	❏	❏	❏	❏
84.	❏	❏	❏	❏
85.	❏	❏	❏	❏
86.	❏	❏	❏	❏
87.	❏	❏	❏	❏
88.	❏	❏	❏	❏
89.	❏	❏	❏	❏
90.	❏	❏	❏	❏
91.	❏	❏	❏	❏
92.	❏	❏	❏	❏
93.	❏	❏	❏	❏
94.	❏	❏	❏	❏
95.	❏	❏	❏	❏
96.	❏	❏	❏	❏
97.	❏	❏	❏	❏
98.	❏	❏	❏	❏
99.	❏	❏	❏	❏
100.	❏	❏	❏	❏
101.	❏	❏	❏	❏
102.	❏	❏	❏	❏
103.	❏	❏	❏	❏
104.	❏	❏	❏	❏
105.	❏	❏	❏	❏
106.	❏	❏	❏	❏
107.	❏	❏	❏	❏
108.	❏	❏	❏	❏
109.	❏	❏	❏	❏
110.	❏	❏	❏	❏

	A	B	C	D			A	B	C	D
111.	❏	❏	❏	❏		122.	❏	❏	❏	❏
112.	❏	❏	❏	❏		123.	❏	❏	❏	❏
113.	❏	❏	❏	❏		124.	❏	❏	❏	❏
114.	❏	❏	❏	❏		125.	❏	❏	❏	❏
115.	❏	❏	❏	❏		126.	❏	❏	❏	❏
116.	❏	❏	❏	❏		127.	❏	❏	❏	❏
117.	❏	❏	❏	❏		128.	❏	❏	❏	❏
118.	❏	❏	❏	❏		129.	❏	❏	❏	❏
119.	❏	❏	❏	❏		130.	❏	❏	❏	❏
120.	❏	❏	❏	❏		131.	❏	❏	❏	❏
121.	❏	❏	❏	❏						

7

Pharmacology

1. Any chemical substance that when taken into a living organism produces a biologic response affecting one or more of that organism's processes or functions is a:

   a. solution.
   b. drug.
   c. antigen.
   d. antibody.

2. The term for the study of how a drug is altered as it travels through the body is:

   a. pharmacokinetics.
   b. pharmacodynamics.
   c. pharmaceutics.
   d. antagonism.

3. The study of how and why a drug works, specifically its biochemical and physiologic effects is called:

   a. pharmacodynamics.
   b. pharmaceutics.
   c. pharmacokinetics.
   d. pharmacopoeia.

4. The chemical breakdown of a drug while in the body is called:

   a. absorption.
   b. distribution.
   c. elimination.
   d. biotransformation.

5. The general properties of a drug include all the following, *except*:

   a. therapeutic.
   b. prophylactic.
   c. diagnostic.
   d. research.

6. Drug induced physiologic changes on a body function or process are known as a (an):

   a. drug action.
   b. side effect.
   c. half-life.
   d. idiosyncrasy.

7. A drug that stimulates a receptor is called a (an):

   a. agonist.
   b. antagonist.
   c. sympatholytic.
   d. sympathomimetic.

8. The major mechanism by which a drug affects the body is by joining with receptors located on the:

   a. red blood cells.
   b. target organs or tissues.
   c. white blood cells.
   d. mast cells.

9. Drugs that mimic the functions of the sympathetic nervous system are called:

   a. agonist.
   b. antagonist.
   c. sympatholytic.
   d. sympathomimetic.

10. An example of an emergency use drug that is also a sympathetic nervous system neurotransmitter is:

    a. dopamine.
    b. isoproterenol.
    c. dobutamine.
    d. procainamide.

11. ACLS drugs such as epinephrine, dopamine, and isoproterenol belong to a group of drugs called:

    a. fibrins.
    b. ionospheres.
    c. sympatholytics.
    d. sympathomimetics.

12. Antiadrenergic drugs that block the function of the sympathetic nervous system are called:

    a. fibrins.
    b. ionospheres.
    c. sympatholytics.
    d. sympathomimetics.

13. Cholinergic receptors respond to the neurotransmitter:

    a. acetylcholine.
    b. epinephrine.
    c. norepinephrine.
    d. nortriptyline.

14. Drugs that block cholinergic receptors and parasympathetic response are called parasympatholytics. In the prehospital setting the most commonly used parasympatholytic is:

    a. metaprolol.
    b. atenolol.
    c. dobutamine.
    d. atropine.

15. For a drug to get inside a cell or body part, the two primary means of transportation are active and passive transport. The difference between the two is that active transport requires:

    a. energy produced through a chemical reaction.
    b. a change in homeostasis.
    c. the formation of genetic repressors.
    d. energy to produce and displace phosphatide.

16. When repeated doses of a drug lead to toxicity in a patient, this condition is known as a:

    a. side effect.
    b. habituation.
    c. hypersensitivity.
    d. cumulative effect.

17. When a patient takes a medication and has an unexpected response that most patients would *not* have, this is called a/an:

    a. idiosyncrasy.
    b. side effect.
    c. toxicity.
    d. cumulative effect.

18. A physiologic blockade that protects the brain from exposure to various drugs is called:

    a. cerebral spinal fluid.
    b. blood-brain barrier.
    c. meninges.
    d. collateral barrier.

19. The name of a drug that is assigned by the U.S. Adopted Name Council is the _____ name.

    a. official
    b. generic
    c. trade
    d. brand

20. ACE inhibitors work primarily by inhibiting:

    a. renin from releasing sodium.
    b. angiotensin I from converting angiotensin II.
    c. sodium and water retention.
    d. acetylcholine.

21. Chemical assay is a test that determines a drug's:

    a. ingredients.
    b. reliability.
    c. half-life
    d. mechanism of injury.

22. The Pure Food and Drug Act of 1906 required drug manufacturers to:

    a. test a drug for effectiveness.
    b. test a drug for safety.
    c. label all ingredients.
    d. label all dangerous ingredients in drug products.

23. The FDA is responsible for all the following, *except*:

    a. testing of drugs.
    b. marketing of drugs.
    c. availability of drugs.
    d. drug enforcement.

24. Which of the following routes of drug administration injects the medication under the dermis into connective tissue or fat?

    a. subcutaneous
    b. intramuscular
    c. enteral
    d. epidural

25. A drug's ability to join with a receptor is known as:

    a. affinity.
    b. ability.
    c. selective response.
    d. agonist.

26. A drug that joins partially with a receptor and prevents a reaction is called a(an):

    a. partial antagonist.
    b. partial agonist.
    c. agonist.
    d. antagonist.

27. The two types of sympathetic receptors in the body are:

    a. dopaminergic and adrenergic.
    b. adrenergic and cholinergic.
    c. iatrogenic and dopaminergic.
    d. cholinergic and inhibitoric.

28. All the following are means of passive transport of a solute through or across a cell membrane *except*:

    a. diffusion.
    b. filtration.
    c. osmosis.
    d. precipitation.

29. The pressure that develops when two solutions of different concentrations are separated by a semipermeable membrane is called _____ pressure.

    a. osmotic
    b. hydrostatic
    c. hypertonic
    d. hypotonic

30. The term for the combined effect of drugs taken at the same time altering the expected therapeutic effect of each is known as:

    a. systemic action.
    b. therapeutic antagonism.
    c. drug interaction.
    d. mechanism of action.

31. When two drugs are used together to produce a desired effect that is much better than only one drug alone could produce is what type of synergism?

    a. additive effect
    b. potentiation
    c. competitive effect
    d. physiologic effect

32. You are interviewing a patient and find that the patient has been taking barbiturates regularly. Today he has also been drinking alcohol. What type of synergistic effect would you expect to find in this patient?

    a. additive
    b. potentiation
    c. competitive
    d. therapeutic

33. A patient who has ingested poison was given activated charcoal. The charcoal will bind and absorb to toxins present in the GI tract to inactivate and then excrete them. This chemical process is known as:

    a. loading dose.
    b. tolerance.
    c. hypersensitivity.
    d. antagonism.

34. A paramedic is about to administer adenosine to a patient experiencing SVT. The paramedic chooses a large venous access and will administer this medication in a *rapid* IV push, followed by a rapid flush, to achieve the correct therapeutic effect. Which of the following terms best refers to the specific reason for this therapeutic effect?

    a. idiosyncrasy
    b. adverse reaction
    c. half-life
    d. side effect

35. Which of the following legislative acts required drug manufactures for the first time to label certain dangerous ingredients on the packages?

    a. The Pure Food and Drug Act of 1906
    b. The Sherely Amendment of 1912
    c. The Kefauver-Harris Amendment in 1962
    d. The Harrison Narcotic Act

36. Controlled substances are divided into five schedules depending on their potential for abuse. Which of the following schedules would a cough preparation containing an opioid be listed in?

    a. I
    b. II
    c. IV
    d. V

37. For a drug product liability to exist it must meet three criteria. Which of the following is *not* one of those criteria?

    a. The paramedic administered the improper dose.
    b. The defect caused harm.
    c. The defect occurred before it left the manufacturer.
    d. The product is defective or not fit for its intended reasonable uses.

38. The injection of a drug into the spinal canal on or outside the dura mater that surrounds the spinal column is called a (an):

    a. subdural.
    b. epidural.
    c. intrapleural.
    d. intravenous.

39. When a drug is administered to be dissolved between the cheek and gum, what type of route is this?

    a. buccal
    b. sublingual
    c. ingestion
    d. intra-atricular

40. When diazepam is administered per rectum, what route of administration has this drug been given?

    a. transdermal
    b. subcuatenous
    c. enteral
    d. parenteral

41. One of the primary advantages for giving drugs by parenteral route in emergencies is that:

    a. IV access is always available.
    b. it is convenient.
    c. it is the most economical.
    d. absorption effects are more predictable.

42. You are assessing a patient with an altered mental status (AMS) and you find that the patient takes lasix, potassium and colace. The potassium bottle is old and empty. Based on the medications of the patient only, what might be the cause of the patient's AMS?

    a. dehydration
    b. hypertension
    c. diabetes
    d. thyroid

43. A 66-year-old female patient is experiencing severe side effects (slow heart rate and low blood pressure) from a new medication. Her past medical history includes stroke, COPD, kidney failure and diverticulitis. Based on her PMH, which of the following is the probable cause of the side effects?

    a. decreased pulmonary function
    b. decreased renal function
    c. neurologic dysfunction
    d. decreased GI motility

44. A drug reference and the only official book of drug standards in the United States that only lists drugs that have met high standards of quality, purity and strength is the:

    a. Physician's Desk References (PDR).
    b. US Pharmacopoeia.
    c. Hospital Formulary (HF).
    d. The FDA's Drug Reference.

45. Because the stomach has a pH of approximately 1.4 and the small intestine a pH of 5.3, a drug's chemical acidity will determine where it is absorbed. Which drugs will be better absorbed in the stomach than in the intestine?

    a. all drugs are absorbed in the intestine
    b. drugs that are neutral
    c. drugs with a weak base.
    d. drugs with weak acidity

46. IM drug administration should be avoided in the patient suspected of having an AMI because:

    a. the pain of injection may worsen the MI.
    b. it may elevate diagnostic enzyme levels.
    c. the drug will not be absorbed fast enough to be of benefit.
    d. total drug volumes are too large for cardiac patients.

47. You are administering an aerosolized medication to a patient for an asthma attack. How can you avoid inhaling the medication yourself?

    a. Have the patient take deep breaths and hold them.
    b. Wear a facemask.
    c. Ask the patient to exhale in a direction away from you.
    d. Plug the end of the nebulizer oxygen tubing.

48. Drugs are metabolized in the body by various organs and tissues. Which of the following is not involved in this process?

    a. liver
    b. lungs
    c. heart muscle
    d. intestinal mucosa

49. The adverse mental or physical condition affecting a patient through the outcome of treatment by a practitioner is called:

    a. iatrogenic.
    b. assay.
    c. disregard.
    d. identity crises.

50. The method for making sure a drug dosage and reliability are accurate is called:

    a. standardization.
    b. classification.
    c. cataloging.
    d. bioassay.

Test #7 Answer Form

	A	B	C	D		A	B	C	D
1.	❏	❏	❏	❏	26.	❏	❏	❏	❏
2.	❏	❏	❏	❏	27.	❏	❏	❏	❏
3.	❏	❏	❏	❏	28.	❏	❏	❏	❏
4.	❏	❏	❏	❏	29.	❏	❏	❏	❏
5.	❏	❏	❏	❏	30.	❏	❏	❏	❏
6.	❏	❏	❏	❏	31.	❏	❏	❏	❏
7.	❏	❏	❏	❏	32.	❏	❏	❏	❏
8.	❏	❏	❏	❏	33.	❏	❏	❏	❏
9.	❏	❏	❏	❏	34.	❏	❏	❏	❏
10.	❏	❏	❏	❏	35.	❏	❏	❏	❏
11.	❏	❏	❏	❏	36.	❏	❏	❏	❏
12.	❏	❏	❏	❏	37.	❏	❏	❏	❏
13.	❏	❏	❏	❏	38.	❏	❏	❏	❏
14.	❏	❏	❏	❏	39.	❏	❏	❏	❏
15.	❏	❏	❏	❏	40.	❏	❏	❏	❏
16.	❏	❏	❏	❏	41.	❏	❏	❏	❏
17.	❏	❏	❏	❏	42.	❏	❏	❏	❏
18.	❏	❏	❏	❏	43.	❏	❏	❏	❏
19.	❏	❏	❏	❏	44.	❏	❏	❏	❏
20.	❏	❏	❏	❏	45.	❏	❏	❏	❏
21.	❏	❏	❏	❏	46.	❏	❏	❏	❏
22.	❏	❏	❏	❏	47.	❏	❏	❏	❏
23.	❏	❏	❏	❏	48.	❏	❏	❏	❏
24.	❏	❏	❏	❏	49.	❏	❏	❏	❏
25.	❏	❏	❏	❏	50.	❏	❏	❏	❏

Medication Administration

1. You are working the v-fib algorithm on a patient in cardiac arrest, you have intubated, started an IV, given three shocks and administered 1 mg epinephrine and now you call medical control for further direction. Up to this point all the skills you have performed have been done as:

   a. direct orders of medical control.
   b. indirect orders of medical control.
   c. quality management.
   d. quality improvement.

2. The "six rights of medication administration" are used by health care providers as an effort to:

   a. avoid making medication administration errors.
   b. gain patient consent for emergency treatment.
   c. assure the patient is informed of his rights.
   d. remember when to document a PCR.

3. A chemical product designed for topical application to kill bacteria is a (an):

   a. antimicrobiotic.
   b. antibiotic.
   c. antiseptic.
   d. disinfectant.

4. A chemical or physical agent approved by the EPA to prevent infection by killing bacteria is a (an):

   a. antimicrobiotic.
   b. antibiotic.
   c. antiseptic.
   d. disinfectant.

5. All the following are examples of a sharp *except* a(an):

   a. used bristojet injector.
   b. open ampule.
   c. used angio catheter.
   d. open vial.

6. Which of the following is the most common complication associated with drawing blood samples?

   a. local infection
   b. systemic infection
   c. nerve or muscle damage
   d. miscannulation of an artery instead of a vein

7. You are looking at a patient's prescription medication bottle and the dose reads 40 mg b.i.d. How often should the medication be taken?

   a. once a day
   b. four times a day
   c. twice a day
   d. twice a night

8. Common sites for IM injection of medication include all the following *except*:

   a. medial malleolus.
   b. deltoid muscle.
   c. gluteus muscle.
   d. vastus lateralis.

9. The three systems of measure used for drug administration include the metric system, the apothecary system, and the _____ method.

   a. household
   b. English
   c. Mayan
   d. Egyptian

10. In the metric system of measure the basic unit of mass (weight) is the:

   a. kilo.
   b. ounce.
   c. gram.
   d. pound.

11. You are adjusting your drip rate to run approximately one drop every two seconds. This is the standard rate used when an IV is kept in place for purposes other than replacing fluids and is often referred to as:

   a. KVO.
   b. TKO.
   c. either KVO or TKO.
   d. neither KVO or TKO.

12. Change 44% into a decimal.

   a. 0.04
   b. 0.44
   c. 04.4
   d. 44.0

13. Change 7.8 into a percent.

    a. 7.8%
    b. 78%
    c. 780%
    d. 7800%

14. What is 25% of 0.66?

    a. 0.17
    b. 16.50
    c. 2.64
    d. 1.70

15. What is 250% of 30?

    a. 7500
    b. 0.12
    c. 8.33
    d. 75

16. What is 35.5% of 70?

    a. 1.97
    b. 24.85
    c. 248.5
    d. 197.18

17. Convert 1.5 to percent.

    a. 15%
    b. 150%
    c. 1500%
    d. 1.50%

18. Change the following improper fraction to a mixed number and reduce it to lowest terms, 32/12 = _____.

    a. 2 2/3
    b. 2 8/12
    c. 2.67
    d. 2 4/6

19. Multiply the following fractions and reduce to lowest terms, 3/10 x 8/16 = _____.

    a. 3/5
    b. 24/40
    c. 24/160
    d. 3/20

20. Divide the following fractions and reduce to lowest terms, 3/8 ÷ 2/3 = _____.

    a. 1/4
    b. 9/18
    c. 3/6
    d. 4 1/2

21. You need to administer 1.5 mg/kg of lidocaine to your patient who weighs 176 pounds. The drug comes packaged as 100 mg in 10 ml. How much lidocaine do you need to administer?

    a. 265 mg
    b. 120 mg
    c. 100 mg
    d. 80 mg

22. In reference to the previous question, how many milliliters of the lidocaine will you need to administer to deliver 1.5 mg/kg?

    a. 20.65
    b. 12
    c. 10
    d. 4

23. Medical control gives you an order to administer a 300 ml bolus over 30 minutes using a 10 gtt drip set. How many drops per minute will it take to infuse the bolus?

    a. 10 gtt/min
    b. 100 gtt/min
    c. 30 gtt/min
    d. 300 gtt/min

24. You are to administer D-50 to an unresponsive diabetic patient. The D-50 comes in a 50 cc (preload) syringe and you will administer all of it. How many grams of dextrose will you administer?

    a. 5
    b. 25
    c. 50
    d. 500

25. Medical control advises you to administer D-25 to a diabetic pediatric patient. The only dextrose you have on hand is D-50. What do you need to do to administer the proper concentration?

    a. Hang a drip of D-50.
    b. Infuse half the dose of D-50 without diluting.
    c. Dilute the D-50 by one-half, then administer.
    d. Tell medical control you cannot help the patient.

26. Following a bolus of lidocaine, you now need to set up an IV drip of 3 mg per minute. You have 200 mg of lidocaine, a 50 cc bag of normal saline, and a 60 gtt drip set. How many drops (gtts) per minute will you need to run to administer a 3 mg/min drip?

    a. 15 gtts
    b. 30 gtts
    c. 45 gtts
    d. 60 gtts

27. You are given an order to administer 5 mg of morphine sulfate to a patient. You have on hand two vials each containing 4 mg in 2 ml. How many ml of the drug will you have remaining after administering the correct dose?

    a. 0.5 ml
    b. 1 ml
    c. 1.5 ml
    d. 2 ml

28. You were just given a report on a patient and were told that the patient's temperature is 101.6° Fahrenheit. What is the patient's temperature in Celsius?

    a. 38.7°
    b. 39.5°
    c. 40.1°
    d. 41.3°

29. A drug package that is a small glass container with a rubber stopper by which the drug is withdrawn by a needle and syringe is a(an):

    a. ampule.
    b. vial.
    c. pre-loaded cartridge.
    d. small volume nebulizer.

30. Which of the following medications is administered enterally in the prehospital setting?

    a. epinephrine
    b. nitro paste
    c. nitro spray
    d. ASA

31. Which of the following is not true about medication administration by (PO) oral route?

    a. The absorption rate is fast.
    b. The absorption rate is slow.
    c. NPO in the field is common due to nausea and vomiting.
    d. PO medications are easy to take.

32. Which of the following is true about medication administration by (PR) rectal route?

    a. PR is the preferred route for pediatric medications.
    b. PR is the preferred route for seizure patients.
    c. PR allows for rapid absorption.
    d. The absorption rate is unpredictable.

33. While reviewing your paperwork you realize you made an error while charting a medication administration dose. The proper way to correct this error is to:

    a. erase the error and rewrite the correct dose.
    b. use a single line to mark out the error, make the change, and initial it.
    c. write over the error to fix it.
    d. never change or correct medications errors.

34. When using a blood pressure cuff as a tourniquet to start an IV, the cuff is inflated to occlude venous blood flow, but not arterial flow. What is the appropriate range of inflation for this procedure?

    a. 140–160 mmHg
    b. 120–130 mmHg
    c. 90–110 mmHg
    d. 70–80 mmHg

35. You have administered 25 mg of Benadryl® IVP to a patient experiencing an allergic reaction to a bee sting. Suddenly the patient becomes hypotensive. The hypotension is probably a result of:

    a. an incorrect dose of Benadryl®.
    b. a reaction from the bee sting.
    c. the incorrect route of medication administration.
    d. a potentiation effect of the medication.

36. Which of the following metric units is the largest prefix?

    a. kilo
    b. deka
    c. centi
    d. milli

37. Medical control has given you an order to administer 30 ml of ipecac to your patient who has ingested a poison. How many ounces do you administer to complete the order?

    a. one
    b. two
    c. three
    d. four

38. Given the same order for 30 ml of ipecac, how many tablespoons would you administer to complete the order?

    a. one
    b. two
    c. three
    d. four

39. You are setting up a Bretylium drip and you have 500 mg in 10 cc and a 50 cc bag of normal saline. When you combine the two, what is the concentration per cc?

    a. 10 mg/cc
    b. 20 mg/cc
    c. 30 mg/cc
    d. 40 mg/cc

40. Medical control gives you an order to run a dopamine drip at 5 mcg/kg/min. The patient weighs 100 kg and you have a concentration of 1600 mcg/ml mixed in a 250 ml bag with a micro drip set. How many drips per minute do you run?

    a. 19
    b. 30
    c. 45
    d. 63

41. Medical control gives you the order to administer 0.02 mg/kg of atropine to a child who weighs 12 pounds. The minimum loading dose of atropine is 0.1 mg. What is the correct dose for this child?

    a. 0.1 mg
    b. 0.15 mg
    c. 1.0 mg
    d. 1.5 mg

42. You are running a micro drip at one drop every two seconds. How many minutes will it take for a 50 ml bag of normal saline to run out completely?

    a. 25
    b. 30
    c. 50
    d. 100

43. You are running a one-liter bag of normal saline through a 10-gtts administration set at 60 gtts/min. During a 20 minute transport time to the hospital, how much fluid will be infused?

    a. 10 ml
    b. 20 ml
    c. 60 ml
    d. 120 ml

44. You are going to administer 5 mg/kg of Bretylium® to a 198-pound patient. The Bretylium® comes packaged in a vial of 500 mg in 10 ml. What is the smallest size syringe you can use to administer all the dose in one injection.

    a. 1 cc
    b. 5 cc
    c. 10 cc
    d. 15 cc

45. You are going to administer 150 mg of Amiodarone® over ten minutes. How many mg per minute will you infuse?

    a. 10
    b. 15
    c. 1.0
    d. 1.5

46. A male patient is bleeding from a traumatic injury and has lost 3.5 pints of blood. If his total blood volume is 6 quarts, what percent of his blood volume has he lost?

    a. 10
    b. 20
    c. 25
    d. 30

47. You have started an IV with a macro drip set at 10 gtt/ml. Medical control tells you to give one liter bag at a rate of 250 ml/hr. How many drops per minute will you need to infuse?

    a. 4 gtts/min
    b. 10 gtts/min
    c. 33 gtts/min
    d. 42 gtts/min

48. You are administering oxygen via a non-rebreather mask to a patient at 12 lpm. The tank contained 350 liters of oxygen when you began. How many minutes can you continue at the current rate before running completely out of oxygen?

    a. 25
    b. 29
    c. 33
    d. 39

49. You are going to give a subcutaneous injection to a patient. Which of the following needles would be the most appropriate for this administration?

    a. 19-ga and 1.5 inch needle
    b. 23-ga and 0.5 inch needle
    c. 18-ga angio
    d. 20-ga biopsy needle

Test #8 Answer Form

	A	B	C	D		A	B	C	D
1.	❏	❏	❏	❏	26.	❏	❏	❏	❏
2.	❏	❏	❏	❏	27.	❏	❏	❏	❏
3.	❏	❏	❏	❏	28.	❏	❏	❏	❏
4.	❏	❏	❏	❏	29.	❏	❏	❏	❏
5.	❏	❏	❏	❏	30.	❏	❏	❏	❏
6.	❏	❏	❏	❏	31.	❏	❏	❏	❏
7.	❏	❏	❏	❏	32.	❏	❏	❏	❏
8.	❏	❏	❏	❏	33.	❏	❏	❏	❏
9.	❏	❏	❏	❏	34.	❏	❏	❏	❏
10.	❏	❏	❏	❏	35.	❏	❏	❏	❏
11.	❏	❏	❏	❏	36.	❏	❏	❏	❏
12.	❏	❏	❏	❏	37.	❏	❏	❏	❏
13.	❏	❏	❏	❏	38.	❏	❏	❏	❏
14.	❏	❏	❏	❏	39.	❏	❏	❏	❏
15.	❏	❏	❏	❏	40.	❏	❏	❏	❏
16.	❏	❏	❏	❏	41.	❏	❏	❏	❏
17.	❏	❏	❏	❏	42.	❏	❏	❏	❏
18.	❏	❏	❏	❏	43.	❏	❏	❏	❏
19.	❏	❏	❏	❏	44.	❏	❏	❏	❏
20.	❏	❏	❏	❏	45.	❏	❏	❏	❏
21.	❏	❏	❏	❏	46.	❏	❏	❏	❏
22.	❏	❏	❏	❏	47.	❏	❏	❏	❏
23.	❏	❏	❏	❏	48.	❏	❏	❏	❏
24.	❏	❏	❏	❏	49.	❏	❏	❏	❏
25.	❏	❏	❏	❏					

9

Basic Cardiac Life Support Resuscitation Issues

1. The care provided in the first few minutes of a life-threatening emergency is called:

   a. CPR.
   b. FHPE.
   c. basic life support.
   d. ongoing assessment.

2. Basic life support is often used interchangeably with the term(s):

   a. BCLS.
   b. BLS.
   c. CPR.
   d. Any of the above are correct.

3. The general term now used to describe the spectrum of disease from acute angina to myocardial infarction is:

   a. heart attack.
   b. acute coronary syndrome.
   c. unstable angina.
   d. coronary illness.

4. Where do the International Guidelines 2000 come from?

   a. The United Nations
   b. The home office in Stockholm
   c. Consensus of the AHA and International Resuscitation Committee
   d. *The New England Journal of Medicine*

5. In which medical journal dated August 22, 2000 can you find the unabridged version of the Guidelines 2000 printed?

   a. *Annals of Emergency Medicine*
   b. *Circulation*
   c. *JEMS*
   d. *JAMA*

6. Guidelines that are supported by excellent, definitive evidence of effectiveness in humans would be considered class:

   a. I
   b. IIA
   c. IIB
   d. Indeterminate

7. The goal of the Guidelines 2000 was to develop widely accepted international resuscitation guidelines that were:

   a. based on a majority vote.
   b. based on the least cost to implement.
   c. based on scientific evidence.
   d. easy to read and explain.

8. Guidelines that are supported by very good evidence of effectiveness and safety in humans are class:

   a. I
   b. IIA
   c. IIB
   d. III

9. Guidelines supported by fair to good evidence of effectiveness and safety in humans with evidence of harm are class:

   a. I
   b. IIA
   c. IIB
   d. III

10. Actions or interventions with insufficient evidence to support a final recommendation for clinical use are placed into class:

    a. IIA
    b. IIB
    c. III
    d. Indeterminate

11. Each of the following is a Class IIA guideline *except*:

    a. no longer teaching lay rescuers the pulse check.
    b. early defibrillation capability for first responders.
    c. use of AED in patients under 8 years old.
    d. biphasic waveform defibrillation.

12. Leaving the non-traumatic cardiac arrest victim, after an adequate trial of BLS and ALS has been done, to support the survivors would be an example of a Class _____ guideline.

    a. I
    b. IIA
    c. IIB
    d. III

13. That all health care providers with a duty to perform CPR should be trained, equipped, and authorized to perform defibrillation is a class _____ guideline.

    a. I
    b. IIA
    c. IIB
    d. III

14. Changing the ratio to 15 compressions and 2 ventilations for both one and two rescuer adult CPR is a class _____ guideline.

    a. I
    b. IIA
    c. IIB
    d. Indeterminate

15. The recommendation that citizens in the work place be trained in the use of an AED is a class _____ guideline.

    a. I
    b. IIA
    c. IIB
    d. Indeterminate

16. When research strongly suggests the probability of harm, a guideline is called class:

    a. I
    b. IIB
    c. Indeterminate
    d. III

17. The use of abdominal thrusts in infants is considered a class _____ guideline.

    a. IIB
    b. IIA
    c. III
    d. Indeterminate

18. When an individual executes his right of self-determination and declares he does not want to be resuscitated if he becomes unresponsive, this is referred to as a/an:

    a. unrecognized determination.
    b. DNAR order.
    c. termination order.
    d. finale rite.

19. The Guidelines 2000 are considered:

    a. the legal standard of care.
    b. national regulations.
    c. consensus standards.
    d. international law.

20. For a patient to have undergone a successfully executed prehospital resuscitation and death pronouncement in the field, each of the following is necessary *except*:

    a. effective oxygenation and ventilation.
    b. VF has been shocked when present.
    c. appropriate medications were administered for the ECG dysrhythmia.
    d. the patient was unable to be tubed.

21. Who should pronounce death?

    a. whoever your state authorizes
    b. the paramedic on scene
    c. the EMT–basic on scene
    d. all of the above

22. If a patient received an adequate trial of ALS in the field, in which circumstance should you continue the arrest and transport to the local ED?

    a. a lengthy downtime
    b. the patient has a mortal injury
    c. A low body temperature
    d. rigor mortis is apparent

23. According to the Guidelines 2000, in order to assist the family of a deceased patient, the EMS provider should know all the following *except*:

    a. how to help the family accept non-transport of the patient.
    b. the fastest route to each funeral home.
    c. how to properly transfer the body to a funeral home.
    d. how to call a chaplain or family minister for grief counseling.

24. Of all the interventions available to the cardiac arrest patient, which has the most scientific evidence in its favor?

    a. CPR
    b. defibrillation
    c. compressions
    d. high dose epinephrine

25. The use of the AED is encouraged for all patients over the age of:

    a. 50
    b. 15
    c. 8
    d. 4

26. Where is the best "bang for the buck" in saving cardiac arrest patients?

    a. adding more ALS units
    b. expanding the use of fibrinolytics
    c. removing barriers to implementing PAD
    d. training EMT–Bs to intubate

27. Why do we phone fast instead of phone first in children less than 8 years of age?

    a. the biphasic defibrillator needs time to warm up
    b. these children need the medications first
    c. respiratory events are the most common cause of cardiac arrest
    d. defibrillation would be ineffective

28. In what situation should you phone first instead of phone fast?

    a. a child with previous ACS
    b. a child who may have drowned
    c. a child with a possible airway obstruction
    d. when you are not near a phone

29. In adults, when should the rescuer consider phoning fast instead of phoning first?

    a. cardiac arrest caused by electrical shock
    b. preexisting ACS
    c. poisoning or drug overdose
    d. patients over 60 years old

30. Why is the BVM now being emphasized for all health care providers learning CPR?

    a. The new BVMs insert the ventilations more quickly.
    b. When oxygen is used, the volume is less than previously thought.
    c. The new BVMs require one hand to use.
    d. The new BVMs provide higher airway pressures.

31. When using a BVM, the rescuer should:

    a. enlist a second rescuer to help squeeze the bag.
    b. use the "C"/"E" clamp hand position.
    c. provide slow breaths.
    d. all of the above.

32. Where is the best position for the ventilator when using a BVM on a supine patient?

    a. at the patient's side
    b. about 18" above the head of the patient
    c. straddling the patient
    d. lying flat on your stomach

33. Which statement is not correct?

    a. Proper use of the BVM requires practice.
    b. The jaw thrust can be used for one rescuer BVM, technique on a trauma patient.
    c. Tidal volumes of 400 to 600 ml can be given over one second.
    d. The BVM should be attached to 100% oxygen.

34. When smaller tidal volumes are used with the BVM, the:

    a. patient should be hyperventilated.
    b. breaths need to be given faster.
    c. breaths need to be more forceful.
    d. chest should rise visibly.

35. If a rescuer is unable to cover both the mouth and nose of an infant with his/her own mouth, it is acceptable to:

    a. do mouth to nose breathing.
    b. skip the ventilations.
    c. defibrillate the patient.
    d. use a Combitube®.

36. What is a false negative error?

    a. A positive finding
    b. type II
    c. type I
    d. an error that always occurs

37. What evidence helped researchers recommend dropping the pulse check step for laypersons?

    a. no one checks it anyway
    b. the patient often still has a faint pulse
    c. it takes too much time to teach
    d. they were frequently wrong in their assessment

38. What should the lay rescuer check to assess circulation?

 a. Listen for a cough
 b. Look for movement of the body
 c. Look for normal breathing
 d. All of the above

39. If a foreign body airway obstruction is suspected in an adult patient, the health care provider should:

 a. call for the defibrillator.
 b. reposition the neck and reattempt to ventilate.
 c. simply give chest compressions.
 d. perform a blind finger sweep.

40. In the United States, there are approximately _____ people who die each year from choking.

 a. 3,000
 b. 6,000
 c. 30,000
 d. 60,000

41. If a person has a FBAO and is an adult:

 a. do not do chest compressions.
 b. chest compression may be helpful.
 c. reach down their throat to remove the object.
 d. ventilate twice as fast.

42. Where are the hands placed to do CPR compressions on an adult?

 a. on the bottom of the breastbone
 b. at the top of the breastbone
 c. on the 7th intercostal space
 d. in the center of the chest between the nipples

43. At what rate should the chest be compressed for an adult patient?

 a. 60
 b. 80
 c. 100
 d. 120

44. The chest compression rate was changed in the Guidelines 2000 for all the following reasons except:

 a. frequent interruptions in compression reduce blood flow.
 b. the patient's blood volume increases at this rate.
 c. rescuers will eventually fatigue and slow down.
 d. the faster rate is better for blood pressure.

45. What is the compression to ventilation ratio in adults?

 a. 15:2
 b. 1:5
 c. 2:15
 d. 5:1

46. A faster, more forceful, ventilation increases the risk of:

 a. gastric inflation.
 b. aspiration.
 c. regurgitation.
 d. all of the above.

47. The first choice technique for chest compression in an infant when there are two rescuers is to do the:

 a. two thumb encircling hands chest technique.
 b. two fingers at the center of the chest.
 c. one-handed technique.
 d. none of the above.

48. If the public is unwilling to do the ventilations of CPR, they should be taught:

 a. to not offer assistance.
 b. to keep reassessing the breathing.
 c. compression-only CPR.
 d. to call first with all patients.

49. Under certain clinical conditions the evidence shows that:

 a. the LMA is superior to an ET tube.
 b. the LMA and Combitube® are better than BVM.
 c. the Combitube® is a dangerous device.
 d. all EMT–Bs should be trained in the use of the Combitube®.

50. Who should decide if EMT–Basics are trained to use the LMA?

 a. the training officer
 b. the International Resuscitation Committee
 c. the AHA
 d. the Medical Director

Test #9 Answer Form

	A	B	C	D			A	B	C	D
1.	❏	❏	❏	❏		26.	❏	❏	❏	❏
2.	❏	❏	❏	❏		27.	❏	❏	❏	❏
3.	❏	❏	❏	❏		28.	❏	❏	❏	❏
4.	❏	❏	❏	❏		29.	❏	❏	❏	❏
5.	❏	❏	❏	❏		30.	❏	❏	❏	❏
6.	❏	❏	❏	❏		31.	❏	❏	❏	❏
7.	❏	❏	❏	❏		32.	❏	❏	❏	❏
8.	❏	❏	❏	❏		33.	❏	❏	❏	❏
9.	❏	❏	❏	❏		34.	❏	❏	❏	❏
10.	❏	❏	❏	❏		35.	❏	❏	❏	❏
11.	❏	❏	❏	❏		36.	❏	❏	❏	❏
12.	❏	❏	❏	❏		37.	❏	❏	❏	❏
13.	❏	❏	❏	❏		38.	❏	❏	❏	❏
14.	❏	❏	❏	❏		39.	❏	❏	❏	❏
15.	❏	❏	❏	❏		40.	❏	❏	❏	❏
16.	❏	❏	❏	❏		41.	❏	❏	❏	❏
17.	❏	❏	❏	❏		42.	❏	❏	❏	❏
18.	❏	❏	❏	❏		43.	❏	❏	❏	❏
19.	❏	❏	❏	❏		44.	❏	❏	❏	❏
20.	❏	❏	❏	❏		45.	❏	❏	❏	❏
21.	❏	❏	❏	❏		46.	❏	❏	❏	❏
22.	❏	❏	❏	❏		47.	❏	❏	❏	❏
23.	❏	❏	❏	❏		48.	❏	❏	❏	❏
24.	❏	❏	❏	❏		49.	❏	❏	❏	❏
25.	❏	❏	❏	❏		50.	❏	❏	❏	❏

10

Life Span Development

1. The average weight of a newborn at birth is:

    a. 2.5–3.0 kg.
    b. 3.0–3.5 kg.
    c. 4.0–4.5 kg.
    d. 4.5–5.0 kg.

2. During the first week of life a baby will lose _____ percent of its body weight due to excretion of extracellular fluid present at birth.

    a. 2–5
    b. 5–10
    c. 10–15
    d. 15–20

3. The average weight of an infant is double its birth weight by what age?

    a. One year
    b. 3 months
    c. 4–6 months
    d. 9–12 months

4. When an infant has made the shift from fetal circulation to normal infant circulation, all the following statements are true, *except* the:

    a. ductus arteriosus opens.
    b. ductus arteriosus closes.
    c. ductus venosus closes.
    d. foramen ovale closes.

5. Infants are primarily obligate nose breathers until what age?

    a. 4 weeks
    b. 3 months
    c. 6 weeks
    d. 6 months

6. Of the following statements about the infant's pulmonary system, which is true?

    a. Diaphragmatic breathing causes the airways to be more easily obstructed.
    b. Accessory muscles of respiration are prone to barotraumas.
    c. The alveoli are numerous with increased collateral ventilation.
    d. The ribs are positioned horizontally, causing diaphragmatic breathing.

7. At what age do the posterior fontanelles close on an infant?

    a. 3 months
    b. 6 months
    c. 12 months
    d. 18 months

8. At what age do the anterior fontanelles usually close on an infant?

    a. 3–6 months
    b. 6–9 months
    c. 9–18 months
    d. 2 years

9. Which of the following factors does not influence bone growth?

    a. General health
    b. Parathyroid hormone
    c. Sleep cycle
    d. Thyroid hormone

10. What is the average annual weight gain, in kilograms, for children from one to five years of age?

    a. One
    b. Two
    c. Three
    d. Four

11. A four-year-old boy puts on his father's golf shoes and attempts to take a few practice swings with one of his father's golf clubs. In psychologic terms, what type of behavior is the child displaying?

    a. magical thinking
    b. modeling
    c. separation anxiety
    d. sibling rivalry

12. In which age group do children primarily develop self-esteem?

    a. toddler
    b. preschool
    c. school age
    d. adolescence

13. When a young teenage male experiences a change in voice quality, this is an example of a typical stage of:

    a. primary sexual development.
    b. secondary sexual development.
    c. a growth spurt.
    d. menarche.

14. Which of the following statements is true about endocrine system changes that take place during adolescence?

    a. Gonadotropins released by the pituitary gland promote the production of testosterone.
    b. Interstitial cell-stimulating hormone causes acne.
    c. Muscle mass increases from the release of lutenizing hormone.
    d. Body fat decreases from the release of follicle stimulating hormone.

15. Changes that occur during late adulthood within the respiratory system that lead to decreased respiratory function include a(an):

    a. decrease in elasticity of the diaphragm.
    b. increase in chest wall resolution.
    c. decrease in alveolar pressures.
    d. increase in pulmonic vascular strength.

16. The elderly often have an ineffective cough reflex caused by:

    a. exposure to cigarette smoke.
    b. weakening of the chest wall.
    c. lower production of cortisol.
    d. atrophy of the pituitary gland.

17. A major change in the endocrine system function during late adulthood is a(an):

    a. increased insulin production.
    b. decreased insulin production.
    c. increased thyroid hormone production.
    d. decrease in RBC production.

18. Older adults are often prescribed medications in lower doses than younger adults because of changes in metabolism caused by:

    a. increased acid reflux.
    b. increase in GI obstruction.
    c. vitamin deficiencies.
    d. changes in renal function.

19. Major changes in the gastrointestinal system that occur during late adulthood include all the following, *except*:

    a. a decrease in normal peristalsis.
    b. muscle sphincters become less effective.
    c. mineral deficiencies are common.
    d. salivary enzymes increase causing increased acid reflux.

20. Which of the following statements about adolescent growth spurts is most accurate?

    a. More boys than girls experience growth spurts.
    b. Growth spurts begin with enlargement of the chest and trunk.
    c. Growth spurts begin with enlargement of the feet and hands.
    d. Most boys are finished growing before most girls.

21. In which age group are the kidneys unable to concentrate urine?

    a. Infancy
    b. Toddler
    c. Adolescence
    d. Late adulthood

22. The "startle" reflex is a normal reflex in the first year of life. It consists of a rapid abduction and extension of the arms, followed by adduction of the arms. This reflex is also known as what reflex?

    a. Moro
    b. Palmar grasp
    c. Suckling
    d. Rooting

23. At birth, the infant immune system is relatively unde-veloped. Antibodies transferred from the mother main-tain passive immunity through what age?

    a. Six months
    b. One year
    c. Eighteen months
    d. Two years

24. A heart rate of less than _____ bpm in a newborn is abnormal.

    a. 140
    b. 120
    c. 110
    d. 100

25. You have just assisted in the delivery of a newborn, the respiratory rate after one minute is 20. This is consid-ered a/an _____ finding.

    a. normal
    b. abnormal
    c. critical
    d. insignificant

26. You are assessing an infant that is 11 months old. You do not know the child's exact weight, but you can es-timate that the child's weight is _____ its birth weight.

    a. double
    b. triple
    c. quadruple
    d. five times

27. Baby teeth begin to erupt at _____ months.

    a. 1 to 3
    b. 5 to 7
    c. 12 to 18
    d. 18 to 24

28. During the shift from fetal circulation to normal infant circulation, which of the following occurs?

    a. The ductus venosus closes.
    b. The foramen ovale opens.
    c. The ductus arteriosus opens.
    d. The lungs develop expectorants.

29. What is the leading cause of death among early adults?

    a. cancer
    b. Accidents
    c. AMI
    d. Suicide

30. In what age group does cardiovascular disease become a major concern?

    a. Adolescent
    b. Early adulthood
    c. Middle adulthood
    d. Late adulthood

31. The _____ syndrome occurs when all of a parent's children become old enough to leave home.

    a. biological clock
    b. desolation
    c. life span
    d. empty nest

32. _____ is the total duration of one life from birth to death.

    a. Life expectancy
    b. Life profile
    c. Development
    d. Life span

33. With the affects of aging, the baroreceptors within blood vessels lose their sensitivity. As a result, late adults are more sensitive to _____ changes.

    a. climate
    b. orthostatic
    c. elevation
    d. nutritional

34. It is not uncommon for a blood pressure reading to be falsely high in late adults because of the effects of:

    a. arteriosclerosis.
    b. postural hypotension.
    c. orthostatic changes.
    d. gravity.

35. As the heart ages, the myocardium is less able to re-spond to exercise because the muscle is:

    a. dehydrated.
    b. hypertrophied.
    c. less elastic.
    d. more elastic.

36. Degeneration of the cardiac conduction system may lead to a combination of brady and tachydysrhythmias, often called "tachy–brady" syndrome or _____ syn-drome.

    a. Wolff–Parkinson–White
    b. Sick–sinus
    c. Wilson–Mikety
    d. Witzelsucht

37. With aging there is a decreased functional blood volume and a decrease in the levels of RBCs caused by:

    a. polypharmacy.
    b. poor nutrition and malabsorption.
    c. dehydration.
    d. hypothyroidism.

38. _____ decreases the oxygen-carrying capacity of the blood, thus worsening an already tenuous cardiac function in the late adult.

    a. Atrial valve disease
    b. Diabetes
    c. Anemia
    d. Cardiomegaly

39. Which of the following statements is true about the changes in the respiratory system in late adulthood?

    a. There is an increase in generalized lung capacity.
    b. They have a decrease in upper respiratory infections.
    c. There is an increase of normal mucous membrane linings.
    d. They have a loss of normal mucous membrane linings.

40. Because of a decrease in _____ in the late adult, the development of serious diseases with very few clinical signs or symptoms may occur.

    a. pain perception
    b. kinesthetic sense
    c. visual acuity
    d. proprioception

41. Normal changes in the nervous system during late adulthood result in disturbances of the:

    a. sleep–wake cycle.
    b. myelin sheath.
    c. psychosomatic process.
    d. leukapheresis cycle.

42. Major psychosocial challenges of late adulthood include all the following, *except*:

    a. decreased self-worth.
    b. declining well-being.
    c. developing better relations with family.
    d. death or dying of friends.

43. In which age group do the changes in the respiratory system reach mature levels?

    a. school-age
    b. adolescence
    c. early adulthood
    d. middle adulthood

44. In which age group do the changes in the endocrine and reproductive systems reach adult levels?

    a. school-age
    b. adolescence
    c. early adulthood
    d. middle adulthood

45. At what age does the hearing sense reach peak (maturity) levels?

    a. 1 to 2 years
    b. 3 to 4 years
    c. 5 to 6 years
    d. 7 to 8 years

46. Normal behavioral "milestones" for the school-age child include all the following, *except* develops:

    a. self-concept.
    b. self-identity.
    c. self-esteem.
    d. morals.

47. Normal behavioral "milestones" for the toddler and preschool child include all the following, *except*:

    a. develops basics of language.
    b. understanding cause and effect.
    c. understanding of body image.
    d. television may affect behavior.

48. _____ is a term for normal hearing loss caused by aging.

    a. Tympanitis
    b. Otomylitis
    c. Kinesthesia
    d. Presbycusis

49. The late adult is less equipped to handle bodily stresses such as severe infection because of:

    a. an increase in thyroid hormone production.
    b. an increase in insulin production.
    c. a decrease in cortisol production.
    d. a decrease in financial status.

50. Changes in the myocardium in the late adult include:

    a. loss of normal cardiac pacemaker cells.
    b. enhanced automaticity.
    c. increased syncytium.
    d. decreased syncytium.

Test #10 Answer Form

	A	B	C	D		A	B	C	D
1.	❏	❏	❏	❏	26.	❏	❏	❏	❏
2.	❏	❏	❏	❏	27.	❏	❏	❏	❏
3.	❏	❏	❏	❏	28.	❏	❏	❏	❏
4.	❏	❏	❏	❏	29.	❏	❏	❏	❏
5.	❏	❏	❏	❏	30.	❏	❏	❏	❏
6.	❏	❏	❏	❏	31.	❏	❏	❏	❏
7.	❏	❏	❏	❏	32.	❏	❏	❏	❏
8.	❏	❏	❏	❏	33.	❏	❏	❏	❏
9.	❏	❏	❏	❏	34.	❏	❏	❏	❏
10.	❏	❏	❏	❏	35.	❏	❏	❏	❏
11.	❏	❏	❏	❏	36.	❏	❏	❏	❏
12.	❏	❏	❏	❏	37.	❏	❏	❏	❏
13.	❏	❏	❏	❏	38.	❏	❏	❏	❏
14.	❏	❏	❏	❏	39.	❏	❏	❏	❏
15.	❏	❏	❏	❏	40.	❏	❏	❏	❏
16.	❏	❏	❏	❏	41.	❏	❏	❏	❏
17.	❏	❏	❏	❏	42.	❏	❏	❏	❏
18.	❏	❏	❏	❏	43.	❏	❏	❏	❏
19.	❏	❏	❏	❏	44.	❏	❏	❏	❏
20.	❏	❏	❏	❏	45.	❏	❏	❏	❏
21.	❏	❏	❏	❏	46.	❏	❏	❏	❏
22.	❏	❏	❏	❏	47.	❏	❏	❏	❏
23.	❏	❏	❏	❏	48.	❏	❏	❏	❏
24.	❏	❏	❏	❏	49.	❏	❏	❏	❏
25.	❏	❏	❏	❏	50.	❏	❏	❏	❏

11

Airway Management and Ventilation

1. The upper airway consists of all the following structures, *except*:

   a. alveoli.
   b. thyroid cartilage.
   c. cricoid ring.
   d. vocal cords.

2. In the pediatric patient, the smallest diameter of the airway is located at the:

   a. epiglottis.
   b. pyriform fossae.
   c. ring in the trachea.
   d. cricothyroid membrane.

3. Which of the following is not correct about differences between adult and pediatric airways?

   a. The epiglottis of an infant or child is large and floppy.
   b. The epiglottis of infants and children is more rigid and firm.
   c. The mouth and nose of an infant or child is more easily obstructed.
   d. Infants and children have a softer, more flexible trachea than adults.

4. Which of the following is most correct about the tongues of infants and children?

   a. The tongue is difficult to manipulate during intubation.
   b. The tongue is easy to manipulate during intubation.
   c. They are proportionately smaller and take up less space in the mouth.
   d. They are proportionately larger and take up more space in the mouth.

5. Which of the following is not a component of the lower airway?

   a. Trachea
   b. Carina
   c. Bronchi
   d. Pyriform fossae

6. The function of the upper airway is to:

   a. warm, filter, and humidify the air we breathe.
   b. facilitate oxygenation at the cellular level.
   c. service pulmonary circulation through ventilation.
   d. exchange oxygen and carbon dioxide in the nares.

7. The function of the lower airway is to:

   a. warm, filter, and humidify the air we breathe.
   b. facilitate conversion of oxygen to energy.
   c. exchange oxygen and carbon dioxide at the cellular level.
   d. equalize pulmonary pressures.

8. _____ is the movement of carbon dioxide out of the lungs, and _____ is the movement of oxygen into the lungs.

   a. Ventilation; oxygenation
   b. Ventilation; perfusion
   c. Perfusion; ventilation
   d. Oxygenation; ventilation

9. The combined pressure of all atmospheric gases is the total pressure. At sea level the pressure, measured in torr, should add up to _____ torr and the percentage should equal _____ %.

   a. 100; 100
   b. 100; 760
   c. 760; 100
   d. 760; 760

10. The partial pressure of oxygen in the atmosphere at sea level is _____ torr.

   a. 597.0
   b. 159.0
   c. 3.7
   d. 0.3

11. Which of the following is correct about the difference between the concentration of alveolar and atmospheric gas?

    a. There is less nitrogen and oxygen in the alveolar gas.
    b. There is more nitrogen and oxygen in the alveolar gas.
    c. There is less water and carbon dioxide in the alveolar gas.
    d. There is no difference in concentrations.

12. The major controlling factors of the respiratory rate are the CNS and the:

    a. patient's mental status.
    b. patient's metabolic status.
    c. age of the patient.
    d. patient's heart rate.

13. What area in the CNS is the primary involuntary respiratory center?

    a. medulla
    b. vagus nerve
    c. chemoreceptor
    d. baroreceptor

14. The pons has the secondary control center of respirations called the _____ center.

    a. secondary
    b. backup
    c. chemoreceptor
    d. apneustic

15. Chemoreceptors control respiration by measuring the pH of the blood and:

    a. surfactant.
    b. pulmonary pressure.
    c. CSF.
    d. blood pressure.

16. Chemoreceptors are most plentiful in the carotid sinus and:

    a. aortic arch.
    b. medulla.
    c. pons.
    d. pneumotaxic center.

17. Normally the primary stimulus to breathe is a _____ in the blood.

    a. low concentration of carbon dioxide
    b. high concentration of carbon dioxide
    c. low concentration of oxygen
    d. high concentration of oxygen

18. In chronic COPD patients the normal stimulus to breathe may fail because of:

    a. the use of steroids.
    b. excessive mucus production.
    c. trapped or retained CO_2.
    d. excessive surfactant production.

19. Which of the following is not correct about COPD patients with hypoxic drive?

    a. These patients are very difficult to wean from ventilators.
    b. Long-term use of high flow oxygen is not harmful to these patients.
    c. The risk of underoxygenating a sick patient is usually greater than the risk of suppressing the stimulus to breathe.
    d. Only a small percentage of COPD patients are chronic CO_2 retainers.

20. The rate of respiration can be increased by any of the following factors, *except*:

    a. fever.
    b. drugs.
    c. acidosis.
    d. hypertension.

21. The condition that is characterized by a lack of oxygen in the tissues of the body is called:

    a. anaerobic metabolism.
    b. anoxia.
    c. hypoxemia.
    d. hypoxia.

22. _____ is a lack of oxygen in the blood.

    a. Anaerobic metabolism
    b. Anoxia
    c. Hypoxemia
    d. Hypoxia

23. The paramedic should consider any patient with a neurologic emergency to be _____ until proven otherwise.

    a. hyperventilating and alkalotic
    b. hypoventilating and hypoxemic
    c. obstructed
    d. acidotic

24. Common causes of laryngeal spasm include all the following, *except*:

    a. an overly aggressive intubation attempt.
    b. postextubation.
    c. cold water drowning.
    d. CVA.

25. Laryngeal edema can be caused by exposure to all the following, *except* inhaling:

    a. sea water.
    b. smoke.
    c. superheated gases.
    d. toxic substances.

26. Which of the following is not a complication associated with aspiration?

    a. FBAO
    b. severe allergic reaction
    c. destruction of lung tissue
    d. exposure of pathogens into the lungs

27. The bulb syringe, V-Vac® or foot pump unit are all examples of _____ devices.

    a. battery-powered airway
    b. oxygen-powered suction
    c. manual suction
    d. AC- or DC-powered suction

28. Oxygen-powered suction units work well but the biggest disadvantage is that they:

    a. are difficult to clean.
    b. are expensive.
    c. are heavy and difficult to carry.
    d. deplete your oxygen source rapidly.

29. Sterile suction technique is necessary when:

    a. performing any type of patient suctioning.
    b. suctioning the nose only.
    c. suctioning the tracheobronchial region.
    d. the patient has an OPA in place.

30. Suctioning can cause vagal stimulation by:

    a. changing the intrathoracic pressure.
    b. tickling the back of the throat.
    c. creating a hypoxic state.
    d. irritating the carotid sinuses.

31. Oral airways are hard plastic tubes designed to:

    a. prevent the tongue from obstructing the glottis.
    b. facilitate oral suctioning.
    c. facilitate oral tracheal intubation.
    d. guarantee that the airway will remain open.

32. The advantages of using a nasal airway include all the following, *except*:

    a. you can suction through them.
    b. they provide a patent airway.
    c. they can be used on a conscious patient.
    d. they cannot be used on a conscious patient.

33. Which of the following is correct about the bevel on the end of a nasal airway?

    a. The bevel helps to facilitate suctioning.
    b. The bevel is designed to face the nasal septum.
    c. The bevel is a measuring device.
    d. The bevel follows the natural curvature of the nasopharynx.

34. Only water-soluble jelly is used when lubricating airway tubes, because other products are not biodegradable and can:

    a. cause laryngeal edema.
    b. cause excessive slipping of the airway adjuncts.
    c. collect in the lung tissue causing a chemical aspiration pneumonia.
    d. interfere with surfactant production.

35. Pulsus paradoxus is present when the _____ BP drops more than 10 mmHg with _____

    a. systolic; inspiration.
    b. systolic; expiration.
    c. diastolic; inspiration.
    d. diastolic; expiration.

36. Pulsus paradoxus is seen in COPD patients and patients with pericardial tamponade, and may occur:

    a. in an allergic reaction.
    b. during an asthma attack.
    c. with pneumonia.
    d. with a URI.

37. All the following are examples of protective reflexes used by patients to modify their respirations, *except* a:

    a. cough.
    b. sneeze
    c. burp.
    d. hiccup.

38. _____ is an involuntary deep breath that increases opening of alveoli preventing atelectasis. This occurs, on average, once every hour.

    a. Coughing
    b. Sighing
    c. Hiccuping
    d. A gag reflex

39. Which of the following is not an example of an abnormal breathing pattern?

    a. Agonal
    b. Biot's
    c. Central neurogenic hyperventilation
    d. Eupnea

40. All the following are modified forms of respiration, *except*:

    a. sniffing position.
    b. Fowler's position.
    c. Trendelenburg position.
    d. tripod position.

41. Gastric distention results when a rescuer is giving too much ventilatory volume or when the:

    a. patient has an inspiratory effort.
    b. airway is not properly opened.
    c. patient aspirates.
    d. patient is not intubated.

42. Gastric distention increases the risk of regurgitation and potential for aspiration, as well as:

    a. creating resistance to bag-valve-mask ventilation.
    b. making an intubation more difficult.
    c. increasing the potential for laryngospasm.
    d. increasing the potential for bronchospasm.

43. The non-invasive method for managing gastric distention includes being prepared for the patient to vomit and:

    a. slowly applying pressure to the epigastric region.
    b. rapidly suctioning the hypopharynx until the patient is relieved.
    c. stimulating the gag reflex with the rigid suction tip.
    d. performing cricoid pressure and pressing on the stomach.

44. Which of the following statements about the use of a gastric tube is incorrect?

    a. It can be tolerated well by a conscious patient.
    b. It is only for use on unconscious patients.
    c. It does not interfere with intubation.
    d. It mitigates recurrent gastric distention and nausea.

45. Disadvantages of the use of a gastric tube include all the following, *except*:

    a. the patient can still talk.
    b. it may cause the patient to vomit.
    c. it may cause bradycardia.
    d. it interferes with a mask seal.

46. While inserting a naso-gastric tube in a patient with severe gastric distention, you observe that the patient's heart rate is decreased significantly. Which of the following would be appropriate to correct the problem?

    a. Terminate the procedure.
    b. Continue the procedure and then hyperventilate the patient.
    c. Ask the patient to stop talking.
    d. Administer phenergan for nausea.

47. If your efforts to correct the bradycardia in the patient described in question 46 have not worked and the heart rate remains low, your next step would include:

    a. administering atropine.
    b. terminating the procedure.
    c. administering phenergan for nausea.
    d. asking the patient to cough.

48. Managing the airway of a patient can be a hazard because of the:

    a. potential for a spinal injury.
    b. potential for breaking teeth.
    c. patient might bring a law suit when harm is done.
    d. exposure to body fluids.

49. Oxygen tanks are pressurized vessels that can be very dangerous if dropped. The weakest point is the _____, which could break and send the pressurized vessel flying like a missile.

    a. bottom of the tank
    b. valve stem
    c. hydrostate plate
    d. spine of the tank

50. Oxygen cylinders need to be hydrostatically tested every five years. However, if the tank has a star after the test date it is good for a(an) _____ year period.

    a. 8
    b. 10
    c. 12
    d. 15

51. When handling oxygen cylinders, the use of adhesive tape to mark or label tanks is not recommended because the materials in these products:

    a. may react with the oxygen and cause a fire.
    b. may react with the oxygen and cause an explosion.
    c. may cause the pressurized vessel to fly like a missile.
    d. makes the tank sticky and difficult to handle.

52. Which of the following statements about oxygen tank pressure and regulators is incorrect?

    a. The pressure of the tank is usually around 2,200 PSI.
    b. High pressure regulators are needed to deliver oxygen to patients.
    c. High pressure must be reduced to low pressure so that it is legal for ambulance use.
    d. Therapy regulators in ambulances are generally set at 50 PSI.

53. The maximum pressure recommended for positive pressure ventilation should not exceed _____ cm H_2O.

    a. 15
    b. 30
    c. 50
    d. 100

54. Which of the following oxygen delivery devices is also used to deliver medication?

    a. Partial-rebreather
    b. Venturi mask
    c. BiPAP
    d. Small volume nebulizer

55. Which of the following statements about the care of a laryngectomy patient is not correct?

    a. When doing rescue breathing, you ventilate into the stoma.
    b. When ventilating a partial laryngectomy patient, you need to cover the mouth.
    c. When ventilating a complete laryngectomy patient, you need to cover the mouth.
    d. In a laryngectomy patient, the airway may be attached to the end of a stoma in the neck.

56. What is the potential hazard of using a BVM with a pop-off valve?

    a. Pop-off valves are difficult to close and open.
    b. Pop-off valves are difficult to size to patients.
    c. Ventilations can exit the pop-off valve without getting air into the patient.
    d. It is more difficult to get a mask seal.

57. After a cervical collar is applied to a patient, it can be removed for intubation or to correct a problem in the airway only when:

    a. two hands provide manual in-line stabilization.
    b. a second paramedic is available to assist.
    c. the head is taped to a long backboard.
    d. the front of a collar is removed.

58. Which of the following is an indication for the use of intermittent positive pressure breathing (IPPB)?

    a. When a patient is noncompliant or combative.
    b. When a patient has poor tidal volume.
    c. When a patient needs a high volume of high concentration oxygen.
    d. When the patient is a small child.

59. One of the advantages of using IPPB is:

    a. that it allows for an easy mask seal.
    b. it reduces the risk of overinflation.
    c. there is no chance for barotrauma.
    d. there is no chance for gastric distention.

60. Which of the following is a contraindication for the use of a demand-valve?

    a. Tachypnea
    b. Bradypnea
    c. Apnea
    d. Dyspnea

61. All the following are advantages of an automatic transport ventilator (ATV), except they:

    a. are lightweight and portable.
    b. can minimize airway pressures.
    c. can reduce the risk of distension.
    d. can eliminate the risk of aspiration.

62. Which of the following is not a contraindication for the use of an ATV?

    a. Conscious patients that are combative.
    b. Patient with an obstructed airway.
    c. Patient with a pneumothorax.
    d. Conscious patients who are sedated.

63. _____ refers to positive pressure ventilation in a patient using either a tight-fitting nasal or face mask, but without endotracheal intubation.

    a. Continuous inflation flow
    b. Esophageal obturator
    c. Noninvasive ventilation
    d. Noninvasive transthoracic perfusion

64. The major advantage to the use of CPAP and BiPAP devices is that:

    a. intubation may be avoided where it may have previously been required.
    b. there is no wasting of oxygen.
    c. it is available to all prehospital providers.
    d. it does not require continuing education.

65. Collapse of the smaller airways and alveoli caused by hypoventilation or obstruction is called:

    a. pneumotaxis.
    b. atelectasis.
    c. hemotaxis.
    d. pneumothorax.

66. Which of the following patients are at risk for the condition described in question 65?

    a. A person with a history of deep vein thrombosis (DVT).
    b. A child on a ventilator.
    c. A patient who just had abdominal surgery.
    d. A COPD patient on BiPAP.

67. Why is the ET tube more likely to slide into the right mainstem bronchus than the left?

    a. The left mainstem is harder to see.
    b. The left mainstem is often occuled with mucus.
    c. The right mainstem bronchus is straighter.
    d. The right mainstem is more rigid than the left.

68. The _____ is used to help visualize the vocal cords during intubation with a laryngoscope.

    a. Berman maneuver
    b. Rothberg maneuver
    c. tripod position
    d. sniffing position

69. The patient you have intubated, because of a near respiratory arrest, appears to be improving and attempting to remove the ET tube. Which of the following is appropriate for the paramedic to manage the patient?

    a. Be prepared to suction the patient.
    b. Anticipate the need to reintubate the patient.
    c. Consider physical and chemical restraint in consult with Medical Control.
    d. All of the above.

70. Which of the following is not a significant risk associated with patients attempting to extubate themselves?

    a. Trauma to the airway
    b. Aspiration
    c. Hypoxia
    d. Protocol violation

71. What is the complication associated with performing the Sellick maneuver?

    a. When pressure is applied improperly, airway obstruction results.
    b. When performed improperly, atelectasis may develop.
    c. The early release of pressure can result in obstruction.
    d. The late release of pressure can result in aspiration.

72. When performing the Sellick maneuver, pressure is applied on the _____ of the cartilages and maintained until after the ET tube is inserted and _____

    a. lateral edge; the tube is measured.
    b. top edge; the cuff is inflated.
    c. bottom edge; and the tube is measured.
    d. lateral edge; the cuff is inflated.

73. All the following airway devices are considered indirect methods of airway control, *except* a/an:

    a. EOA.
    b. PTL.
    c. LMA.
    d. ETT.

74. The laryngeal mask airway, or LMA, can be used on all the following patients, *except*:

    a. children.
    b. chest trauma.
    c. cardiac arrest.
    d. elderly.

75. Digital or tactile intubation is a technique that may be helpful when:

    a. there is a suspected cervical spine injury.
    b. the tongue is extra large.
    c. secretions are copious.
    d. bleeding into the airway is uncontrolled.

76. Which of the following statements about retrograde intubation is not correct?

    a. It involves placing a needle through the cricothyroid membrane.
    b. It involves the use of a guidewire.
    c. It is a surgical procedure.
    d. It should only be performed by properly trained providers.

77. Pulse oximetry is a noninvasive technique that uses a/an _____ light beam to measure the oxygen saturation of the blood.

    a. effervescent
    b. luminescent
    c. infrared
    d. ultraviolet

78. The principle of pulse oximetry assumes all the following, *except* normal:

    a. capillary blood flow.
    b. hemoglobin concentration.
    c. hemoglobin molecule.
    d. venous blood flow.

79. Pulse oximetry would most likely be unreliable in all the following conditions, *except*:

    a. asthma attack.
    b. cardiac arrest.
    c. hypovolemia.
    d. hypothermia.

80. Which of the following devices is used for detection of exhaled CO_2 via the paper filter method?

    a. Pulse oximetry
    b. Colorimetric
    c. Capnography
    d. Capnometer

81. Before obtaining an accurate end-tidal CO_2 reading, it is recommended that the patient be ventilated 5–6 times to:

    a. wash out any residual $EtCO_2$ that may be present in the esophagus.
    b. rule out the presence of a pulmonary embolism.
    c. give the meter a chance to warm up.
    d. make sure the patient is hyperoxygenated.

82. The most common conditions for false capnography readings include all the following, *except*:

    a. non-perfusing patients.
    b. premature neonates.
    c. presence of a pulmonary embolism.
    d. ingestion of fruits prior to obtaining a reading.

83. A/An _____ is a syringe-like device that is helpful in verifying tracheal, versus esophageal, intubation.

    a. esophageal-gastric tube airway
    b. esophageal intubation detector
    c. Beck airway flow monitor
    d. esophageal obturator airway

84. During transport to the hospital with a cardiac arrest patient, you observe that the patient has become difficult to ventilate. Which of the following should you check first?

    a. Verify lung sounds.
    b. Check the pulse oximeter reading.
    c. Check the capnograph reading.
    d. Check the pulse.

85. Advantages of nasotracheal intubation include all the following, *except* the:

    a. technique does not require the use of a laryngoscope.
    b. patient cannot bite the tube.
    c. tube placement is more easily verified.
    d. tube is more easily secured.

86. The major disadvantage of nasotracheal intubation is that it:

    a. is a blind technique for breathing patients.
    b. is more difficult to verify tube placement.
    c. does not work with spinal cord injured patients.
    d. often has false-positive capnography readings.

87. Devices such as the Beck Airway Airflow Monitor (BAAM) and the Endotrol® tube are effective in facilitation of:

    a. orotracheal intubation.
    b. nasotracheal intubation.
    c. sterile suctioning.
    d. CO_2 monitoring.

88. _____ is a last resort airway technique when a patient has a complete airway obstruction or in whom tracheal intubation is otherwise impossible.

    a. LMA
    b. Needle decompression
    c. Needle cricothyrotomy
    d. Rapid sequence intubation

89. Translaryngeal cannula ventilation (TLCV) is a means of providing ventilation through a large-bore needle that is directly inserted:

    a. through the cricothyroid membrane.
    b. in the second intercostal space on the midclavicular chest.
    c. in the fifth intercostal space on the midaxillary chest.
    d. in the laryngectomy patient's stoma.

90. The neuromuscular blocking agent succinylcholine (SUX) is contraindicated in patients with massive tissue injury because of the:

    a. side effects associated with hypovolemia.
    b. effects of prolonged muscular tremors.
    c. risk of hypokalemia.
    d. risk of hyperkalemia.

91. Your patient is a two-year-old infant in respiratory arrest. Your partner is ventilating with a BVM while you prepare to intubate the child. You choose an uncuffed tube for this intubation because:

    a. cuffed tubes make visualization of the vocal cords more difficult.
    b. uncuffed tubes are easier to place than cuffed tubes.
    c. the cricoid cartilage narrows the trachea, and serves as a functional cuff.
    d. it is easier to verify tube placement with an uncuffed tube.

92. The patient you are evaluating for a syncopal event has started to seize and his teeth are clenched. Which of the following airway devices are appropriate for this patient?

    a. LMA
    b. Nasotracheal intubation
    c. Nasal airway
    d. Nasogastric tube

93. Which of the following lubrication products do you apply to the airway device used for the patient in question 92?

    a. an aloe-based product
    b. Vasoline®.
    c. Surgilube®.
    d. Valvoline®.

94. Research in the Guidelines 2000 has it acceptable to ventilate a person with a BVM _____ provided the BVM is attached to 100% oxygen.

    a. at lower volumes
    b. at the same volumes
    c. with a pop-off device
    d. that is smaller than previously used

95. Which of the following situations would most likely invite a paramedic to the courtroom?

    a. Use of the wrong size LMA that resulted in laryngitis.
    b. Use of a pediatric pop-off device that prevented adequate oxygenation of a patient.
    c. Recognition of a misplaced endotracheal tube, which was subsequently extubated in the field by the paramedic in charge.
    d. Documentation of a normal pulse oximetry reading by the paramedic on a patient who was really sick.

96. When the preintubation assessment of a patient indicates that endotracheal tube placement is going to be difficult, which of the following should the paramedic be prepared for?

    a. Do not attempt the intubation.
    b. Wait for the supervisor.
    c. Prepare a backup adjunct such as the LMA.
    d. Call Medical Control for instructions on performing a retrograde intubation.

97. Which of the following is not used to verify endotracheal tube placement?

    a. Pulse oximetry
    b. Capnography
    c. EID
    d. Digital intubation

98. Upon arrival at the scene of a MVC, you find that the driver is slumped over the steering wheel. You manually stabilize his cervical spine and see that he struck his neck on the rim of the steering wheel. Which of the following airway problems can you expect with this patient?

    a. Laryngeal edema
    b. Fractured larynx
    c. Laryngeal spasm
    d. All of the above

99. Further evaluation of the patient described in question 98 reveals that he has slow, shallow, stridorous respirations at a rate of 10 bpm. You begin to ventilate the patient with a BVM and consider using which of the following airway devices?

    a. OPA
    b. NPA
    c. LMA
    d. Combitube®

100. Which of the following patients is an ideal candidate for rapid sequence intubation?

    a. A patient with exacerbation of chronic COPD who has an altered mental status.
    b. A skier with a head injury who is conscious, but combative.
    c. Victim of a motor vehicle collision who has an altered mental status and severe facial trauma.
    d. A severely burned victim from a house fire.

Test #11 Answer Form

	A	B	C	D		A	B	C	D
1.	❏	❏	❏	❏	27.	❏	❏	❏	❏
2.	❏	❏	❏	❏	28.	❏	❏	❏	❏
3.	❏	❏	❏	❏	29.	❏	❏	❏	❏
4.	❏	❏	❏	❏	30.	❏	❏	❏	❏
5.	❏	❏	❏	❏	31.	❏	❏	❏	❏
6.	❏	❏	❏	❏	32.	❏	❏	❏	❏
7.	❏	❏	❏	❏	33.	❏	❏	❏	❏
8.	❏	❏	❏	❏	34.	❏	❏	❏	❏
9.	❏	❏	❏	❏	35.	❏	❏	❏	❏
10.	❏	❏	❏	❏	36.	❏	❏	❏	❏
11.	❏	❏	❏	❏	37.	❏	❏	❏	❏
12.	❏	❏	❏	❏	38.	❏	❏	❏	❏
13.	❏	❏	❏	❏	39.	❏	❏	❏	❏
14.	❏	❏	❏	❏	40.	❏	❏	❏	❏
15.	❏	❏	❏	❏	41.	❏	❏	❏	❏
16.	❏	❏	❏	❏	42.	❏	❏	❏	❏
17.	❏	❏	❏	❏	43.	❏	❏	❏	❏
18.	❏	❏	❏	❏	44.	❏	❏	❏	❏
19.	❏	❏	❏	❏	45.	❏	❏	❏	❏
20.	❏	❏	❏	❏	46.	❏	❏	❏	❏
21.	❏	❏	❏	❏	47.	❏	❏	❏	❏
22.	❏	❏	❏	❏	48.	❏	❏	❏	❏
23.	❏	❏	❏	❏	49.	❏	❏	❏	❏
24.	❏	❏	❏	❏	50.	❏	❏	❏	❏
25.	❏	❏	❏	❏	51.	❏	❏	❏	❏
26.	❏	❏	❏	❏	52.	❏	❏	❏	❏

	A	B	C	D		A	B	C	D
53.	❏	❏	❏	❏	77.	❏	❏	❏	❏
54.	❏	❏	❏	❏	78.	❏	❏	❏	❏
55.	❏	❏	❏	❏	79.	❏	❏	❏	❏
56.	❏	❏	❏	❏	80.	❏	❏	❏	❏
57.	❏	❏	❏	❏	81.	❏	❏	❏	❏
58.	❏	❏	❏	❏	82.	❏	❏	❏	❏
59.	❏	❏	❏	❏	83.	❏	❏	❏	❏
60.	❏	❏	❏	❏	84.	❏	❏	❏	❏
61.	❏	❏	❏	❏	85.	❏	❏	❏	❏
62.	❏	❏	❏	❏	86.	❏	❏	❏	❏
63.	❏	❏	❏	❏	87.	❏	❏	❏	❏
64.	❏	❏	❏	❏	88.	❏	❏	❏	❏
65.	❏	❏	❏	❏	89.	❏	❏	❏	❏
66.	❏	❏	❏	❏	90.	❏	❏	❏	❏
67.	❏	❏	❏	❏	91.	❏	❏	❏	❏
68.	❏	❏	❏	❏	92.	❏	❏	❏	❏
69.	❏	❏	❏	❏	93.	❏	❏	❏	❏
70.	❏	❏	❏	❏	94.	❏	❏	❏	❏
71.	❏	❏	❏	❏	95.	❏	❏	❏	❏
72.	❏	❏	❏	❏	96.	❏	❏	❏	❏
73.	❏	❏	❏	❏	97.	❏	❏	❏	❏
74.	❏	❏	❏	❏	98.	❏	❏	❏	❏
75.	❏	❏	❏	❏	99.	❏	❏	❏	❏
76.	❏	❏	❏	❏	100.	❏	❏	❏	❏

12

Therapeutic Communications and History Taking

1. Like many professions, _____ is an integral component of the EMS profession.

    a. encoding
    b. communication
    c. sign language
    d. diet

2. Which of the following is not a form of communication used in the EMS profession?

    a. written
    b. verbal
    c. non-verbal
    d. prayer

3. During the patient interview the paramedic should be able to determine all the following, *except* if the patient is:

    a. conversing normally.
    b. responding reasonably to questions.
    c. hypertensive.
    d. oriented.

4. A _____ history is all the medical events and conditions that have ever occurred to the patient.

    a. complete health
    b. focused
    c. past medical
    d. SAMPLE

5. A focused history is the chronologic history of the patient's:

    a. surgeries.
    b. present illness.
    c. medication use.
    d. family history.

6. The paramedic should attempt to obtain all the following information about a patient's current event, *except*:

    a. Is this similar to any previous events?
    b. How many times has an event like this happened?
    c. When was the last event?
    d. Will a similar event occur in the future?

7. The acronym OPQRST is used to remember the set of questions used to obtain information about the patient's:

    a. past medical history.
    b. complete health history.
    c. use of OTC medications.
    d. present illness or injury.

8. Use the acronym SAMPLE to remember the set of questions used to obtain information about the patient's:

    a. past medical history.
    b. focused history.
    c. childhood history.
    d. present illness or injury.

9. Which of the following pieces of patient information is irrelevant to the paramedic in the field?

    a. recent surgery
    b. recent illness
    c. change in daily living activities
    d. tonsillectomy in childhood

10. All the following should be asked about a patient's medications, *except* have they:

    a. started taking any new ones.
    b. stopped taking any new ones.
    c. changed from name brand to generic label.
    d. modified any current doses.

11. Why is it important for the paramedic to be empathetic when obtaining a health history?

    a. Showing empathy helps to obtain more cooperation from the patient.
    b. Empathy helps the family to trust you with the patient.
    c. It is a way of showing respect to the patient.
    d. It helps the patient to communicate with the next health care provider.

12. Which of the following is a disrespectful use of terms for the patient?

    a. using the patient's proper name
    b. calling the patient honey
    c. using the patient's nickname with permission
    d. using the patient's first name with permission

13. Although paramedics are taught to ask direct questions of the patient, which of the following is an example of a good open-ended question to ask a patient?

    a. What do you for relaxation?
    b. Why did you call us here today?
    c. How does that make you feel?
    d. Why do you feel that your doctor is unable to help you?

14. When you are not getting the answer to questions that appear obvious, consider that the patient may be:

    a. pregnant.
    b. falsely reassured.
    c. not ill or injured.
    d. embarrassed.

15. In order to maintain privacy for the patient, examples of questions that you should not ask the patient in public include all the following, *except*:

    a. Are you pregnant?
    b. Do you have a psychiatric illness?
    c. Do you have chest pain?
    d. Have you been raped?

16. When is it better to ask direct questions of the patient?

    a. when a behavioral problem is suspected
    b. when specific information is required
    c. when the patient's family is present
    d. when the patient has no specific complaint

17. Which of the following cultures may consider direct eye contact during an interview to be impolite or aggressive?

    a. Italians
    b. Germans
    c. Native Americans
    d. New Yorkers

18. Why should the paramedic avoid providing false reassurance when the situation is serious?

    a. The patient will sue if they find out the truth.
    b. The patient will suffer harm.
    c. The paramedic could lose his/her certification.
    d. The paramedic could lose the patient's trust.

19. Which of the following is an example of a leading question?

    a. Do you have sharp chest pain?
    b. Are you pregnant?
    c. Do you have a history of diabetes?
    d. When did you last take your medication?

20. Which of the following is an example of a condescending question to be avoided during an interview?

    a. How much did you have to drink tonight?
    b. You don't smoke, do you?
    c. Do you take your medications every day?
    d. When was your last menstrual period?

21. During an interview with a patient, all the following are to be avoided, *except*:

    a. the use of complicated medical terminology.
    b. explaining what is happening to the patient.
    c. talking down to the patient.
    d. the use of leading questions.

22. Which of the following is not an example of negative non-verbal communications?

    a. sitting close to the patient
    b. inattentiveness
    c. arms crossed
    d. standing over the patient

23. _____ is the way you speak, and how your posture and your actions are used to encourage the patient to say more.

    a. Empathy
    b. Confrontation
    c. Facilitation
    d. Reflection

24. To repeat or echo the patient's own words as a way of encouraging the flow of conversation without interrupting the patient's concentration is referred to as:

    a. interpretation.
    b. clarification.
    c. facilitation.
    d. reflection.

25. _____ is reasoning based not on what you observed from the patient, but what you have concluded from the information you have compiled.

   a. Interpretation
   b. Clarification
   c. Empathy
   d. Silence

26. Which of the following medications can be found in a patient's refrigerator?

   a. Epi-pen®
   b. Insulin
   c. Vial-of-life®
   d. Nitroglycerin

27. A rolled piece of paper in a plastic container, which contains medical information about a patient, is a/an:

   a. Medic alert tag®.
   b. Prescription bottle.
   c. Vial of life®.
   d. Emergency lifeline®.

28. While treating a patient that only speaks a foreign language that you do not, and no interpreter is immediately available, which of the following can you do to best facilitate care?

   a. use positive body language while you begin care
   b. wait for a translator before initiating care
   c. ask police for assistance
   d. call the paramedic supervisor

29. While caring for a blind patient, it is appropriate to announce yourself, explain as much as possible and to:

   a. secure the seeing eye dog for your protection.
   b. speak while facing the patient.
   c. interact with the patient the same as with a seeing patient.
   d. ask permission to touch the patient before actually touching him or her.

30. You are caring for a patient who is very angry and is taking his anger out on you. Which of the following should you avoid doing?

   a. getting angry in return
   b. do a quick pat down for weapons
   c. keep the situation calm
   d. request police

31. Sleep disorders, appetite disturbances, the inability to concentrate, and lack of energy are all signs of:

   a. fear.
   b. confusion
   c. depression.
   d. abuse.

32. When interviewing a patient who is extremely talkative, but is not providing you with the information you need, which of the following techniques might be useful in obtaining what you need?

   a. Ignore the patient.
   b. Ask the patient to stop talking and listen.
   c. Try using diversion tactics.
   d. Try using direct yes or no questions.

33. _____ and history taking are a significant portion of the patient interview.

   a. Dispatch information
   b. A rapid response time
   c. Establishing a rapport with the patient
   d. Professional appearance

34. Getting a good history can be difficult for each of the following reasons, *except*:

   a. the patient is a poor historian.
   b. unconsciousness.
   c. the patient is blind.
   d. the patient is a nursing home resident.

35. Which of the following is not considered part of a health history?

   a. religious beliefs
   b. career status
   c. daily living activities
   d. current vital signs

36. Information obtained from the patient or bystanders about the current event, including what led up to it is called:

   a. chief complaint.
   b. focused history.
   c. signs and symptoms.
   d. positive feedback.

37. Communication techniques that may be useful during the patient interview include all the following, *except*:

   a. silence.
   b. encoding.
   c. listening
   d. explanation.

38. _____ may be found on necklaces, bracelets and anklets and provide vital medical information such as a medical condition or reaction.

   a. Dog tags®
   b. Lucky charms®
   c. Medic alert tags®
   d. Coils

39. Once you have arrived at the ED with a hearing impaired patient, the _____ requires that the hospital provide a sign interpreter within 30 minutes of the patient's arrival.

   a. ADA
   b. VA
   c. CDC
   d. ASL bill

40. When caring for a hearing impaired patient be sure to face the patient when you are speaking and to:

   a. speak very slowly.
   b. use a family member to communicate.
   c. exaggerate your speech.
   d. look to see if his/her hearing aid is on.

Test #12 Answer Form

	A	B	C	D			A	B	C	D
1.	❏	❏	❏	❏		21.	❏	❏	❏	❏
2.	❏	❏	❏	❏		22.	❏	❏	❏	❏
3.	❏	❏	❏	❏		23.	❏	❏	❏	❏
4.	❏	❏	❏	❏		24.	❏	❏	❏	❏
5.	❏	❏	❏	❏		25.	❏	❏	❏	❏
6.	❏	❏	❏	❏		26.	❏	❏	❏	❏
7.	❏	❏	❏	❏		27.	❏	❏	❏	❏
8.	❏	❏	❏	❏		28.	❏	❏	❏	❏
9.	❏	❏	❏	❏		29.	❏	❏	❏	❏
10.	❏	❏	❏	❏		30.	❏	❏	❏	❏
11.	❏	❏	❏	❏		31.	❏	❏	❏	❏
12.	❏	❏	❏	❏		32.	❏	❏	❏	❏
13.	❏	❏	❏	❏		33.	❏	❏	❏	❏
14.	❏	❏	❏	❏		34.	❏	❏	❏	❏
15.	❏	❏	❏	❏		35.	❏	❏	❏	❏
16.	❏	❏	❏	❏		36.	❏	❏	❏	❏
17.	❏	❏	❏	❏		37.	❏	❏	❏	❏
18.	❏	❏	❏	❏		38.	❏	❏	❏	❏
19.	❏	❏	❏	❏		39.	❏	❏	❏	❏
20.	❏	❏	❏	❏		40.	❏	❏	❏	❏

13
Techniques of Physical Examination

1. All the following are examples of *cognitive* skills used by paramedics, *except*:

    a. assessing mental status.
    b. assessing vital signs.
    c. obtaining a focused history.
    d. making a priority treatment decision.

2. Putting on gloves and wearing a face mask and a gown are examples of:

    a. taking standard precautions.
    b. performing an assessment.
    c. components of a physical examination.
    d. patient contact priorities.

3. Which technique of physical examination is the best to use when assessing a patient's chest wall for symmetry?

    a. auscultation
    b. visual inspection
    c. percussion
    d. palpation

4. An example of a patient's specific characteristic that is apparent on visual inspection is:

    a. wheezing.
    b. personal hygiene.
    c. bruits.
    d. crepitus.

5. Listening skills that a paramedic should hone with frequent practice include all the following, *except*:

    a. lung sounds.
    b. heart sounds.
    c. bruits.
    d. ambient noises.

6. One step that the paramedic can take to reduce a patient's anxiety, fear and muscle tensing prior to palpation is:

    a. warm hands before touching the patient.
    b. establish medical control.
    c. begin transport and turn the lights down low.
    d. apply oxygen by non-rebreather.

7. Evaluating the patient for level of distress, age, gender and skin color, temperature, and condition are examples of things the paramedic looks for to determine:

    a. the patient's chief complaint.
    b. the general appearance of the patient.
    c. when to question a patient's family about history.
    d. how to recognize a sensory dysfunction.

8. When auscultating for heart sounds the paramedic should place the bell of the stethoscope at the:

    a. fifth intercostal space at the midclavicular line on the left chest.
    b. mid-axillary line at the fourth intercostal space on the left chest.
    c. just above the left nipple line.
    d. two inches to the left of the suprasternal notch.

9. An EMT–B is assessing a blood pressure on a patient who is morbidly obese, you notice that the blood pressure cuff is too small for the patient's arm. What reading would you expect to get under this circumstance?

    a. an accurate reading
    b. inaccurately high reading
    c. inaccurately low reading
    d. no reading

10. While taking a blood pressure, the sounds heard with a stethoscope that indicate the systolic and diastolic readings are called:

    a. pulse pressures.
    b. pulsus paradoxus.
    c. apical pulse.
    d. Korotkoff sounds.

11. When taking a blood pressure by palpation, the paramedic will palpate a distal pulse while first inflating and then deflating the cuff in order to obtain a _____ pressure.

   a. pulse
   b. systolic
   c. diastolic
   d. mean arterial

12. The method of obtaining a blood pressure by palpation is often used because:

   a. ambient noise is too loud to hear pulse sounds.
   b. the paramedic is too lazy to use a stethoscope.
   c. taking a blood pressure by auscultation takes too long.
   d. a trained provider is not available to take it.

13. A paramedic is about to take a blood pressure on a patient's right arm when she tells him that she has had a mastectomy on the right side. The paramedic now takes the blood pressure on the left arm because taking a blood pressure on the right arm may be painful for the patient, as well as:

   a. cause the patient to experience a TIA.
   b. precipitate a blood clot.
   c. cause an inaccurate reading.
   d. give the patient a reason to sue the paramedic.

14. While assessing a patient's legs for the presence of edema, the paramedic notes that edema is severe and pitting +4. The paramedic recognizes that this condition is significant and indicates a problem with patient's heart, lungs or:

   a. spleen.
   b. kidneys.
   c. gall bladder.
   d. liver.

15. Assessing the elasticity of the skin (turgor) can indicate the patient's state of hydration. Another possible reason for having an increased skin turgor is that the patient has:

   a. obesity.
   b. ingested methanol.
   c. Cushing's syndrome.
   d. connective tissue disease.

16. The presence of JVD in a patient sitting at a 90° position is an abnormal finding and may indicate serious pathology such as severe right heart failure, pericardial tamponade or:

   a. tension pneumothorax.
   b. thyroid storm.
   c. hypertensive crises.
   d. hypovolemia.

17. The presence of unilateral JVD is abnormal and may indicate which of the following conditions?

   a. liver disease
   b. excessive alcohol use
   c. local vein blockage or restriction
   d. congestive heart failure

18. To assess the hepatojugular reflex on a patient, the paramedic begins by placing the patient in which position?

   a. trendelenburg position
   b. semi-fowlers with the head at the 30° angle
   c. high-fowlers with the head at a 10° angle
   d. semi-recumbent

19. While assessing a patient's hepatojugular reflex, the paramedic notes an increase of 1.5 cm in JVD. This finding may indicate right heart failure or:

   a. an AMI.
   b. unstable angina.
   c. stable angina.
   d. fluid overload.

20. A device consisting of a light source projected through a cone shaped device that is placed into an orifice to visualize the inner structures is called a/an:

   a. otoscope.
   b. ophthalmoscope.
   c. penlight.
   d. Doppler.

21. A device consisting of a light source and several lenses that is used to look at the eye is called a/an:

   a. otoscope.
   b. ophthalmoscope.
   c. penlight.
   d. Doppler.

22. Pulse oximetry is used to assess the oxygen saturation of a patient's:

    a. hematocrit.
    b. central venous pressure.
    c. capillary venous pressure.
    d. hemoglobin.

23. A patient who is in a shock may have pulse oximetry readings that are:

    a. indicative of an AMI.
    b. consistent with altered mental status.
    c. falsely low.
    d. falsely high.

24. When percussing the chest of a patient with a disease, such as the accumulation of fluid in the lungs, the paramedic may expect to hear what type of sound?

    a. dull or flattened tone
    b. hyperresonance
    c. intonation
    d. sonority

25. A paramedic is assessing a patient for carotid bruits and hears them on the patient's left side. The paramedic knows that the left carotid artery is occluded at least:

    a. one-quarter to one-half.
    b. one-half to two-thirds.
    c. one-third.
    d. twenty percent.

26. The most helpful finding the paramedic can provide to the ED about a patient's bowel sounds is which of the following?

    a. hyperactive sounds
    b. hypoactive sounds
    c. absence of sounds
    d. normal sounds

27. After performing deep palpation on a patient's abdomen, the paramedic reported to the ED that the patient was positive for Murphy's sign. Which of the following conditions did the paramedic find during her examination?

    a. tenderness of the gallbladder
    b. enlarged liver
    c. enlarged spleen
    d. tenderness of the appendix

28. In which of the following cases would the pulse oximetry reading be most useful to the paramedic?

    a. SpO_2 96% in a 65-year-old female complaining of exertional dyspnea and who has a history of COPD.
    b. SpO_2 88% in a 3 year old having an asthma attack.
    c. SpO_2 98% in a 30-year-old female complaining of weakness and a history of anemia.
    d. SpO_2 100% in a 19-year-old male who just attempted suicide by CO exposure.

29. Whenever possible, avoid taking a blood pressure on an extremity that is:

    a. painful or injured.
    b. cool to the touch.
    c. wet or diaphoretic.
    d. presenting with pitting edema.

30. A _____ is a turbulent noise that sounds like swishing, which can be heard over arteries in the body that have become occluded.

    a. crackle
    b. bruit
    c. tic
    d. murmur

31. You are assessing a 74-year-old patient complaining of shortness of breath, with a history of COPD and CHF. She is at home in bed and states she has been unable to get up to take her medications for two days. During your physical examination, you look for the presence of edema. What area would be prominent with edema?

    a. ankles
    b. feet
    c. hands
    d. sacral area

32. Which of the following is a sign of a distressed patient?

    a. A baby with grunting respirations.
    b. A teenager with loud bilateral bowel sounds.
    c. A toddler screaming after falling out of a shopping cart.
    d. A sleepy baby after having a febrile seizure.

33. _____ is an irregular body texture characterized by air trapped under the skin.

    a. Edema
    b. Crepitus
    c. Tenting
    d. Subcutaneous emphysema

34. In which of the following patients would a head to toe exam be the preferred method of physical examination?

    a. 2-year-old infant with respiratory distress.
    b. 18-year-old male in a motorcycle accident.
    c. 48-year-old female with abdominal pain.
    d. 72-year-old with fears of being sent to a nursing home by her son.

35. You are transporting a patient from a nursing home to the hospital for evaluation. On the chart you read that the patient has had rhinorrhea for two days. What clinical finding would this indicate?

    a. watery discharge from the nose
    b. bloody nose
    c. csf seeping from the ear canal
    d. excessive drooling without control

36. In the prehospital setting the most common site to auscultate for bruits is over the:

    a. carotid artery.
    b. abdomen.
    c. upper chest.
    d. brachial artery.

37. To accurately assess a patient for the presence of JVD, the patient should be placed in which position?

    a. supine with legs dangling
    b. sitting upright at 90°
    c. sitting up at 45°
    d. trendelenburg position

38. To listen for vesicular breath sounds place the diaphragm over the:

    a. second intercostal space at the midclavicular line.
    b. second intercostal space at the midaxillary line.
    c. fifth anterior axillary line and midaxillary line at the fifth rib level.
    d. fifth posterior axillary line and midclavicular line.

39. Muffled or distant heart sounds may indicate the presence of:

    a. trapped air.
    b. fluid.
    c. bruits.
    d. a broken stethoscope.

40. All the following are normal findings during examination of the abdomen, *except*:

    a. muscle tensing on palpation.
    b. non-tender on palpation.
    c. presence of bowel sounds.
    d. absence of bowel sounds.

41. A term for local or generalized abnormal accumulation of fluids in body tissues is:

    a. bloat.
    b. tenting.
    c. subcutaneous emphysema.
    d. edema.

42. When assessing a patient with bruising, the most significant clinical feature of the bruise is:

    a. the color or age.
    b. the shape.
    c. how he/she got it.
    d. how long will it last.

43. HEENT is an acronym used to recall all the areas to be examined about the:

    a. extremities.
    b. trunk.
    c. airway.
    d. head.

44. The most significant clinical finding about a person's hearing is:

    a. the absence of hearing.
    b. the presence of tinnitus.
    c. acute changes in hearing.
    d. the use of a hearing aide.

45. Common abnormal findings about the head include all the following, *except*:

    a. muscle tics.
    b. facial drooping.
    c. decreased skin turgor.
    d. unrestricted ROM.

46. Which of the following devices would you use to inspect a patient's eyes?

    a. otoscope
    b. ophthalmoscope
    c. hydroscope
    d. doppler

47. An $EtCO_2$ device measures the amount of _____ during each breath at the end of _____.

    a. carbon dioxide: inspiration.
    b. carbon monoxide: inspiration.
    c. carbon dioxide: exhalation.
    d. carbon monoxide: exhalation.

48. _____ is a term used when assessing a patient's skin for state of hydration.

    a. Hydrolysis
    b. Edema
    c. Turgor
    d. Rigidity

49. The bell of the stethoscope is best used for listening to _____ sounds.

    a. normal heart
    b. abnormal heart
    c. bowel
    d. breath

50. The presence of ascites upon physical examination is an abnormal finding on which area of the body?

    a. head
    b. neck
    c. abdomen
    d. extremities

Test #13 Answer Form

	A	B	C	D		A	B	C	D
1.	❏	❏	❏	❏	26.	❏	❏	❏	❏
2.	❏	❏	❏	❏	27.	❏	❏	❏	❏
3.	❏	❏	❏	❏	28.	❏	❏	❏	❏
4.	❏	❏	❏	❏	29.	❏	❏	❏	❏
5.	❏	❏	❏	❏	30.	❏	❏	❏	❏
6.	❏	❏	❏	❏	31.	❏	❏	❏	❏
7.	❏	❏	❏	❏	32.	❏	❏	❏	❏
8.	❏	❏	❏	❏	33.	❏	❏	❏	❏
9.	❏	❏	❏	❏	34.	❏	❏	❏	❏
10.	❏	❏	❏	❏	35.	❏	❏	❏	❏
11.	❏	❏	❏	❏	36.	❏	❏	❏	❏
12.	❏	❏	❏	❏	37.	❏	❏	❏	❏
13.	❏	❏	❏	❏	38.	❏	❏	❏	❏
14.	❏	❏	❏	❏	39.	❏	❏	❏	❏
15.	❏	❏	❏	❏	40.	❏	❏	❏	❏
16.	❏	❏	❏	❏	41.	❏	❏	❏	❏
17.	❏	❏	❏	❏	42.	❏	❏	❏	❏
18.	❏	❏	❏	❏	43.	❏	❏	❏	❏
19.	❏	❏	❏	❏	44.	❏	❏	❏	❏
20.	❏	❏	❏	❏	45.	❏	❏	❏	❏
21.	❏	❏	❏	❏	46.	❏	❏	❏	❏
22.	❏	❏	❏	❏	47.	❏	❏	❏	❏
23.	❏	❏	❏	❏	48.	❏	❏	❏	❏
24.	❏	❏	❏	❏	49.	❏	❏	❏	❏
25.	❏	❏	❏	❏	50.	❏	❏	❏	❏

14

Overview: Patient Assessment

1. The components of the paramedic's patient assessment begin with the:

   a. initial assessment.
   b. focused history.
   c. scene size-up.
   d. general impression.

2. Components of the initial assessment include mental status (MS), ABCs, and:

   a. vital signs.
   b. scene safety.
   c. scene size-up.
   d. general impression.

3. All the following are considered baseline vital signs, *except*:

   a. pulse rate.
   b. temperature.
   c. blood pressure.
   d. respiratory effort.

4. The patient's MS, emotional state, physical condition, and _____ may change the usual progression of the assessment.

   a. location of the call
   b. DNAR status
   c. the presence of a health care proxy
   d. gender

5. Because of the dynamics of pre-hospital assessment, clinical judgement and experience will direct when specific steps should be:

   a. redefined.
   b. overhauled.
   c. omitted, deferred, or repeated.
   d. developed.

6. Which of the following is a component of scene size-up?

   a. assessing the need for appropriate PPE
   b. performing initial extrication
   c. assessing the patient's level of distress
   d. estimating the patient's age

7. While forming a general impression of the patient, the paramedic should include:

   a. a determination of the MOI.
   b. the call for extrication assistance.
   c. an observation of the patient's environment.
   d. assessing the need for PPE.

8. The components of forming a general impression of the patient include all the following, *except* determining the patient's:

   a. gender.
   b. approximate age.
   c. health history.
   d. level of distress.

9. The initial assessment guides the decision making for the remaining steps in evaluation, treatment, and:

   a. ongoing assessment.
   b. focused history and physical examination.
   c. detailed physical examination.
   d. transportation.

10. The standard assessment is the _____ format.

    a. toe to head
    b. head to toe
    c. focused exam
    d. vectored exam

11. The detailed physical examination is another name for the:

    a. ABCDE.
    b. head to toe exam.
    c. toe to head exam.
    d. vectored physical exam.

12. On which of the following patients would you perform the detailed physical examination?

    a. pediatric asthma patient
    b. geriatric isolated extremity injury
    c. trauma patient with significant MOI
    d. responsive medical patient

13. For which of the following patients should spinal precautions be taken?

    a. asymptomatic patient after a trip and fall
    b. wrist pain after falling from a standing position
    c. asymptomatic after a fall of approximately 3 times the patient's height
    d. a fall while skiing with isolated knee pain

14. All the following are criteria for significant MOI, for which spinal precautions should be taken, *except*:

    a. an explosion within a confined space.
    b. motor vehicle rollover.
    c. asymptomatic after ejection from a car.
    d. minor damage to the front end of a car where the airbag deployed.

15. _____ is the process of obtaining a baseline assessment, repeating the assessment, and then using the information to reevaluate the patient's condition or modify treatment.

    a. Trending
    b. Diagnosis
    c. Toiling
    d. Scooping

16. The components of the _____ are directed at a quick and gross head to toe assessment of the body, similar to the detailed physical examination, yet not as thorough.

    a. initial assessment
    b. rapid trauma assessment
    c. focused physical examination
    d. ongoing exam

17. Diagnostic information such as ECG, SpO_2, $EtCO_2$, and _____ become even more essential to the assessment process when caring for the unresponsive patient.

    a. DNAR status
    b. PO intake
    c. blood glucose
    d. Doppler

18. Each patient will require a different level of ongoing assessment based on:

    a. the advanced directives.
    b. local protocol.
    c. the age of the patient.
    d. severity of the specific complaint.

19. All the following are legal and ethical components of patient assessment, *except*:

    a. respecting patient confidentiality.
    b. good documentation.
    c. obtaining consent for treatment.
    d. not documenting equipment failure.

20. Which of the following is not considered part of the patient assessment?

    a. obtaining vital signs
    b. reporting physical findings to the ED
    c. obtaining consent from the patient
    d. observation of the patient's personal hygiene

21. You are assessing a patient with an isolated ankle injury. Which of the following exams would be most appropriate for this patient?

    a. Focused trauma examination
    b. Rapid trauma examination
    c. Detailed physical examination
    d. Head to toe exam

22. The purpose of the initial assessment is to _____ and find and manage any life-threatening conditions.

    a. assess for potential hazards
    b. determine the patient's mental status
    c. obtain baseline vital signs
    d. obtain patient consent

23. You are evaluating a patient who has a chief complaint of respiratory distress. On which of the following body systems, besides the respiratory system, should you focus your exam?

    a. Neurologic and cardiac
    b. Cardiac and musculoskeletal
    c. Gastric and behavioral
    d. Endocrine and musculoskeletal

24. To evaluate the mental status of an unconscious patient, check for deep pain response and:

    a. pulse.
    b. ECG.
    c. reflexes.
    d. glucose.

25. Good documentation of the patient on the run report is part of the _____ component of patient assessment.

    a. legal
    b. moral
    c. ethical
    d. protocol

Test #14 Answer Form

	A	B	C	D			A	B	C	D
1.	❑	❑	❑	❑		14.	❑	❑	❑	❑
2.	❑	❑	❑	❑		15.	❑	❑	❑	❑
3.	❑	❑	❑	❑		16.	❑	❑	❑	❑
4.	❑	❑	❑	❑		17.	❑	❑	❑	❑
5.	❑	❑	❑	❑		18.	❑	❑	❑	❑
6.	❑	❑	❑	❑		19.	❑	❑	❑	❑
7.	❑	❑	❑	❑		20.	❑	❑	❑	❑
8.	❑	❑	❑	❑		21.	❑	❑	❑	❑
9.	❑	❑	❑	❑		22.	❑	❑	❑	❑
10.	❑	❑	❑	❑		23.	❑	❑	❑	❑
11.	❑	❑	❑	❑		24.	❑	❑	❑	❑
12.	❑	❑	❑	❑		25.	❑	❑	❑	❑
13.	❑	❑	❑	❑						

15

Scene Size-up and the Initial Assessment

1. The second component of an assessment in the field is:

   a. scene size-up.
   b. initial assessment.
   c. open the airway.
   d. provide high flow oxygen.

2. One step the paramedic can take to make a scene safe is to:

   a. look for hazards.
   b. maintain c-spine stabilization.
   c. notify dispatch of arrival.
   d. suction the patient.

3. All the following are examples of significant MOI, *except*:

   a. GSW.
   b. fall from a height of 30 feet.
   c. near drowning.
   d. trip and fall from a standing position.

4. The injury pattern commonly seen in children who have been hit by a motor vehicle includes injury to the legs, chest, and head is known as:

   a. Waddell's triad.
   b. Chusing's blow.
   c. Warren's impact.
   d. Humphrey's reflex.

5. Getting a general impression of a patient is sometimes referred to as:

   a. the look test.
   b. patient interview.
   c. prioritizing.
   d. nature of illness.

6. The acronym AVPU is used in the initial assessment to:

   a. determine the patient's mental status.
   b. obtain an airway.
   c. assess the need for an additional ambulance.
   d. determine the MOI.

7. The first and foremost priority on calls for the paramedic is:

   a. dispatch information.
   b. the patient's chief complaint.
   c. recognizing hazards.
   d. the MOI.

8. Which of the following clues indicate there may be hazardous materials involved in the incident?

   a. The family pet dog is barking at the front door.
   b. Three out of four family members are complaining of headache.
   c. Power lines are down on the scene of a motor vehicle collision.
   d. There is advance notice of infestation at the scene of a call.

9. What does the term "secure" scene mean?

   a. The area is closed off to the public.
   b. The media is barred from entering the scene.
   c. The area is a crime scene.
   d. A potentially violent scene is safe for EMS.

10. Which of the following examples is a potential threat to the paramedic in a typical residential area?

    a. A nighttime response to a house, which has no lights on.
    b. A response to a house with no one to let you in, but a woman is calling out "I can't get up."
    c. A standby at a fire scene of a fully involved structure fire.
    d. A response to a suicide attempt with PD on scene.

11. Things a paramedic can do at the scene to help keep it a safe scene include all the following, *except*:

    a. always bring the portable radio into the call.
    b. scan the room for real or potential weapons.
    c. never rely on your gut instinct.
    d. always leave yourself an exit.

12. Before a scene is secure, where should EMS respond?

    a. staging area
    b. standby in quarters
    c. to get restock at the nearest station to the call
    d. to the nearest police department

13. Which of the following is an example of a potentially infectious process at the scene that may involve a hazard to the paramedic?

    a. a crying baby
    b. a patient with a bad cough
    c. the odor of vomitus at the scene
    d. the presence of insulin syringes at the scene

14. Which of the following is an example of an unstable scene that the paramedic can easily stabilize, if recognized?

    a. put out a small engine fire with a fire extinguisher
    b. engage the emergency brake on a car that has been left in neutral
    c. disarm a perpetrator at a crime scene
    d. stand between a wife and her abusive husband

15. What is one of the most common and greatest hazards to the paramedic?

    a. needle stick injuries
    b. exposure to TB
    c. exposure to hazardous materials
    d. working in traffic at the scene of a collision

16. Which one of the following is not an example of a common MOI?

    a. sports related injuries
    b. assault
    c. nose bleed
    d. abuse

17. All the following are examples of common "nature of illness" complaints for medical problems, *except*:

    a. suicide attempt.
    b. seizure.
    c. poisoning.
    d. altered mental status.

18. When the paramedic understands about the _____, he/she can make some predictions or be more attuned to specific injury patterns.

    a. past medical history
    b. chief complaint
    c. mechanism of injury
    d. nature of illness

19. The _____ is your first impression of the patient as you approach him/her and has been referred to as the "assessment from the doorway."

    a. scene size-up
    b. general impression
    c. initial assessment
    d. MOI

20. While working in an incident command situation, which of the following is not appropriate for the paramedic to do?

    a. Report to the incident commander upon arrival.
    b. Obtain a quick report and assignment for your crew.
    c. Complete the assignment and search for the next patient.
    d. Complete the assignment and report back to command.

21. Which of the following acronyms are used to determine a patient's initial mental status?

    a. AVPU
    b. SAMPLE
    c. GCS
    d. OPQRST

22. While assessing a patient for a painful response, which of the following is an appropriate response?

    a. withdraw from pain
    b. no response
    c. flexing the arm
    d. extending the arm

23. The level of consciousness or mental status of an infant is best assessed by:

    a. calling medical control to consult for advice.
    b. using the Broslow tape for pediatrics.
    c. how loud they cry.
    d. asking the parent or caregiver to determine if the response is normal.

24. _____ is the degree of alertness, wakefulness, or arousibility of the patient.

   a. Mental response
   b. Level of consciousness
   c. Emotion
   d. Reaction

25. Decerebrate neurologic posturing is illustrative of _____ brain functioning.

   a. absence of
   b. low level
   c. mid level
   d. high level

26. Neurologic posturing is most commonly caused by herniation and compression of the brainstem or:

   a. the effects of advanced Alzheimer's.
   b. metabolic causes.
   c. hyperventilation by the patient.
   d. injury to the lumbar spine.

27. Even if a patient is responsive and alert, he/she may still have serious airway compromise, such as a/an:

   a. broken jaw.
   b. abscessed tooth.
   c. cervical spine injury.
   d. postnasal drip.

28. Anytime a patient has received a high energy impact from the clavicles or superior to the clavicles, the paramedic must consider the possibility of:

   a. low blood sugar.
   b. hypoxia.
   c. neck injury.
   d. hypovolemia.

29. _____ is the appropriateness of the patient's thinking.

   a. Mental status
   b. Level of response
   c. Emotion
   d. Reaction

30. _____ volume is the amount of gas inspired or expired in a minute.

   a. Adequate
   b. Inadequate
   c. Tidal
   d. Minute

31. The neck of an infant should not be hyper-extended when opening the airway as this can:

   a. cause the infant to swallow the tongue.
   b. close the airway.
   c. interfere with nose breathing.
   d. cause cervical spinal injury.

32. During the initial assessment of an unconscious child, the pulse is taken at the _____ for the "quick check" to determine if the patient has a pulse.

   a. radial artery
   b. brachial artery
   c. carotid artery
   d. carotid vein

33. Assessing the _____ pulse is more useful in the initial assessment of a patient because it gives information about the effectiveness of the _____ circulation.

   a. radial; distal
   b. brachial; central
   c. carotid; central
   d. femoral; core

34. What is assessed in the patient's skin during the initial assessment?

   a. color and pigmentation
   b. color, temperature, and condition
   c. pulse oximetry
   d. the presence of urticaria

35. Which of the following is not an abnormal skin color?

   a. pale
   b. lentigo
   c. blue
   d. red

36. Skin color is assessed by looking at the:

   a. face and neck.
   b. nail beds, lips, and eyes.
   c. hands and ankles.
   d. tongue and eyes.

37. In which of the following is capillary refill a reliable sign?

   a. 55-year-old male with COPD
   b. 25-year-old female with anemia
   c. 14-year-old male with hypothermia
   d. 3-year-old asthmatic

38. Which of the following is not a system used to prioritize a patient?

    a. High/low classification
    b. CUPS
    c. Priority 1, 2, 3
    d. Triage A, B, C

39. Where is severe trauma stabilized?

    a. on scene
    b. in the ambulance
    c. in the ED
    d. in the OR

40. Which of the following steps may be skipped or expedited during the care of a critical trauma patient?

    a. use of a short board immobilization device
    b. use of a long board immobilization device
    c. bleeding control for life-threatening external bleeding
    d. airway control

41. The _____ assessment is a name for what is done in the ambulance enroute to the hospital and includes reassessment of vital signs and interventions.

    a. detailed
    b. focused
    c. ongoing
    d. vectored

42. A (an) _____ exam is an examination that attempts to look at a specific patient problem and not examine every body part, which could take a long time and not be in the patient's best interest.

    a. detailed
    b. focused
    c. ongoing
    d. initial

43. The initial assessment is repeated in the ongoing assessment in cases where the patient's:

    a. condition may be changing rapidly.
    b. condition shows an improved mental status from the baseline.
    c. condition includes a non-significant MOI.
    d. blood glucose returns to normal.

44. _____ is establishing a pattern of assessment findings, which will help the paramedic determine if the patient's condition is getting worse or better.

    a. Diagnosing
    b. Trending
    c. Documenting
    d. Prioritizing

45. Medical patients are classified into two groups within the medical category of assessment-based management. These two groups are:

    a. significant and non-significant.
    b. conscious and unconscious.
    c. critical and non-critical.
    d. adult and child.

46. Trauma patients are classified into two groups within the trauma category of assessment-based management. These two groups are _____ MOI.

    a. significant and non-significant
    b. conscious and unconscious
    c. adult and child
    d. alpha and delta

47. When a patient has both a medical and trauma problem, which is treated first?

    a medical
    b. trauma
    c. any threat to life
    d. medical control decides

48. What is the best treatment the paramedic can provide for the patient with internal bleeding?

    a. start two large bore IVs
    b. apply MAST pants and inflate
    c. administer analgesia for pain
    d. provide rapid transport to an OR

49. All the following are examples of critical patients, *except*:

    a. respiratory failure.
    b. isolated ankle injury.
    c. compensated shock.
    d. rising ICP.

50. All the following are examples of stable patients, *except*:

    a. low-grade fever.
    b. minor illness.
    c. significant MOI with neck injury.
    d. minor isolated injury.

Test #15 Answer Form

	A	B	C	D			A	B	C	D
1.	❑	❑	❑	❑		26.	❑	❑	❑	❑
2.	❑	❑	❑	❑		27.	❑	❑	❑	❑
3.	❑	❑	❑	❑		28.	❑	❑	❑	❑
4.	❑	❑	❑	❑		29.	❑	❑	❑	❑
5.	❑	❑	❑	❑		30.	❑	❑	❑	❑
6.	❑	❑	❑	❑		31.	❑	❑	❑	❑
7.	❑	❑	❑	❑		32.	❑	❑	❑	❑
8.	❑	❑	❑	❑		33.	❑	❑	❑	❑
9.	❑	❑	❑	❑		34.	❑	❑	❑	❑
10.	❑	❑	❑	❑		35.	❑	❑	❑	❑
11.	❑	❑	❑	❑		36.	❑	❑	❑	❑
12.	❑	❑	❑	❑		37.	❑	❑	❑	❑
13.	❑	❑	❑	❑		38.	❑	❑	❑	❑
14.	❑	❑	❑	❑		39.	❑	❑	❑	❑
15.	❑	❑	❑	❑		40.	❑	❑	❑	❑
16.	❑	❑	❑	❑		41.	❑	❑	❑	❑
17.	❑	❑	❑	❑		42.	❑	❑	❑	❑
18.	❑	❑	❑	❑		43.	❑	❑	❑	❑
19.	❑	❑	❑	❑		44.	❑	❑	❑	❑
20.	❑	❑	❑	❑		45.	❑	❑	❑	❑
21.	❑	❑	❑	❑		46.	❑	❑	❑	❑
22.	❑	❑	❑	❑		47.	❑	❑	❑	❑
23.	❑	❑	❑	❑		48.	❑	❑	❑	❑
24.	❑	❑	❑	❑		49.	❑	❑	❑	❑
25.	❑	❑	❑	❑		50.	❑	❑	❑	❑

16

Focused History and Physical Examination: Medical Patient

1. The focused history and physical examination of the medical patient are performed:

    a. immediately after the scene size-up has been performed.
    b. after the initial assessment has been completed.
    c. before the ABCs are managed.
    d. before the chief complaint has been attained.

2. The objective of the focused physical examination is to direct the assessment to:

    a. the patient's ABCs.
    b. gather a SAMPLE history.
    c. the patient's chief complaint.
    d. establish consent to treat the patient.

3. Your patient fell and possibly experienced a loss of consciousness while coming out of the bathroom. She is alert and oriented when you perform your initial assessment, but she tells you that when she was on the floor she could not move or cry out for help. You suspect that the patient may have experienced a:

    a. TIA.
    b. AMI.
    c. hypertensive event.
    d. hypoglycemic event.

4. In the absence of trauma and a MOI, the patient will most often have a (an):

    a. medical complaint.
    b. concurrent medical problem.
    c. need for a rapid physical examination.
    d. presumptive diagnosis.

5. While gathering a SAMPLE history on a medical patient, the paramedic asks about all the following, *except*:

    a. allergies.
    b. medications.
    c. pertinent blood loss.
    d. events leading up to this episode.

6. While obtaining the focused history from a patient, the paramedic should gather a SAMPLE history, a history of the present illness (HPI), and:

    a. a list of the patient's possessions that they will be taking to the hospital.
    b. positive findings and pertinent negatives.
    c. a history of childhood vaccinations.
    d. the date of the patient's last tetanus shot.

7. A paramedic interviewing a patient has asked about chest pain associated with breathing, orthopnea, prolonged bed rest and activity at onset. Based on these questions, what is most likely the patient's chief complaint?

    a. dizziness
    b. nausea and vomiting
    c. chest tightness
    d. difficulty breathing

8. A diabetic patient is presenting with an altered mental status and a low blood sugar reading. Which of the following pieces of information from the SAMPLE history obtained in the focused history is most important to the paramedic immediately?

    a. A—allergies
    b. M—medications
    c. P—past medical history
    d. L—last meal

9. The acronym "AEIOU-TIPS" is helpful to the paramedic when considering the causes of:

    a. chest pain.
    b. altered mental status.
    c. abdominal pain.
    d. shortness of breath.

10. While obtaining a focused history and physical examination on an elderly patient, it is not uncommon to discover:

 a. traumatic injury.
 b. measles.
 c. concurrent medical problems.
 d. poisoning.

11. When a medical patient is discovered to be unconscious, the paramedic performs an initial assessment followed by the:

 a. rapid physical examination.
 b. focused history.
 c. ongoing assessment.
 d. SAMPLE history.

12. A 54-year-old male has shortness of breath and chest pain with deep inspiration. His skin color, temperature and condition are pale, warm, and moist. Auscultation of the lungs reveals clear and dry sounds in all fields. Vitals are: pulse 100 bpm and slightly irregular, blood pressure 130/68 and respiratory rate of 30 and labored. The paramedic begins treatment for this patient by providing high flow oxygen and a(an):

 a. diuretic.
 b. nitrate.
 c. bronchodilator.
 d. analgesic.

13. Examples of pertinent negatives include all the following, *except*:

 a. absence of chest pain.
 b. no loss of consciousness.
 c. history of COPD.
 d. history of a non-productive cough.

14. The frequency of performing ongoing assessments is usually based on:

 a. medical versus trauma patient.
 b. good clinical judgement and experience.
 c. age of patient.
 d. past medical history.

15. During the patient interview, the patient admitted to having a fever and productive cough for two days in addition to a chief complaint of chest pain. This information aside from the chief complaint, is referred to as:

 a. the SAMPLE history.
 b. provocation.
 c. associated signs and symptoms.
 d. stimulus.

16. During a patient interview, the EMS provider discovered that the patient's chief complaint was dizziness felt only when he moved his head. This piece of information most likely indicates that the patient is experiencing a(an):

 a. TIA.
 b. stroke.
 c. hypoglycemia.
 d. inner ear problem.

17. Establishing a rapport with a patient is necessary for all the following reasons *except* to:

 a. gain consent for treatment.
 b. show respect and professionalism to the patient.
 c. physically examine a patient.
 d. gain trust and cooperation from the patient.

18. The revised DOT EMT–Basic and Paramedic curriculum differentiates medical patients by:

 a. responsiveness.
 b. stable versus critical.
 c. young versus old.
 d. chief complaint.

19. A 78-year-old female is complaining of weakness, dizziness and nausea. She denies having chest pain or shortness of breath and is not diabetic. Which of the following body systems should the paramedic focus on first?

 a. gastrointestinal
 b. genitourinary
 c. cardiac
 d. neurologic

20. The components of the dynamic focused physical examination are guided by:

 a. scene size-up and baseline vital signs.
 b. priority dispatch, scene size-up and the presence of a DNAR.
 c. initial assessment and absence of a DNAR.
 d. chief complaint, initial assessment and the focused PE findings.

21. In many cases making a precise diagnosis in the field is difficult; therefore, the paramedic should strive to recognize emergent signs and symptoms and then:

 a. begin transport and initiate treatment enroute.
 b. stabilize and transport.
 c. transport to the nearest facility.
 d. contact medical control and transport.

22. During an initial assessment of a patient complaining of "chest tightness and feeling weak," you see that he looks pale, but his skin is warm and dry. You apply oxygen to the patient and begin your focused physical examination on which area of the patient?

    a. cardiothoracic
    b. abdominal
    c. neurologic
    d. airway

23. In reference to the previous question, the paramedic would most likely auscultate which area(s) of the patient's body?

    a. lungs
    b. abdomen
    c. carotid arteries
    d. PMI

24. The components of the medical patient assessment include all the following, *except*:

    a. scene size-up.
    b. initial assessment.
    c. establishing medical control.
    d. ongoing assessment.

25. A paramedic is assessing a patient that has had a loss of bowel control, decreased sensation in the legs bilaterally and impaired coordination. Based on these problems what type of medical problem might this patient be further evaluated for?

    a. cardiac
    b. neurologic
    c. behavioral disorder
    d. respiratory

26. A paramedic is assessing a patient who has a chief complaint of headache, nausea and dizziness. The focused history revealed that the patient has had these symptoms for several days and that the spouse and children have had similar complaints but less severe. From the information obtained in the focused history, the paramedic should consider these to be associated symptoms of:

    a. food poisoning.
    b. possible CO poisoning.
    c. the presence of pets in the home.
    d. family history of mental disorders.

27. When assessing a patient, the mnemonic DCAP-BTLS is used to help the paramedic remember to look for specific information about the patient's:

    a. skin.
    b. mental status.
    c. respiratory effort.
    d. trauma status.

28. In which of the following cases would the paramedic most likely perform a rapid physical examination?

    a. an unresponsive 40-year-old male
    b. a 55-year-old female with crushing chest pain
    c. an 18-month-old who is post ictal after a seizure and crying
    d. a 16-year-old experiencing an acute asthma attack

29. The components of the focused physical examination are guided by the chief complaint of the patient and:

    a. the dispatch information.
    b. findings from the initial assessment.
    c. the status of a patient's DNAR.
    d. all of the above.

30. When the paramedic assesses a patient for weakness or the inability of the patient to move a body part, which focused assessment is the EMS provider examining?

    a. behavioral
    b. neurologic
    c. cardiac
    d. trauma

31. Common causes of vertigo include all the following, *except*:

    a. traumatic brain injury (TBI).
    b. alcohol.
    c. viruses.
    d. syncope.

32. The difference between vertigo and dizziness is that:

    a. vertigo is a vestibular disorder.
    b. there is no difference.
    c. only adults experience vertigo.
    d. vertigo is not associated with nausea.

33. The patient is complaining of lower back pain and dysuria. Which of the following body systems should the paramedic focus on first?

   a. gastrointestinal
   b. genitourinary
   c. cardiac
   d. neurologic

34. The body's vomiting reflex can be stimulated by:

   a. morphine sulfate.
   b. migraine headache.
   c. stress.
   d. all of the above.

35. Which statement best describes the difference between vomiting and regurgitation?

   a. There is no difference.
   b. Vomiting is an active process in conscious patients and regurgitation is not.
   c. Vomiting is a passive process in unconscious patients and regurgitation is not.
   d. Regurgitation is an active process in unconscious patients and vomiting is not.

36. Sensory receptors that stimulate the vomiting reflex can be found in the:

   a. aortic arch.
   b. rectum.
   c. heart.
   d. stomach.

37. You respond to a residence for a 29-year-old male who fell in the bathroom. He has a laceration on the back of his head with active bleeding. His wife tells you that he was shaving when she heard him fall, and that he was unconscious for about 90 seconds. The first treatment step is to:

   a. take c-spine precautions.
   b. stop the bleeding.
   c. administer oxygen.
   d. start an IV.

38. In reference to the previous question, the patient denies having chest pain or shortness of breath, but states he felt dizzy just before passing out. The most likely cause of the fall may be from what type of syncope?

   a. pharmacologic
   b. neurologic
   c. vasovagal
   d. respiratory

39. All the following are cardiac causes of syncope, *except*:

   a. heart block.
   b. hemorrhage.
   c. sick sinus syndrome.
   d. angina.

40. One of the most common drug classifications causing syncope are:

   a. beta-blockers.
   b. cold medications.
   c. antacids.
   d. antibiotics.

41. A patient is complaining of a severe headache after experiencing a seizure for the first time. There is no apparent trauma visible from the seizure, pulse is 80 and regular and respirations are 20 and non-labored. The patient stated he checked his sugar 30 minutes ago and the blood sugar was 110 mg/dl. In continuing with the focused history and physical examination, what should the paramedic consider next?

   a. focused history
   b. ECG
   c. breath sounds
   d. blood pressure

42. Vomiting in itself is not a medical diagnosis; however, prolonged or frequent vomiting can lead to serious complications such as:

   a. GI bleeding.
   b. limbic system disorders.
   c. cardiac stress.
   d. endogenous infections.

43. Cardiac patients are often medicated to prevent vomiting for the following reason:

   a. to prevent discomfort.
   b. vagus stimulation.
   c. dehydration.
   d. hypoxia.

44. One of the most common rooms in the home in which a patient becomes ill or injured is the:

   a. bathroom.
   b. garage.
   c. basement.
   d. attic.

45. During a detailed physical examination of a patient complaining of "almost passing out," the paramedic identifies a life-threatening condition. Which of the following did the paramedic most likely identify?

    a. temperature of 104°F
    b. blood sugar of 80 mg/dl
    c. heart block
    d. CABG scarring on the patient's chest

46. When obtaining a history about the patient who has experienced a syncopal event, the paramedic should specifically ask about:

    a. pre-syncope information, such as position of patient.
    b. post-syncope information, such as duration of LOC.
    c. history of any similar events.
    d. all of the above.

47. The most common causes of syncope are vasovagal faint, positional orthostatic hypotension and:

    a. cardiac dysrhythmias.
    b. micturition.
    c. neurologic induced.
    d. dehydration.

48. Orthostatic hypotension is a common symptom in which of the following circumstances:

    a. prolonged bed rest.
    b. hypovolemia with a blood loss of >1000 cc.
    c. certain medications cause this condition.
    d. all of the above.

49. Orthostatic vitals signs are not always significant or reliable because most people will normally have subtle vital sign changes when going from a supine or sitting position to a standing position. A more significant finding is:

    a. an abnormal pulse oximetry reading.
    b. positional symptoms.
    c. the age of the patient.
    d. the presence of edema.

50. After interviewing a patient with a chief complaint of chest pain increasing with movement and palpation of the chest, the paramedic obtained a history that included smoking, lack of exercise and a family history of hypertension. Based on this information the paramedic should plan to treat the patient for:

    a. AMI.
    b. pleurisy.
    c. pneumonia.
    d. pericarditis.

Test #16 Answer Form

	A	B	C	D			A	B	C	D
1.	❏	❏	❏	❏		26.	❏	❏	❏	❏
2.	❏	❏	❏	❏		27.	❏	❏	❏	❏
3.	❏	❏	❏	❏		28.	❏	❏	❏	❏
4.	❏	❏	❏	❏		29.	❏	❏	❏	❏
5.	❏	❏	❏	❏		30.	❏	❏	❏	❏
6.	❏	❏	❏	❏		31.	❏	❏	❏	❏
7.	❏	❏	❏	❏		32.	❏	❏	❏	❏
8.	❏	❏	❏	❏		33.	❏	❏	❏	❏
9.	❏	❏	❏	❏		34.	❏	❏	❏	❏
10.	❏	❏	❏	❏		35.	❏	❏	❏	❏
11.	❏	❏	❏	❏		36.	❏	❏	❏	❏
12.	❏	❏	❏	❏		37.	❏	❏	❏	❏
13.	❏	❏	❏	❏		38.	❏	❏	❏	❏
14.	❏	❏	❏	❏		39.	❏	❏	❏	❏
15.	❏	❏	❏	❏		40.	❏	❏	❏	❏
16.	❏	❏	❏	❏		41.	❏	❏	❏	❏
17.	❏	❏	❏	❏		42.	❏	❏	❏	❏
18.	❏	❏	❏	❏		43.	❏	❏	❏	❏
19.	❏	❏	❏	❏		44.	❏	❏	❏	❏
20.	❏	❏	❏	❏		45.	❏	❏	❏	❏
21.	❏	❏	❏	❏		46.	❏	❏	❏	❏
22.	❏	❏	❏	❏		47.	❏	❏	❏	❏
23.	❏	❏	❏	❏		48.	❏	❏	❏	❏
24.	❏	❏	❏	❏		49.	❏	❏	❏	❏
25.	❏	❏	❏	❏		50.	❏	❏	❏	❏

17

Focused History and Physical Examination: Trauma Patient

1. What are life-threatening conditions that require immediate intervention?

   a. any head injury
   b. any burn injury
   c. any injury that interferes with the ABCs
   d. all motorcycle collision injuries

2. Critical trauma patients have the best chance for survival if they can be stabilized in a surgical suite within _____ of the onset of injury.

   a. 30 minutes
   b. 1 hour
   c. 2 hours
   d. 6 hours

3. The maximum time the paramedic should spend on-scene with a critical trauma patient, barring any lengthy extrication, is _____ minutes.

   a. 10
   b. 15
   c. 20
   d. 30

4. For the non-critical trauma patient the concerns are similar to the critical trauma patient; however, _____ may not be required.

   a. determination of MOI
   b. the initial assessment
   c. assessment of the ABCs
   d. rapid transport

5. Proper evaluation of the _____ by the paramedic can help predict injuries that may or may not be readily apparent.

   a. ABCs
   b. MOI
   c. CTC
   d. vital signs

6. _____ is the abbreviation used to remember what is assessed about the patient's soft tissue.

   a. BTLS
   b. DCAP-BTLS
   c. GCS
   d. MOI

7. _____ physical examination is a complete head to toe exam for non-life or limb threatening injuries or significant MOI enroute to the hospital.

   a. Detailed
   b. Focused
   c. Ongoing
   d. Rapid trauma

8. When should transport of the critical trauma patient be delayed while waiting for ALS to arrive?

   a. when the patient is unconscious
   b. only when the patient is fully immobilized
   c. only after MAST have been inflated
   d. transportation should not be delayed while waiting for ALS to arrive

9. The transportation decision is usually made after the scene assessment for MOI and the _____ has been completed.

   a. cervical collar application
   b. initial assessment
   c. radio report
   d. immobilization

10. A cervical collar should be applied in all the following cases, *except*:

    a. the presence of an MOI.
    b. when the patient complains of neck pain.
    c. when an unconscious patient has no MOI.
    d. an unconscious patient with unknown MOI.

11. How often should the ongoing assessment of the non-critical trauma patient be repeated?

    a. every 5 minutes
    b. every 15 minutes
    c. only when a change in MS is noted
    d. only when the patient becomes critical

12. A Level _____ trauma center may be a clinic rather than a hospital where the goal is to provide initial stabilization of the patient and then transfer to a higher level trauma center.

    a. I
    b. II
    c. III
    d. IV

13. A level _____ trauma center is a regional center that serves as a leader in trauma care for a specific geographic area.

    a. I
    b. II
    c. III
    d. IV

14. Which one of the following patients should be transported to the nearest hospital even if it is not a Level I trauma center?

    a. severe burns
    b. pediatric trauma
    c. pregnant trauma patient
    d. traumatic cardiac arrest

15. All the following are criteria for air-medical transport, *except*:

    a. access to remote areas.
    b. traumatic cardiac arrest.
    c. access to personnel with specialty skills.
    d. access to specialty equipment.

16. The _____ is a numeric grading system that combines the GCS and measurements of cardiopulmonary function as a gauge of the severity of injury and a predictor of survival after blunt injury to the head.

    a. Cincinnati score
    b. Trauma Score
    c. CUPS
    d. TBI Scale

17. If a patient fell from a height of 20 feet and landed feet first, which of the following injuries could you predict the patient might have?

    a. fractures of the heels, ankles, hips
    b. fractures of the heels, ankles and clavicles
    c. lower extremity fractures and head injury
    d. lower and upper extremity fractures

18. Which of the following steps cannot be skipped or omitted during the care of a critical trauma patient?

    a. full spinal immobilization
    b. short board spinal immobilization
    c. bleeding control for venous bleeding
    d. hand fracture immobilization

19. Trauma is the number one killer of _____ in the United States.

    a. men
    b. women
    c. children
    d. geriatrics

20. Special considerations for assessment of the elderly trauma patient include all the following, *except*:

    a. a minor injury can worsen a preexisting medical condition.
    b. a preexisting medical condition may have precipitated a traumatic injury.
    c. decreased body fat minimizes the body's padding (protection) against traumatic injury.
    d. cardiac stroke volume decreases slowing any bleeding from a traumatic injury.

21. _____ is the most common cause of death in children.

    a. Spinal cord injury
    b. Head injury
    c. Abdominal trauma
    d. Chest trauma

22. The most common MOI in children is:

    a. falls.
    b. bicycle accidents.
    c. MVC.
    d. auto–pedestrian collisions.

23. Special considerations for assessment of the pediatric trauma patient include all the following, *except*:

    a. airways that are easily prone to obstruction.
    b. airways that are less prone to obstruction.
    c. the presence of rib fractures is a critical finding.
    d. the abdomen is large and exposed.

24. Slowed peristalsis creates a full stomach in the pregnant trauma patient, and this increases the risk of:

    a. abdominal trauma.
    b. vomiting.
    c. hypotension.
    d. abruptio placenta.

25. In the third trimester pregnant trauma patient a blood loss of _____ can occur before any signs of shock begin to develop.

    a. 10%
    b. 20%
    c. 30%
    d. 40%

26. The MOI is a rapid head first impact, injuries to consider include cranial, cervical spine and:

    a. thoracic aortic disruption.
    b. crushed trachea.
    c. fractured ribs.
    d. fractured sternum.

27. You are assessing the driver of a rapid deceleration MVC in which the patient went down and under the steering column. What predictable injuries should you assess for?

    a. chest and abdominal
    b. knee, femur and hip
    c. facial
    d. head and neck

28. Physical signs on a motor vehicle that lead you to suspect underlying injuries to the patient include all the following, *except*:

    a. cracked windshield.
    b. broken steering wheel.
    c. flat tires.
    d. intrusion into the side of the passenger compartment.

29. Striking one side of the head often causes blunt trauma to the brain in the area that was struck, as well as the opposite area of the brain. What type of injury is this called?

    a. contra coup
    b. coup contra coup
    c. traumatic brain ischemia
    d. contra coup constriction

30. _____ is an injury pattern in children when struck by a vehicle involving the legs, chest and head.

    a. Waddell's triad
    b. SCIWORA
    c. Crushing
    d. Whipple's triad

31. The momentary acceleration of tissue laterally away from the projectile tract of a bullet in the body, which explains why exit wounds are usually larger than entrance wounds, is called:

    a. tumble.
    b. fragmentation.
    c. profile.
    d. cavitation.

32. It is estimated the chance of a spinal injury increases up to _____ times by being ejected from a vehicle while not wearing a seat belt.

    a. 30
    b. 300
    c. 1,300
    d. 3,000

33. Striking the "temples" of the cranium with a blunt object can cause the middle meningeal artery to bleed and a/an _____ to develop.

    a. neoplasm
    b. leak of CSF in the ears
    c. subdural hematoma
    d. epidural hematoma

34. Secondary injuries from a MVC where the driver went up and over the steering column/dash, include:

    a. face and head.
    b. head and neck.
    c. chest and abdomen.
    d. cervical spine.

35. You are caring for a critical trauma patient. Which of the following can be used to move the patient safely, quickly and minimize scene time?

    a. long backboard
    b. KED
    c. short backboard
    d. blanket

36. Paradoxical motion, crepitation and asymmetry are all abnormal findings the paramedic may find on the:

    a. head.
    b. chest.
    c. abdomen.
    d. pelvis.

37. Criteria for the designated transportation destination of trauma patients for a specific EMS agency can usually be found in:

    a. regional protocols.
    b. EMT-B and paramedic texts.
    c. hospital rules.
    d. state law.

38. Children have all the following unique physiologic responses to trauma, *except* they:

    a. compensate for shock better than adults in early shock.
    b. decompensate quicker in shock then adults.
    c. decompensate slower in shock then adults.
    d. appear better than they actually are.

39. Which of the following statements about pediatric trauma is not true?

    a. Children can sustain spinal cord injuries without the same visible injuries that would be seen in an adult.
    b. When long bone injuries occur, growth plate injuries must be ruled out in the ED.
    c. Rib fractures occur frequently in chest trauma.
    d. Large tongues and anterior airway structures make the airway prone to obstruction.

40. Which of the following statements about trauma in the elderly is false?

    a. Aging immune systems put the elderly at risk for system infections.
    b. The use of MAOIs can interfere with the body's normal response to pain.
    c. Decreases in brain mass leave the brain at risk for injury from rapid deceleration forces.
    d. The use of beta-blockers can mask the signs of shock.

41. You are assessing a belted passenger involved in a moderate speed MVC. Initially the patient had no complaint of injury or pain. Twenty minutes after the collision the patient states he feels dizzy and looks pale and diaphoretic. What do you suspect the patient has?

    a. potential spinal injury
    b. head injury
    c. intra-abdominal hemorrhage
    d. neurogenic shock

42. While responding to a call for a self-inflicted GSW, dispatch advises that the injury was to the head and face as reported by police. What do you anticipate will be the priority of care for this patient?

    a. complicated airway
    b. blood loss
    c. rapid transport
    d. spinal immobilization

43. A patient who was burned in a house fire sustained multiple injuries. Which of the following is the primary concern for the paramedic?

    a. third degree burns on both hands
    b. first and second degree burns on the face and neck
    c. clothing is charred into the chest and back
    d. wheezing is present with a hoarse voice

44. After responding to the scene of a diving accident you are treating a male patient who is unable to move any part of his body below the neck. You have him fully immobilized and are ready for transport. Where should you take him?

    a. to the nearest hospital
    b. level I trauma center
    c. level II trauma center
    d. level III trauma center

45. While enroute to the hospital with patient from the previous question, you determine that he has sensation to the shoulders but none below. Where do you suspect the spinal injury is?

    a. C1 and C2
    b. C3 and C4
    c. C6 and C7
    d. T1 and T2

Test #17 Answer Form

	A	B	C	D			A	B	C	D
1.	❏	❏	❏	❏		24.	❏	❏	❏	❏
2.	❏	❏	❏	❏		25.	❏	❏	❏	❏
3.	❏	❏	❏	❏		26.	❏	❏	❏	❏
4.	❏	❏	❏	❏		27.	❏	❏	❏	❏
5.	❏	❏	❏	❏		28.	❏	❏	❏	❏
6.	❏	❏	❏	❏		29.	❏	❏	❏	❏
7.	❏	❏	❏	❏		30.	❏	❏	❏	❏
8.	❏	❏	❏	❏		31.	❏	❏	❏	❏
9.	❏	❏	❏	❏		32.	❏	❏	❏	❏
10.	❏	❏	❏	❏		33.	❏	❏	❏	❏
11.	❏	❏	❏	❏		34.	❏	❏	❏	❏
12.	❏	❏	❏	❏		35.	❏	❏	❏	❏
13.	❏	❏	❏	❏		36.	❏	❏	❏	❏
14.	❏	❏	❏	❏		37.	❏	❏	❏	❏
15.	❏	❏	❏	❏		38.	❏	❏	❏	❏
16.	❏	❏	❏	❏		39.	❏	❏	❏	❏
17.	❏	❏	❏	❏		40.	❏	❏	❏	❏
18.	❏	❏	❏	❏		41.	❏	❏	❏	❏
19.	❏	❏	❏	❏		42.	❏	❏	❏	❏
20.	❏	❏	❏	❏		43.	❏	❏	❏	❏
21.	❏	❏	❏	❏		44.	❏	❏	❏	❏
22.	❏	❏	❏	❏		45.	❏	❏	❏	❏
23.	❏	❏	❏	❏						

18

Assessment Based Management

1. Which of the following is the cornerstone of patient care?

    a. Past medical history
    b. Assessment
    c. Field impression
    d. Scene size-up

2. It is estimated that 80% of a medical diagnosis is based on the:

    a. physical examination.
    b. medications.
    c. history.
    d. chief complaint.

3. All the following can cause a patient to be uncooperative, hindering the field assessment, *except*:

    a. hypoxia.
    b. tunnel vision.
    c. hypovolemia.
    d. head injury.

4. Factors that may impede decision making or proper assessment in the field include all the following, *except*:

    a. distracting injuries.
    b. paramedic attitude.
    c. environment.
    d. gender.

5. Which of the following is an example of "labeling" a patient?

    a. Frequent flyer
    b. Unstable head injury
    c. Gut instinct
    d. Diabetic neuropathy

6. When obtaining a history from a patient the paramedic should focus on the:

    a. organ systems associated with the complaint.
    b. family preference for treatment and hospital destination.
    c. length of time the patient has waited for treatment.
    d. medical conditions his/her family members may have.

7. Which of the following statements about pattern recognition is incorrect?

    a. To become proficient with pattern recognition, a paramedic's knowledge base needs to be similar to a physician's.
    b. Recognition of patterns can help the paramedic to accurately determine a patient's presenting problem.
    c. Continuing education is paramount to the comparison and recognition of patterns of diseases and disorders.
    d. It is the responsibility of the individual paramedic to continually expand his/her knowledge base of diseases and disorders.

8. The field impression of a patient by the paramedic takes into consideration all the following, *except*:

    a. pattern recognition.
    b. the paramedic's gut instinct based on experience.
    c. the family's concern for the patient's welfare.
    d. the plan of action for patient care.

9. It is important for the paramedic to understand that protocols are intended as:

    a. the gold standard and should never be deviated from.
    b. guidelines for care.
    c. the basis of an action plan for all patients.
    d. a cookbook list of what the paramedic must do.

10. Which of the following is a factor that could impede decision making or proper field assessment by the paramedic?

    a. The paramedic has a bias against people who do not have a similar background to him/her.
    b. Having insufficient access to the patient's medical insurance records.
    c. Taking the time to listen to the patient's associated complaints.
    d. Treating distracting injuries after correcting life threats.

11. When the paramedic has _____, he/she may miss vital pieces of information which may short circuit the information gathering process.

    a. insufficient manpower
    b. a partner with less training or experience
    c. a biased or prejudicial "attitude"
    d. concerned family at the scene

12. The team leader is usually the paramedic who will:

    a. talk to the family and bystanders.
    b. act as the triage group leader in an MCI.
    c. drive the crew to the hospital.
    d. accompany the patient through definitive care.

13. Roles of the patient care provider member of the team usually include any of the following, *except*:

    a. obtaining vital signs.
    b. performing skills as designated by the team leader.
    c. acting as the initial EMS command in an MCI.
    d. gathering patient information.

14. Essential equipment that should be brought to the side of every patient includes:

    a. equipment needed to conduct the initial assessment of the patient's priorities.
    b. only the equipment needed to run an ACLS "code."
    c. only what you can carry.
    d. it is best to decide on each call what equipment to bring.

15. Effective oral patient skills are important for all the following reasons, *except*:

    a. They help to establish trust and credibility.
    b. Other health care providers are usually unimpressed by your oral skills regardless.
    c. A good presentation suggests effective patient assessment and care.
    d. A poor presentation suggests poor assessment and patient care.

16. The paramedic's ability to effectively communicate and transfer patient information is done with every patient encounter by all the following means, *except*:

    a. writing on the PCR.
    b. over the radio.
    c. face-to-face.
    d. dispatch information.

17. The paramedic's professional demeanor can be rated by the patient when he/she considers your:

    a. level of training.
    b. people skills and customer service.
    c. medical performance.
    d. amount of equipment you can carry.

18. Helpful aspects of the general approach to a patient include all the following, *except*:

    a. a calm orderly demeanor.
    b. a preplan to avoid the appearance of confusion.
    c. carrying in the least amount of equipment.
    d. obtaining a good initial size-up.

19. _____ is/are the staging of the events and actions of a call so that they happen smoothly.

    a. Choreography
    b. Algorithms
    c. Protocols
    d. Advanced directives

20. An example of how tunnel vision can obstruct the assessment process is:

    a. responding to an anaphylactic call where the patient forgot to administer his Epi-pen®.
    b. seeing a local drug abuser and immediately blaming his disorientation on the drugs rather than looking for a medical problem.
    c. assessing a patient's MS-ABCs before attending to an open femur fracture with gross angulation.
    d. assuming EMS command at the scene of an MCI where the fire department is on scene first.

21. The paramedic must gather information as well as evaluate and synthesize that information. This is in order to:

    a. diagnose a patient's illness.
    b. provide definitive care for the patient.
    c. educate the patient's family on future 9-1-1 calls for assistance.
    d. make the appropriate management decisions.

22. As you proceed through the assessment, it is important to proceed in an organized fashion and to:

    a. explain each step in the examination.
    b. avoid distractions.
    c. concentrate on one step at a time.
    d. All of the above.

23. Following a sequence when performing an assessment of the patient is most efficient because:

    a. the crew will know what they should do next.
    b. the patient will cooperate more easily.
    c. it allows for a complete and smooth assessment.
    d. it is easier to write up on the PCR.

24. Decision making involves a combination of all the following sources of information, *except*:

    a. EMD procedures.
    b. the history.
    c. the physical exam.
    d. existing BLS/ALS treatment protocols.

25. Which of the following affects the quality of the history taken from the patient by the paramedic?

    a. The patient's knowledge about the health care system.
    b. The paramedic's knowledge of a disease and its assessment findings.
    c. Local protocols and patient algorithms of a specific illness.
    d. The Medical Director's level of involvement in QI/QA.

26. What is the value of a complete physical examination?

    a. Performing a complete physical exam will build trust with the patient.
    b. Important information can be missed by performing a cursory physical exam.

    c. The attending physician at the destinating hospital will be impressed by a complete physical exam.
    d. Performing a complete physical exam will keep you from being sued.

27. There is nothing wrong with the "Cookbook Practice" or using local protocol, as long as:

    a. you have a partner to ask advice.
    b. your supervisor trusts your judgment.
    c. there is a "thinking cook."
    d. you know all the protocols by memory.

28. When two paramedics are working as a team there can be simultaneous information gathering and treatment, which is:

    a. more efficient.
    b. less efficient.
    c. confusing to the patient.
    d. a problem for establishing patient rapport.

29. The paramedic can improve scene choreography by:

    a. utilizing distance learning.
    b. taking a course in MCI leadership.
    c. watching training videos.
    d. preplanning and practice with his/her crew.

30. The patient care provider is responsible for providing scene "cover" by:

    a. shutting of the ambulance and taking the keys out of the ignition.
    b. setting up a cover for the crew working in the rain.
    c. watching everyone's back to make sure no one gets hurt.
    d. establishing a rehab sector for fire standbys.

Test #18 Answer Form

	A	B	C	D			A	B	C	D
1.	❑	❑	❑	❑		16.	❑	❑	❑	❑
2.	❑	❑	❑	❑		17.	❑	❑	❑	❑
3.	❑	❑	❑	❑		18.	❑	❑	❑	❑
4.	❑	❑	❑	❑		19.	❑	❑	❑	❑
5.	❑	❑	❑	❑		20.	❑	❑	❑	❑
6.	❑	❑	❑	❑		21.	❑	❑	❑	❑
7.	❑	❑	❑	❑		22.	❑	❑	❑	❑
8.	❑	❑	❑	❑		23.	❑	❑	❑	❑
9.	❑	❑	❑	❑		24.	❑	❑	❑	❑
10.	❑	❑	❑	❑		25.	❑	❑	❑	❑
11.	❑	❑	❑	❑		26.	❑	❑	❑	❑
12.	❑	❑	❑	❑		27.	❑	❑	❑	❑
13.	❑	❑	❑	❑		28.	❑	❑	❑	❑
14.	❑	❑	❑	❑		29.	❑	❑	❑	❑
15.	❑	❑	❑	❑		30.	❑	❑	❑	❑

19

Ongoing Assessment and Clinical Decision Making

1. Which of the following is not a key aspect of the on-going assessment?

   a. Trending
   b. Time constraints
   c. Scene size-up
   d. Manpower

2. The hormonal "fight or flight" response to stress can affect the paramedic in which of the following ways?

   a. Increased concentration
   b. Improved muscular strength
   c. Decreased visual senses
   d. Improved critical thinking

3. All the following are examples of stimulants of the fight or flight response for paramedics, *except*:

   a. lights and sirens.
   b. pagers.
   c. nitro spray.
   d. traffic.

4. Factors that may alter the ongoing assessment include all the following, *except*:

   a. the patient chief complaint.
   b. predictable patterns of injury.
   c. specific disease processes.
   d. the patient's gender.

5. Which of the following statements about repeating the ongoing assessment is not correct?

   a. The ongoing assessment should be repeated every five minutes for the critical trauma patient.
   b. For the non-critical patient, repeating the ongoing assessment can be done every 15 minutes.
   c. The time interval for repeating the ongoing assessment for the critical medical patient is the same as the critical trauma patient.
   d. Ongoing assessment should only be repeated by a paramedic for critical trauma patients.

6. _____ is the process of obtaining a baseline assessment and then repeating the assessment for comparison.

   a. Trending
   b. Palpation
   c. Pairing off
   d. Serial processing

7. During the management of the patient enroute to the hospital, the earliest indicators of deterioration of a patient are often:

   a. subtle changes in the patient's blood pressure.
   b. subtle changes in the patient's mental status.
   c. changes in skin color.
   d. changes in the lung sounds.

8. Which of the following statements about measurements or observations obtained during management of the patient is most accurate?

   a. Isolated measurements are generally less helpful than changes over time.
   b. Isolated observations are significantly more helpful than acute changes over time.
   c. Treatment protocols are specifically designed for patients with acute assessment changes.
   d. Treatment protocols help the paramedic to anticipate observations that identify deterioration of a patient's mental status.

9. The cornerstone of being an effective paramedic is having the ability to:

   a. perform the ongoing examination on a bumpy street.
   b. avoid conflict with family members.
   c. drive all types of emergency vehicles.
   d. think and work under pressure.

10. The essential concepts of clinical decision making include all the following, *except*:

    a. gathering information.
    b. evaluating and processing information.
    c. being a mentor to a new member.
    d. implementing appropriate patient management.

11. Based on the ongoing assessment and evaluation, the paramedic may:

    a. formulate a new management plan.
    b. provide additional interventions.
    c. call Medical Control for consultation.
    d. all of the above.

12. Which of the following is a major difference between patient care in the prehospital setting and hospital setting?

    a. Patients open up more to the ED staff than they do to paramedics.
    b. The hospital is a relatively controlled environment.
    c. Paramedics can perform skills that nurses cannot.
    d. The ongoing assessment is different in the hospital.

13. Which of the following is an example of a non-life-threatening condition the paramedic would address during an ongoing assessment?

    a. CVA.
    b. Fractured femur.
    c. Isolated extremity injury without neurologic compromise.
    d. Concurrent disease presentations.

14. All the following are critical life-threatening conditions the paramedic would address during an ongoing assessment, *except*:

    a. major single system trauma.
    b. AMI.
    c. TIA.
    d. major multisystem trauma.

15. Fundamental elements of critical thinking for the paramedic include all the following, *except*:

    a. achieving and maintaining an adequate body of knowledge.
    b. following the directions of the paramedic supervisor.
    c. recalling contrary situations.
    d. articulating and constructing valid arguments.

16. Which of the following is not an aspect of critical thinking for the paramedic?

    a. Scrutinizing the actions of the first responders.
    b. Differentiating between relevant and non-relevant information.
    c. Identifying and managing medical ambiguity.
    d. Documenting decision-making reasoning.

17. During a call for an allergic reaction you realize that you have forgotten the new standing order dose for Benadryl®. Which of the following is the most appropriate action?

    a. Use the old standing order dose.
    b. Guess the dose, because it is too embarrassing to ask Medical Control.
    c. Look up the correct dose in your protocol book.
    d. Just give the epinephrine and say that you are out of Benadryl®.

18. The stages of critical thinking for the paramedic include all the following, *except*:

    a. collecting information and formulating concepts.
    b. interpretation and processing of information.
    c. application of treatment and management.
    d. consideration of the scene size-up.

19. Benefits of protocols, standing orders, and patient care algorithms include all the following, *except* they:

    a. cover all aspects of the critically ill patient.
    b. promote a standard approach to patient care.
    c. clearly define performance parameters.
    d. provide some legally defensible backup for the paramedic.

20. Which of the following is not a shortfall of protocols, standing orders, and patient care algorithms?

    a. They do not usually cover multisystem failures or non-specific complaints.
    b. They do not usually cover concurrent disease processes.
    c. They can speed the application of critical interventions.
    d. They usually cover the "textbook" patient injury or illness.

21. In reference to clinical decision making, which of the following is not one of the "Six R's" of putting it all together?

    a. Read the patient.
    b. Read the scene.
    c. React
    d. Rephrase

22. When a paramedic is "reading the scene" of an incident, he/she is considering all the following, *except*:

    a. general environmental conditions.
    b. transportation considerations.
    c. immediate surroundings.
    d. mechanism of injury.

23. While a paramedic is "reading the patient," which of the following is not immediately considered?

    a. Observing the patient.
    b. Talking to the patient.
    c. Auscultating the patient.
    d. Getting insurance information.

24. During the re-evaluation of a patient by the paramedic, all the following are considered, *except* the:

    a. review of the performance after the call.
    b. focused history and detailed assessment.
    c. response to initial management.
    d. discovery of less obvious problems.

25. The mental checklist for the paramedic thinking under pressure should include all the following, *except*:

    a. stop and think.
    b. scan the situation.
    c. observe the patient.
    d. decide and act.

26. Behaviors that can aid the paramedic working under pressure include all the following, *except*:

    a. stay calm and do not panic.
    b. be optimistic and plan for the best outcome.
    c. assume and plan for the worst.
    d. maintain a systematic assessment pattern.

27. For the paramedic thinking and working under pressure, data processing and decision making styles include all the following, *except*:

    a. imaginative versus uninspired.
    b. reflective versus impulsive.
    c. divergent versus convergent.
    d. anticipatory versus reactive.

28. In the sequence of critical thinking process for paramedics, the "evaluation" component consists of all the following, *except*:

    a. reassessment of the patient.
    b. reflection in action.
    c. revision of impression.
    d. run critique.

29. In the clinical decision making process, the paramedic should encourage the patient to actively participate in the process by doing any of the following, *except*:

    a. ask the patient to provide information.
    b. encourage the patient to ask questions.
    c. ask the patient for a signature on a billing form.
    d. take advantage of teaching moments.

30. Which of the following is an example of a potential teaching moment for the paramedic?

    a. An unrestrained victim of an MVC sustained facial lacerations on the windshield.
    b. A three-year-old child experiencing an anaphylactic reaction to a bee sting.
    c. A 55-year-old having an acute myocardial infarction.
    d. An asthmatic having a severe asthma attack after three months without an attack.

31. Which of the following acronyms is used to help paramedics determine treatment and transportation priority decisions?

    a. CUPS
    b. ALS
    c. PHTLS
    d. PALS

32. For most, the more an individual is exposed to an experience, the better he/she is able to manage:

    a. similar experiences.
    b. overcoming having a bad day.
    c. avoiding panic.
    d. all of the above.

33. Key aspects of ongoing assessment include:

    a. observing the MOI.
    b. trending mental status and vital signs.
    c. starting an IV.
    d. obtaining a baseline ECG.

34. In the clinical decision making process, one of the "Six R's" is "react" and this means that the paramedic should:

a. call police backup.
b. take a deep breath when experiencing sensory overload.
c. discuss and analyze the call immediately after the call.
d. treat as he/she goes, correcting life threats first.

35. When a paramedic becomes overwhelmed and critical thinking becomes clouded, which of the following is advised:

a. take a deep breath, and use any of the actions on the mental preparation checklist.
b. call for a backup crew to transport the patient.
c. utilize the paramedic supervisor as a mentor.
d. call the paramedic supervisor and request to go home for the day.

Test #19 Answer Form

	A	B	C	D			A	B	C	D
1.	❑	❑	❑	❑		19.	❑	❑	❑	❑
2.	❑	❑	❑	❑		20.	❑	❑	❑	❑
3.	❑	❑	❑	❑		21.	❑	❑	❑	❑
4.	❑	❑	❑	❑		22.	❑	❑	❑	❑
5.	❑	❑	❑	❑		23.	❑	❑	❑	❑
6.	❑	❑	❑	❑		24.	❑	❑	❑	❑
7.	❑	❑	❑	❑		25.	❑	❑	❑	❑
8.	❑	❑	❑	❑		26.	❑	❑	❑	❑
9.	❑	❑	❑	❑		27.	❑	❑	❑	❑
10.	❑	❑	❑	❑		28.	❑	❑	❑	❑
11.	❑	❑	❑	❑		29.	❑	❑	❑	❑
12.	❑	❑	❑	❑		30.	❑	❑	❑	❑
13.	❑	❑	❑	❑		31.	❑	❑	❑	❑
14.	❑	❑	❑	❑		32.	❑	❑	❑	❑
15.	❑	❑	❑	❑		33.	❑	❑	❑	❑
16.	❑	❑	❑	❑		34.	❑	❑	❑	❑
17.	❑	❑	❑	❑		35.	❑	❑	❑	❑
18.	❑	❑	❑	❑						

Communications

1. The basic model of communications includes each of the following steps, *except*:

   a. sender decodes the message.
   b. sender sends the message.
   c. receiver receives the message.
   d. receiver gives feedback.

2. When a citizen driving by a collision notices the patient and calls 9-1-1, this is called:

   a. notification.
   b. response.
   c. detection.
   d. treatment.

3. When the paramedic confers with Medical Control over the field treatment of the patient, this is referred to as:

   a. notification.
   b. treatment.
   c. preparation for the next call.
   d. response.

4. Communication is necessary on an EMS call to:

   a. advise the triage nurse upon arrival at the hospital.
   b. inform Medical Control and destination hospital for medication orders.
   c. inform the EMD of your availability.
   d. all of the above.

5. On an EMS call the paramedic is required to interact with each of the following, *except*:

   a. emergency service personnel at the scene.
   b. the crew members and bystanders.
   c. the patient's family physician.
   d. the ED staff who will be taking over management of the patient.

6. Special radio codes:

   a. lead to a clearer understanding of the message.
   b. are necessary to avoid listeners.
   c. add an unnecessary level of complexity.
   d. should be used in public.

7. Examples of electronic communication used in EMS include:

   a. a glucometer readout.
   b. Palm Pilots®.
   c. an $EtCO_2$ readout.
   d. all of the above.

8. The study of the meaning in language is called:

   a. diction.
   b. semantics.
   c. linguistics.
   d. context.

9. When talking with a child on an EMS call, it is important to:

   a. minimize the technical terms.
   b. stretch the truth so it sounds better.
   c. use buzz words.
   d. use only short words.

10. When speaking on a portable radio, you should depress the microphone for a moment prior to beginning to speak because:

    a. it will get everyone's attention.
    b. it helps avoid cutting off the first few words.
    c. the radio will transmit louder.
    d. the receivers will be ready to hear you.

11. When an emergency occurs, why should the public avoid dialing "0" on their phones?

    a. The 9-1-1 system is more accurate.
    b. The operator may be unfamiliar with your community.
    c. The 7-digit line is easier to remember.
    d. The operator line is usually busy.

12. The EMS is a professional who has been trained in each of the following, except:

    a. telephone interrogation.
    b. triage.
    c. rapid response to calls.
    d. logistics coordination.

13. When the EMD gives instructions in CPR compressions to the family member who called, this is known as:

    a. interrogation.
    b. prearrival instructions.
    c. radio dispatch.
    d. logistics coordination.

14. The EMD is trained in the four cardinal rules of priority dispatching, which include each of the following, *except*:

    a. what the patient's approximate age is.
    b. whether or not the patient is married.
    c. what the patient's chief complaint is.
    d. whether or not the patient is breathing.

15. The time between the receipt of the call and the time the call is given to the emergency unit to respond is called _____ time.

    a. response
    b. alerting
    c. dispatch
    d. queue

16. When analyzing the time segments of a call, it is important to remember:

    a. scene time begins upon arrival at the patient's side.
    b. the scene time may be artificially lengthened.
    c. scene time ends once you load the patient on the stretcher.
    d. most times are usually inaccurate.

17. Examples of factors that may change the scene time include:

    a. heavy traffic conditions.
    b. a lengthy extrication.
    c. the dispatch priority.
    d. a change in transport destination.

18. One example of a difference between 9-1-1 and an enhanced 9-1-1 system is:

    a. in enhanced 9-1-1, a computer displays the caller's phone number.
    b. The 9-1-1 system is no longer used.
    c. The enhanced system costs more money to make the call.
    d. In the enhanced system there are fewer dispatch centers.

19. When called by someone who is in direct contact with the patient, this is referred to as:

    a. first party caller.
    b. second party caller.
    c. third party caller.
    d. none of the above.

20. The new roles of the FCC include:

    a. creating a model agency for the digital age.
    b. managing the electromagnetic spectrum.
    c. promoting competition in all communication markets.
    d. all of the above.

21. Who was the physician credited with the creation of meaningful change in the way dispatchers were trained in the past 20 years?

    a. Adam Cowley, MD
    b. David Boyd, MD
    c. Eugene Nagel, MD
    d. Jeff Clawson, MD

22. What medical breakthrough is referred to as zero-minute response time?

    a. Public Access Defibrillation
    b. Pre-arrival instructions
    c. System status management
    d. Rapid response vehicles

23. A system where the computer is used to assist the EMD in determining which units to deploy, is called a(an):

    a. SSM.
    b. CAD.
    c. ALS.
    d. CSM.

24. The main purpose of a verbal report over the radio to the hospital is to:

    a. document on tape the patient's problem.
    b. document the run on tape for QI purposes.
    c. give them time to prepare for the patient.
    d. assess the need for diversion.

25. The radio report to the hospital should include all the following, *except*:

    a. baseline vital signs.
    b. response to emergency medical care.
    c. the patient's name.
    d. the chief complaint.

26. In addition to the standard radio report, the paramedic report to Medical Control should also include:

    a. drugs administered on standing orders.
    b. a second set of vital signs.
    c. the patient's ETA.
    d. the patient's age.

27. The official listing of ten codes is prepared by:

    a. NFPA.
    b. OSHA.
    c. FEMA.
    d. APCO.

28. When speaking on a portable radio you should:

    a. only use the last names of patients.
    b. be courteous and say please and thank you.
    c. say each digit for clarity when transmitting a number.
    d. speak quickly with your lips about an inch from the microphone.

29. Radio interference is caused by:

    a. 60 cycle interference.
    b. electromagnetic radiation.
    c. standing too close to a fluorescent light.
    d. all of the above.

30. The number of repetitive cycles per second completed by a radio wave is called the:

    a. telemetry.
    b. frequency.
    c. amplitude modulation.
    d. call simplex.

31. When a radio transmits and receives on the same frequency, this is called:

    a. call simplex.
    b. duplex communications.
    c. telemetry.
    d. ultra-high frequency.

32. When the radio power of a portable is not strong enough to reach a base station, this can be improved by the use of a(an):

    a. amplitude modulator.
    b. frequency modulator.
    c. duplex system.
    d. repeater.

33. Radio frequencies between 300 and 3000 mHz are in the _____ band.

    a. AM
    b. VHF
    c. cellular
    d. UHF

34. The _____ band is less susceptible to interference than _____, so it is more frequently used in EMS communications.

    a. cellular; AM
    b. FM; AM
    c. AM; FM
    d. UHF; FM

35. Voice transmission is also referred to as:

    a. simplex.
    b. analog transmission.
    c. digital transmission.
    d. duplex.

Test #20 Answer Form

	A	B	C	D		A	B	C	D
1.	❑	❑	❑	❑	19.	❑	❑	❑	❑
2.	❑	❑	❑	❑	20.	❑	❑	❑	❑
3.	❑	❑	❑	❑	21.	❑	❑	❑	❑
4.	❑	❑	❑	❑	22.	❑	❑	❑	❑
5.	❑	❑	❑	❑	23.	❑	❑	❑	❑
6.	❑	❑	❑	❑	24.	❑	❑	❑	❑
7.	❑	❑	❑	❑	25.	❑	❑	❑	❑
8.	❑	❑	❑	❑	26.	❑	❑	❑	❑
9.	❑	❑	❑	❑	27.	❑	❑	❑	❑
10.	❑	❑	❑	❑	28.	❑	❑	❑	❑
11.	❑	❑	❑	❑	29.	❑	❑	❑	❑
12.	❑	❑	❑	❑	30.	❑	❑	❑	❑
13.	❑	❑	❑	❑	31.	❑	❑	❑	❑
14.	❑	❑	❑	❑	32.	❑	❑	❑	❑
15.	❑	❑	❑	❑	33.	❑	❑	❑	❑
16.	❑	❑	❑	❑	34.	❑	❑	❑	❑
17.	❑	❑	❑	❑	35.	❑	❑	❑	❑
18.	❑	❑	❑	❑					

21

Documentation

1. In a medicolegal case review, poor documentation is:

   a. only a problem with new EMS personnel.
   b. usually an indication of poor assessment.
   c. usually caused by lack of training or supervision.
   d. a sign of laziness.

2. Which of the following statements about the documentation of prehospital care is incorrect?

   a. Documentation serves as a legal record of the incident.
   b. Documentation provides a professional link between the field and in-hospital management.
   c. All documentation of prehospital care contains administrative data, as well as patient data.
   d. Documentation is used for quality improvement.

3. _____ has defined a minimum data set to be included in all prehospital care reports.

   a. NHTSA
   b. DOT
   c. State EMS
   d. DOH

4. Examples of run data include all the following, *except*:

   a. name of the service.
   b. names of the crew members.
   c. name of the patient.
   d. level of training of the crewmembers.

5. All the following are examples of patient data, *except*:

   a. run times.
   b. nature of the call.
   c. MOI.
   d. location of the patient.

6. All the following are names for the prehospital patient documentation prepared by EMS personnel, *except* the:

   a. PCR.
   b. run sheet.
   c. ambulance call report.
   d. DNAR.

7. All the following are examples of patient demographic information, *except* the:

   a. address.
   b. date of birth.
   c. phone number.
   d. chief complaint.

8. Besides being a legal record of patient care, PCRs are used for all the following, *except*:

   a. run reviews.
   b. publishing.
   c. conferences.
   d. medical audits.

9. Which of the following is most accurate about documentation of vital signs?

   a. Vital signs should be documented before and after a medication administration.
   b. Three sets of vital signs should be documented for every patient.
   c. Vital signs should be documented at least every 10 minutes for critical patients.
   d. It is not difficult to make treatment decisions based on one set of vital signs.

10. Standard guidelines for documentation of prehospital assessment and management include:

    a. always use print on the PCR.
    b. being objective, specific and concrete.
    c. minimizing the use of abbreviations.
    d. avoiding the use of quotations.

11. The prefix Celi/o means:

    a. abdomen.
    b. neck.
    c. color.
    d. around.

12. The suffix Dynia means:

    a. to free.
    b. painful condition.
    c. outer.
    d. through.

13. Because the paramedic will not be present to explain his or her findings to all who ultimately read the PCR, the form should be so complete that it:

    a. leaves no doubt about the patient's diagnosis.
    b. contains the patient's entire past medical history.
    c. includes only objective findings by the paramedic.
    d. "speaks for itself."

14. The presence of a complete and accurate record is helpful in:

    a. keeping the patient from harm or embarrassment.
    b. ensuring and maintaining patient confidentiality.
    c. averting further legal action during the "discovery phase" of a lawsuit.
    d. developing a plan for definitive treatment.

15. Examples of extraneous or non-professional statements that should not be written into the documentation of a PCR include all the following, *except*:

    a. "the patient was asking for the beating."
    b. "these people live in filth."
    c. "the patient vomited four times last night."
    d. "the skell just wanted another ride across town."

16. Which of the following prefixes means "joined together, with?"

    a. Sten-
    b. Sym-
    c. Thio-
    d. Uni-

17. Which of the following suffixes means "a suturing or stitching?"

    a. -rhaphy
    b. -sect
    c. -poiesis
    d. -osis

18. _____ findings are information the patient or bystanders tell the paramedic.

    a. Subjective
    b. Neutral
    c. Objective
    d. Biased

19. _____ findings are information the paramedic can measure such as vital signs.

    a. Subjective
    b. Neutral
    c. Objective
    d. Lawful

20. Patients have a right to have their medical records be:

    a. held from third-party billing agencies.
    b. withheld from medical students.
    c. partially restricted from their HMOs.
    d. held in confidence.

21. Any PCR that is used for quality improvement or educational purposes should not include which of the following?

    a. date of the run
    b. times of the run
    c. name of the patient
    d. none of the above

22. During the discovery phase of a lawsuit any of the following can be considered poor documentation, except an _____ record.

    a. inclusive
    b. incomplete
    c. inaccurate
    d. illegible

23. When documentation is anything less than complete or accurate, the presumption is that the paramedic either did not do the proper care or:

    a. had a bad day.
    b. forgot to include something.
    c. had something to hide.
    d. was not trained properly.

24. When a patient has been intubated in the field the paramedic should include all the following information in his/her documentation, *except*:

    a. the size of the tube.
    b. who placed the tube.
    c. the brand name of the tube.
    d. the method of verification of tube placement.

25. The documentation for staring IVs in the field should include all the following information, *except*:

    a. size of the angio used.
    b. who started the IV.
    c. who adjusted the drip rate.
    d. the number of attempts if the first was not successful.

26. Most often there is additional documentation associated with the administration of narcotics. Which of the following is not included in that information?

    a. The patient's name.
    b. The patient's medical insurance information.
    c. The physician who authorized the administration.
    d. What effect the medication had on the patient.

27. Which of the following is often used as the first line of documentation at an MCI?

   a. Donning identification vests
   b. Triage tags
   c. Labeling sectors
   d. Recording transportation destinations

28. Which of the following is an example of a pertinent negative that is documented on a PCR?

   a. A patient struck his head, but had no loss of consciousness.
   b. A patient with chest pain has no shortness of breath.
   c. A diabetic patient feels hypoglycemic, but did not skip a meal.
   d. All of the above.

29. When making corrections of a recorded error on a PCR, which of the following is an incorrect way to make the change?

   a. Initial and date the mistaken entry.
   b. Draw a single line through the entry.
   c. Write "error" above or next to the entry.
   d. Erase the entry.

30. All of the following are examples of unusual situations that the paramedic should record on a PCR, *except*:

   a. a delay in response time caused by traffic.
   b. radio failure delaying contact with Medical Control.
   c. police request to draw blood alcohol samples.
   d. during the transport your ambulance passes a serious MVC.

31. Documentation of which of the following findings is vital in defending your care of a patient with a suspected fracture or dislocation?

   a. Adequacy of the neurovascular supply before and after immobilization.
   b. The manner in which the fracture/dislocation was immobilized.
   c. The type of splint used.
   d. The use of analgesia for pain management.

32. If a patient makes statements to questions that do not appear in a check box on the PCR, the paramedic should:

   a. paraphrase the patient's statement into the narrative.
   b. document the statement in "quotes."
   c. use a special incident form for complete accuracy.
   d. write in additional check boxes.

33. The PCR is a legal document in which the paramedic should assure that the expressions and terms used are:

   a. derogatory.
   b. approved by the DOH.
   c. standardized and professional.
   d. judgment biased.

34. When a paramedic documents information about a patient's medication that is being taken "four times a day," which of the following would he/she use?

   a. q.d.
   b. q.i.d.
   c. t.i.d.
   d. p.r.n.

35. An example of a situation that should not be documented on a PCR is the:

   a. patient had to be restrained.
   b. patient was hostile or abusive.
   c. patient's marital status.
   d. patient's date of birth.

36. Standardization of the data elements to be included in all PCRs helps to make it easier to:

   a. facilitate corroborating testimony in court.
   b. avoid litigation in the future.
   c. compare data from different agencies.
   d. document the disposition of the call.

37. Which of the following is meant by the document should "stand on its own"?

   a. The record contains everything it should in a clear, legible and concise fashion.
   b. The record does not contain unprofessional language.
   c. The record does not contain any pertinent negatives.
   d. There are no documented errors.

38. Two types of narrative formats used in documentation of PCRs are:

   a. SOAP and CHART.
   b. CUPS and AVPU.
   c. PMHx and OPQRST.
   d. SAMPLE and APGAR.

39. Ensuring that your documentation is complete, accurate, and legible is one of the _____ of the paramedic.

    a. standing orders
    b. local protocols
    c. professional responsibilities
    d. state DOH regulations

40. With which of the following are you not allowed to share a patient's medical information?

    a. The healthcare provider continuing care.
    b. A lawyer with a subpoena.
    c. A police officer who is a friend of the patient.
    d. Third-party billing companies.

41. Which of the following situations requires extra attention to detail when documenting on a PCR?

    a. MCI
    b. RMA
    c. correcting an error
    d. all of the above

42. When the paramedic documents a call where the patient refused care or transport, all the following should be recorded, *except*:

    a. competency of the patient.
    b. ruling out a serious injury.
    c. your recommendation for care and transport.
    d. an explanation to the patient about the consequences of refusal.

43. Ideally, the best time for the paramedic to complete a PCR on a patient is:

    a. enroute to the hospital.
    b. while waiting to transfer the patient to a bed.
    c. at the ED, after transfer of the patient to a bed.
    d. after returning to your station from the ED.

44. The part of a PCR which contains the written report that depicts the call is the:

    a. narrative.
    b. addendum.
    c. administrative section.
    d. demographic section.

45. When documenting assessment findings, which of the following is not necessary to record?

    a. pertinent positives
    b. pertinent negatives
    c. normal findings
    d. all findings should be recorded

46. _____ is the writing of false and malicious statements intended to damage a person's character.

    a. Bias
    b. Jargon
    c. Slander
    d. Libel

47. Which of the following statements about documenting PCRs is most correct?

    a. All personnel and resources involved in the call should be recorded.
    b. Using various formats when documenting helps the paramedic to become a proficient narrator.
    c. When documentation is complete, accurate and legible, there is no chance of becoming involved in litigation.
    d. The discovery phase is the only time a lawyer will be able to gain access to your documentation.

48. Which of the following is a standard term used by the paramedic in documenting something that is situated near the surface of the body?

    a. Superior
    b. Sagittal
    c. Efferent
    d. Superficial

49. _____ is a common medical suffix that means stopping or controlling.

    a. - stasis
    b. - stomy
    c. - scopy
    d. - plasty

50. When a paramedic sees the prefix _____ he/she can recognize that the term is referring to the kidney.

    a. Nephr/o
    b. Hepat/o
    c. Gangli/o
    d. Dacry/o

Test #21 Answer Form

	A	B	C	D			A	B	C	D
1.	❏	❏	❏	❏		26.	❏	❏	❏	❏
2.	❏	❏	❏	❏		27.	❏	❏	❏	❏
3.	❏	❏	❏	❏		28.	❏	❏	❏	❏
4.	❏	❏	❏	❏		29.	❏	❏	❏	❏
5.	❏	❏	❏	❏		30.	❏	❏	❏	❏
6.	❏	❏	❏	❏		31.	❏	❏	❏	❏
7.	❏	❏	❏	❏		32.	❏	❏	❏	❏
8.	❏	❏	❏	❏		33.	❏	❏	❏	❏
9.	❏	❏	❏	❏		34.	❏	❏	❏	❏
10.	❏	❏	❏	❏		35.	❏	❏	❏	❏
11.	❏	❏	❏	❏		36.	❏	❏	❏	❏
12.	❏	❏	❏	❏		37.	❏	❏	❏	❏
13.	❏	❏	❏	❏		38.	❏	❏	❏	❏
14.	❏	❏	❏	❏		39.	❏	❏	❏	❏
15.	❏	❏	❏	❏		40.	❏	❏	❏	❏
16.	❏	❏	❏	❏		41.	❏	❏	❏	❏
17.	❏	❏	❏	❏		42.	❏	❏	❏	❏
18.	❏	❏	❏	❏		43.	❏	❏	❏	❏
19.	❏	❏	❏	❏		44.	❏	❏	❏	❏
20.	❏	❏	❏	❏		45.	❏	❏	❏	❏
21.	❏	❏	❏	❏		46.	❏	❏	❏	❏
22.	❏	❏	❏	❏		47.	❏	❏	❏	❏
23.	❏	❏	❏	❏		48.	❏	❏	❏	❏
24.	❏	❏	❏	❏		49.	❏	❏	❏	❏
25.	❏	❏	❏	❏		50.	❏	❏	❏	❏

22

Pulmonary and Respiratory

1. The process where oxygenated blood is pumped to the tissues, and waste products returned to the lungs, is called:

   a. respiration.
   b. ventilation.
   c. diffusion.
   d. perfusion.

2. _____ refers specifically to the exchange of carbon dioxide, while _____ refers only to the exchange of oxygen.

   a. Ventilation: oxygenation
   b. Oxygenation: ventilation
   c. Diffusion: oxygenation
   d. Perfusion: ventilation

3. A shift in the oxyhemoglobin saturation curve indicates a change in the affinity of hemoglobin for oxygen. A(an) _____ shift decreases it, while a _____ shift of the curve increases the binding (affinity) of oxygen to hemoglobin.

   a. upward: rightward
   b. downward: leftward
   c. rightward: leftward
   d. leftward: rightward

4. When a person develops a fever, the cell's metabolic rate increases and so:

   a. a leftward shift of the oxyhemoglobin saturation curve occurs.
   b. does their oxygen need.
   c. does their hemoglobin need.
   d. a downward shift of the oxyhemoglobin saturation curve occurs.

5. Which of the following factors causes a shift in the oxyhemoglobin curve, decreasing the tissue oxygen delivery?

   a. decreased body temperature
   b. increased body temperature
   c. acidosis
   d. increased metabolic rate

6. The pCO_2 measures ventilation (exchange of carbon dioxide). Normal levels of pCO_2 are _____ mmHg.

   a. 7.35–7.45
   b. 7.40–7.50
   c. 35–40
   d. 40–45

7. pCO_2 is a respiratory:

   a. side-effect.
   b. alkali.
   c. basic.
   d. acid.

8. For every 10 mmHg change of the pCO_2, either up or down, the result is a _____ change in the pH in the opposite direction.

   a. 0.1
   b. 1.0
   c. 1.5
   d. 10.0

9. The pO_2 measures oxygenation at sea level and should normally run greater than _____ mmHg.

   a. 30
   b. 50
   c. 70
   d. 80

10. Which of the following statements about blood gases are correct?

    a. Changes in pO_2 always occur when there is a change in pCO_2.
    b. The only predictable and reproducible relation in blood gases is between the pH and the pCO_2.
    c. Hypoventilation leads to decreased pO_2 and decreased pCO_2.
    d. Hyperventilation raises the pCO_2 and the pO_2.

11. In respiratory acidosis, CO_2 retention leads to increased levels of:

    a. O_2.
    b. pO_2.
    c. pCO_2.
    d. SpO_2.

12. A patient that is hypoventilating, because of a heroin overdose, is most likely experiencing which acid-base disorder?

    a. Respiratory acidosis
    b. Respiratory alkalosis
    c. Metabolic acidosis
    d. Metabolic alkalosis

13. All the following are examples of upper airway obstruction, *except*:

    a. epiglottitis.
    b. FBAO.
    c. tonsillitis.
    d. bronchospasm.

14. Which of the following is not a cause of lower airway obstruction?

    a. Empyema
    b. Epiglottitis
    c. Smooth muscle spasm
    d. Obstructive lung disease

15. Which of the following conditions does not directly affect diffusion of gases in the pulmonary circulation?

    a. Near-drowning
    b. Pulmonary hypertension
    c. FBAO
    d. ARDS

16. All the following conditions affect perfusion, *except*:

    a. hypovolemia.
    b. anemia.
    c. pulmonary embolus.
    d. All of the above affect perfusion.

17. Audible stridor is a potentially life-threatening sign of respiratory distress that should alert you to the possibility of any of the following, *except*:

    a. asthma.
    b. croup.
    c. epiglottits.
    d. FBAO.

18. The presence of grunting is usually a sign of respiratory distress that occurs primarily in infants and small toddlers when the child breathes:

    a. in against a partially closed epiglottis.
    b. in against an airway obstruction.
    c. out against a partially closed epiglottis.
    d. out against an airway obstruction.

19. Which of the following are non-specific findings associated with respiratory distress?

    a. grunting and wheezing
    b. pallor and diaphoresis
    c. cyanosis and dyspnea
    d. AMS and confusion

20. All the following are typical chief complaints that a patient with a respiratory problem may present with, *except*:

    a. "My chest is tight."
    b. "I have a bad cough."
    c. "I have been running a fever."
    d. "My stomach hurts."

21. When obtaining a focused history from a patient with a pulmonary disease, history of previous intubation is:

    a. an accurate indicator of severe pulmonary disease.
    b. a nonspecific associated finding with respiratory distress.
    c. an indication that you will need to intubate the patient.
    d. not suggestive that intubation may be required again.

22. Patients who are taking _____ typically have severe pulmonary disease.

    a. MOA inhibitors
    b. decongestants
    c. oral corticosteriods
    d. inhaled steroids

23. When forming a general impression of a patient's condition, the assessment is based on all the following factors, *except*:

    a. position of comfort.
    b. mentation.
    c. pCO_2 reading.
    d. ability to speak.

24. The presence of tachycardia in a patient with respiratory distress may be caused by any of the following, *except*:

    a. diaphoresis.
    b. hypoxemia.
    c. fear.
    d. use of bronchodilators.

25. In the face of a respiratory problem, _____ is an ominous sign of severe hypoxemia and suggests imminent cardiac arrest.

   a. a low SpO_2 reading
   b. tachypnea
   c. tachycardia
   d. bradycardia

26. The respiratory pattern which is characterized by alternating periods of apnea and deep, rapid breathing is called:

   a. eupnea.
   b. central neurogenic hyperventilation.
   c. Kussmaul.
   d. Cheyne-Stokes.

27. The type of breathing characterized by a series of several short inspirations followed by long, irregular periods of apnea and is associated with increased intracranial pressure is called:

   a. central neurogen hyperventilation.
   b. ataxic.
   c. apneustic.
   d. Cheyne-Stokes.

28. The most common types of abnormal respiratory patterns seen in the field include tachypnea, bradypnea, apnea and:

   a. eupnea.
   b. Biot's.
   c. Kussmaul.
   d. Cheyne-Stokes.

29. Many forms of lung disease cause increased resistance to blood flow in the lungs causing the right heart to work harder. The heart compensates initially, but later is unable to maintain compensatory efforts, resulting in:

   a. right heart failure.
   b. left heart failure.
   c. pursed-lip breathing.
   d. decreased pulmonary resistance.

30. Signs and symptoms of the condition described in question 29 include all the following, *except*:

   a. pigeon chest.
   b. venous distention.
   c. peripheral edema.
   d. ascites.

31. The _____ deformity seen in some COPD and asthma patients is caused by _____ expiratory resistance to flow and air-trapping.

   a. barrel chest: increased
   b. pigeon chest: increased
   c. barrel chest: decreased
   d. pigeon chest: decreased

32. Crackles heard when breathing result from fluid in the airways, in the interstitial tissue, or in:

   a. both.
   b. a friction rub.
   c. pleurisy.
   d. pericarditis.

33. _____ spasm is a spasmodic contraction of the hands, wrists, feet and ankles, which is associated with decreased levels of carbon dioxide.

   a. Hypocapopedal
   b. Carbonix
   c. Carpopedal
   d. Carbondorsal

34. Besides anxiety, all the following conditions are associated with hyperventilation, *except*:

   a. pulmonary embolism.
   b. HTN.
   c. DKA.
   d. myocardial infarction.

35. Capnography measures _____ or how much carbon dioxide is exhaled.

   a. end-tidal CO_2
   b. pO_2
   c. pCO_2
   d. peak flow

36. The most common obstructive airway diseases include asthma and:

   a. URI.
   b. COPD.
   c. cystic fibrosis.
   d. legionnaires' disease.

37. Airway obstruction in obstructive lung disease is usually a result of several factors including all the following, *except*:

   a. smooth muscle spasm.
   b. mucus.
   c. cilia.
   d. inflammation.

38. During bronchospasm, the tiny muscle layers surrounding the bronchioles go into spasm and narrow the lumen of the airways, the result is:

   a. irritation.
   b. wheezing.
   c. snoring.
   d. coughing.

39. During an acute asthma attack, mucus production is increased because of _____ in the bronchial airways.

   a. irritation
   b. wheezing
   c. snoring
   d. coughing

40. _____ are the most common asthma triggers.

   a. Chewing tobaccos
   b. Car fumes
   c. Respiratory infections
   d. Flower spores

41. Exercise or fast breathing is a trigger for asthma attacks, especially during _____ weather.

   a. hot
   b. cold
   c. humid
   d. rainy

42. Any condition that leads to _____ may cause carpopedal spasm.

   a. respiratory acidosis
   b. respiratory alkalosis
   c. metabolic acidosis
   d. metabolic alkalosis

43. Examples of emotions that might trigger an asthma attack include all the following, *except*:

   a. crying.
   b. yelling.
   c. laughing.
   d. smiling.

44. _____ is a severe prolonged asthma attack that does not respond to standard medications.

   a. Acute bronchial asthma
   b. Status asthmaticus
   c. Allergy induced asthma
   d. Exercise induced asthma

45. Death rates from asthma continue to soar despite all the current knowledge about asthma. Two factors that underlie the fatal trend include decreased airway sensitivity and:

   a. inadequate use of anti-inflammatory medication.
   b. the lack of peak flow meter use.
   c. increased use of antibiotics.
   d. increased exposure to the Lyme-carrying tick.

46. _____ results from overgrowth of the airway mucus glands and excess secretion of mucus that blocks the airway.

   a. Asthma
   b. Chronic bronchitis
   c. Emphysema
   d. Exacerbation

47. _____ results from destruction of the walls of the alveoli, which leads to a decrease in elastic recoil.

   a. Asthma
   b. Chronic bronchitis
   c. Emphysema
   d. Legionnaires' disease

48. Which of the following is the major cause of COPD?

   a. Air pollution
   b. Cigarette smoking
   c. Tuberculosis
   d. Asbestos

49. Victims of asthma attacks will have symptoms that _____, as compared with persons with COPD.

   a. are wheezing in nature
   b. are associated with smoking
   c. progressively worsen over several days
   d. come on relatively quickly

50. A young child is presenting with acute respiratory distress and audible wheezing. He has no history of asthma and takes no medications. Which of the following do you attempt to rule out first?

   a. FBAO
   b. COPD
   c. Toxic inhalation
   d. Asthma

51. Epinephrine, terbutaline, and albuterol, all have _____ effects, which are potentially useful in the treatment of obstructive lung disease.

   a. bronchoconstricting
   b. bronchodilating
   c. vasoconstricting
   d. anti-inflammatory

52. Steriods are beneficial in the chronic treatment of nearly all asthma patients and many COPD patients because of the _____ effects.

    a. smooth muscle relaxing
    b. bronchodilating
    c. vasoconstricting
    d. anti-inflammatory

53. The inhaled steroids used in the first line in the treatment of asthma and COPD patients result in _____ side effects than the oral preparations.

    a. more
    b. fewer
    c. the same
    d. different

54. Some EMS systems carry steroids, because these drugs:

    a. take at least one or two hours to work.
    b. work immediately.
    c. are of no benefit after the first 30 minutes of intervention of respiratory distress.
    d. are of minimal benefit after the first 30 minutes of intervention of respiratory distress.

55. _____ is/are one of the major inflammation-causing compounds produced in asthma.

    a. Glucocorticoids
    b. Latex
    c. Leukotrienes
    d. Leukocites

56. Magnesium sulfate has been shown to be of some benefit to some asthmatic patients, primarily because of its _____ effects.

    a. smooth muscle relaxing
    b. bronchodilating
    c. vasoconstricting
    d. anti-inflammatory

57. The accumulation of carbon dioxide in blood is the major stimulus that normally causes:

    a. altered mental status.
    b. hormonal secretions.
    c. us to breathe.
    d. fluid retention.

58. Cigarette smoke directly inhibits the normal:

    a. movement of mucus via bronchial cilia out of the lungs.
    b. response to breathe in teens.
    c. immune response in the elderly.
    d. hormonal response in postmenopausal women.

59. Chronic alcoholics have an increased risk of respiratory infections because of:

    a. decreased thermoregulatory systems.
    b. weakened immune systems caused by ethanol.
    c. increased exposure to hypothermia.
    d. decreased hepatic functions.

60. All the following are examples of high risk patients for pneumonia, *except*:

    a. the elderly.
    b. cancer patients.
    c. organ transplant patients.
    d. diabetic patients.

61. Which of the following statements about pneumonia is most correct?

    a. Most pneumonias are caused by viruses.
    b. The clinical approach to viral or bacterial pneumonia is the same.
    c. The clinical approach to viral or bacterial pneumonia is different.
    d. It is possible to tell the difference between viral and bacterial pneumonia in the prehospital setting.

62. A secondary mechanism that stimulates breathing is a lack of oxygen in the blood and is called:

    a. carbon dioxide drive.
    b. hypoxic drive.
    c. bicarboxic force.
    d. bicarbonic influence.

63. All the following are typical findings associated with pneumonia, *except*:

    a. productive cough.
    b. non-productive cough.
    c. pleuritic chest pain.
    d. decreased breath sounds.

64. Atypical symptoms are more common in viral pneumonia, and in the very young or very old. These can include all the following, *except*:

    a. headache.
    b. muscle aches.
    c. sore throat.
    d. syncope.

65. What should be the primary concern for the paramedic when treating a patient who may have pneumonia?

    a. Respiratory distress
    b. Respiratory failure
    c. Exposure to a contagious patient
    d. Severe dehydration

66. Prehospital treatment with drug therapy of _____ may be helpful, especially if the patient has accompanying obstructive lung disease.

    a. albuterol
    b. antibiotics
    c. aspirin
    d. steroids

67. Influenza is a specific type of _____ infection that may affect both the upper and lower respiratory tracts.

    a. viral
    b. bacterial
    c. fungal
    d. spore

68. It is impossible to differentiate viral URI from a bacterial URI without:

    a. a good past medical history.
    b. cultures.
    c. the presence of an elevated temperature.
    d. a visit to the emergency department.

69. Most patients with URI have spontaneous resolution of their symptoms within seven days:

    a. only when they go to the ED.
    b. only when they see their own MD.
    c. with or without antibiotics.
    d. with or without an underlying disease.

70. Viral URI is a common precipitant of all the following conditions, *except*:

    a. CHF.
    b. pneumonia.
    c. exacerbations of asthma and COPD.
    d. respiratory failure.

71. A patient who presents with URI and has had his/her _____ removed is at grave risk for a life-threatening illness.

    a. lung
    b. appendix
    c. spleen
    d. gallbladder

72. The most common cause of primary lung tumors is:

    a. coal miner's lung.
    b. asbestosis.
    c. cigarette smoking.
    d. heredity.

73. Primary lung tumors commonly metastasize to all the following areas, *except* the:

    a. opposite lung.
    b. pleura.
    c. heart.
    d. ribs.

74. A patient who is being treated with chemotherapy for lung cancer, would most likely have which of the following complaints?

    a. nausea, vomiting and weakness
    b. diaphoresis and shortness of breath
    c. chest pain
    d. vision and equilibrium disturbances

75. Side effects associated with radiotherapy for lung cancer most commonly include any of the following, *except*:

    a. dry cough.
    b. being asymptomatic.
    c. shortness of breath.
    d. hypothermia.

76. Some lung tumors lead to abnormal production of parathyroid hormone, which causes bone breakdown, _____ serum _____ levels.

    a. lowering: calcium
    b. raising: calcium
    c. lowering: potassium
    d. raising: potassium

77. Persons with acute pulmonary edema caused by _____ have "severe congestive heart failure," but not all patients with "severe congestive heart failure" have pulmonary edema.

    a. ARDS
    b. scorpion bites
    c. pericarditis
    d. cardiac ischemia

78. The primary difference between pulmonary edema and congestive heart failure is:

   a. Pulmonary edema develops progressively and CHF does not.
   b. Only pulmonary edema is associated with ARDS.
   c. CHF is a spectrum of conditions associated with decreases in cardiac function.
   d. Only CHF can be exacerbated by asthma or COPD.

79. Patients with CHF or PE may have orthopnea because:

   a. the recumbent position increased venous return to the heart.
   b. the recumbent position decreased venous return to the heart.
   c. these patients have a decreased preload mechanism.
   d. these patients are usually obese and this increases pulmonary resistance.

80. The role of nitroglycerine in the treatment of patients with acute pulmonary edema is:

   a. to dilate the veins.
   b. to dilate the arteries.
   c. vasodilation of both veins and arteries.
   d. decreasing lymphatic flow from the lungs.

81. Furosemide has all the following effects in the treatment of acute pulmonary edema, *except*:

   a. vasodilation.
   b. increased lymphatic flow from the lungs.
   c. diuretic effects.
   d. increased cardiac preload.

82. Besides the analgesic effect, morphine sulfate also has which of the following effects on the patient with acute pulmonary edema?

   a. Reduces cardiac preload and afterload.
   b. Increases cardiac preload and afterload.
   c. Increases cerebral diuresis.
   d. Has an amnesic affect.

83. ACE inhibitors have been used to treat hypertension and CHF for years. The way they work is by blocking:

   a. the hormone aldosterone on the kidneys.
   b. the conversion of angiotensin I to angiotensin II in the lungs.
   c. the collapse of portions of the lung and improving overall ventilation.
   d. vasoconstriction of cardiac arteries.

84. The role of simple positive pressure in the treatment of patients with respiratory distress is to:

   a. decrease intrathoracic pressure.
   b. increase intrathoracic pressure.
   c. regulate pulmonary pressures independently.
   d. regulate pulmonary pressure.

85. All the following are causes of pulmonary emboli, *except*:

   a. fat.
   b. amniotic fluid.
   c. tumor tissue.
   d. osteoblasts.

86. Which of the following is not considered a high risk factor for pulmonary embolism?

   a. prolonged bed rest
   b. obesity
   c. pregnancy
   d. IUD contraceptive use

87. The pathology of a pulmonary embolism includes the emboli becoming lodged in:

   a. pulmonary arterial circulation.
   b. pulmonary venous circulation.
   c. deep veins.
   d. the right heart.

88. The occlusion that results from a pulmonary embolism not only results in decreased blood supply to the effected area, but also leads to the release of histamines which causes _____ in the region of the clot.

   a. bronchospasm
   b. AMI
   c. bronchodilation
   d. tissue necrosis

89. Common signs and symptoms associated with a small pulmonary embolis may include any of the following, *except*:

   a. wheezing.
   b. hemoptysis.
   c. pleuritic chest pain.
   d. sudden cardiac death.

90. Which of the following conditions can mimic a pulmonary embolism?

   a. Hypertensive crisis
   b. AMI
   c. Labor
   d. Hypoglycemia

91. Which of the following has more significance in the differential diagnosis of a pulmonary embolism than the others?

   a. The presence or absence of pleuritic chest pain.
   b. History of a recent URI.
   c. Use of diuretics.
   d. Smoking history.

92. The most common physical finding associated with pulmonary embolism includes tachypnea and:

   a. cyanosis.
   b. wheezing.
   c. peripheral edema.
   d. tachycardia.

93. Pulse oximetry readings in patients with acute pulmonary embolism most often are:

   a. low.
   b. high.
   c. normal.
   d. not obtainable.

94. Which of the following profiles is most often associated with spontaneous pneumothorax?

   a. Elderly, obese, male smoker.
   b. Elderly, thin, female smoker.
   c. Young, tall, male smoker.
   d. Young, petite, female smoker.

95. Potential causes of spontaneous pneumothorax include all the following, *except*:

   a. rupture of a congenital bleb.
   b. menstration.
   c. COPD.
   d. hypertension.

96. Typical findings associated with spontaneous pneumothorax may include any of the following, *except*:

   a. acute chest pain on the affected side.
   b. acute chest pain on the unaffected side.
   c. increased respiratory rate.
   d. coughing.

97. The pathology of hyperventilation results in _____ levels of carbon dioxide and _____ the pH.

   a. low: increases
   b. low: decreases
   c. high: increases
   d. high: decreases

98. What is the major risk in caring for a patient presenting with hyperventilation?

   a. Recognizing the patient is hypoxic.
   b. Understanding that hyperventilation is caused by many illnesses.
   c. Assuming the patient is experiencing a simple anxiety attack.
   d. Providing high flow oxygen to a patient in a state of hypocapnea.

99. You are treating a patient experiencing acute pulmonary edema, but the patient is refusing to wear an oxygen mask. Which of the following is most appropriate for the patient?

   a. Insist that the patient needs the oxygen and apply the mask anyway.
   b. Offer the patient a nasal cannula.
   c. Consider the need for a ventilator.
   d. Ask medical control for authorization to perform RSI.

100. Your patient is a 36-year-old male who has a c/c of acute non-exertional dyspnea that is getting progressively worse. Wheezing is heard on auscultation, but there is no PMHx of any obstructive respiratory or cardiac diseases. The only medication he takes is O-T-C Motrin® for pain in the leg from a fracture two months ago. Which of the following conditions do you suspect is causing the dyspnea?

   a. Pulmonary embolism
   b. Spontaneous pneumothorax
   c. Hyperventilation syndrome
   d. Early CHF

101. When considering the pathology for the cause of the dyspnea described in question 100, which of the following is the most likely cause?

   a. fat embolus from bone marrow
   b. ruptured congenital bleb
   c. anxiety
   d. AMI

102. A slender 24-year-old male is complaining of an acute onset of non-exertional sharp chest pain on the right side and shortness of breath. He is a smoker with a history of a non-productive cough for two days. Breath sounds are decreased on the right side and vital signs are R/R 36, H/R 116 and B/P 100/80. Which of the following conditions do you suspect?

    a. Pneumonia
    b. Pulmonary embolus
    c. Spontaneous pneumothorax
    d. AMI

103. You are dispatched to an office building for a 28-year-old female complaining of dizziness and numbness in her hands and legs. Coworkers tell you that the patient has been under a lot of stress, and today she has been especially anxious. The patient denies S.O.B., chest pain or any recent illnesses, and her vital signs are stable. Based on the initial findings, what do suspect is the cause of the patient's extremity numbness?

    a. CVA
    b. TIA
    c. Psychologic
    d. Carpopedal spasm

104. Further information about the patient described in question 103 confirms that the patient was hyperventilating prior to EMS getting there. The patient has a PMHx of asthma, but has not had an attack in months. Your initial management of this patient includes:

    a. providing high flow oxygen and watching for changes in mental status.
    b. withholding oxygen to see if the numbness resolves.
    c. beginning an albuterol treatment.
    d. calling medical control for advice.

Test #22 Answer Form

	A	B	C	D		A	B	C	D
1.	❏	❏	❏	❏	27.	❏	❏	❏	❏
2.	❏	❏	❏	❏	28.	❏	❏	❏	❏
3.	❏	❏	❏	❏	29.	❏	❏	❏	❏
4.	❏	❏	❏	❏	30.	❏	❏	❏	❏
5.	❏	❏	❏	❏	31.	❏	❏	❏	❏
6.	❏	❏	❏	❏	32.	❏	❏	❏	❏
7.	❏	❏	❏	❏	33.	❏	❏	❏	❏
8.	❏	❏	❏	❏	34.	❏	❏	❏	❏
9.	❏	❏	❏	❏	35.	❏	❏	❏	❏
10.	❏	❏	❏	❏	36.	❏	❏	❏	❏
11.	❏	❏	❏	❏	37.	❏	❏	❏	❏
12.	❏	❏	❏	❏	38.	❏	❏	❏	❏
13.	❏	❏	❏	❏	39.	❏	❏	❏	❏
14.	❏	❏	❏	❏	40.	❏	❏	❏	❏
15.	❏	❏	❏	❏	41.	❏	❏	❏	❏
16.	❏	❏	❏	❏	42.	❏	❏	❏	❏
17.	❏	❏	❏	❏	43.	❏	❏	❏	❏
18.	❏	❏	❏	❏	44.	❏	❏	❏	❏
19.	❏	❏	❏	❏	45.	❏	❏	❏	❏
20.	❏	❏	❏	❏	46.	❏	❏	❏	❏
21.	❏	❏	❏	❏	47.	❏	❏	❏	❏
22.	❏	❏	❏	❏	48.	❏	❏	❏	❏
23.	❏	❏	❏	❏	49.	❏	❏	❏	❏
24.	❏	❏	❏	❏	50.	❏	❏	❏	❏
25.	❏	❏	❏	❏	51.	❏	❏	❏	❏
26.	❏	❏	❏	❏	52.	❏	❏	❏	❏

	A	B	C	D
53.	❑	❑	❑	❑
54.	❑	❑	❑	❑
55.	❑	❑	❑	❑
56.	❑	❑	❑	❑
57.	❑	❑	❑	❑
58.	❑	❑	❑	❑
59.	❑	❑	❑	❑
60.	❑	❑	❑	❑
61.	❑	❑	❑	❑
62.	❑	❑	❑	❑
63.	❑	❑	❑	❑
64.	❑	❑	❑	❑
65.	❑	❑	❑	❑
66.	❑	❑	❑	❑
67.	❑	❑	❑	❑
68.	❑	❑	❑	❑
69.	❑	❑	❑	❑
70.	❑	❑	❑	❑
71.	❑	❑	❑	❑
72.	❑	❑	❑	❑
73.	❑	❑	❑	❑
74.	❑	❑	❑	❑
75.	❑	❑	❑	❑
76.	❑	❑	❑	❑
77.	❑	❑	❑	❑
78.	❑	❑	❑	❑

	A	B	C	D
79.	❑	❑	❑	❑
80.	❑	❑	❑	❑
81.	❑	❑	❑	❑
82.	❑	❑	❑	❑
83.	❑	❑	❑	❑
84.	❑	❑	❑	❑
85.	❑	❑	❑	❑
86.	❑	❑	❑	❑
87.	❑	❑	❑	❑
88.	❑	❑	❑	❑
89.	❑	❑	❑	❑
90.	❑	❑	❑	❑
91.	❑	❑	❑	❑
92.	❑	❑	❑	❑
93.	❑	❑	❑	❑
94.	❑	❑	❑	❑
95.	❑	❑	❑	❑
96.	❑	❑	❑	❑
97.	❑	❑	❑	❑
98.	❑	❑	❑	❑
99.	❑	❑	❑	❑
100.	❑	❑	❑	❑
101.	❑	❑	❑	❑
102.	❑	❑	❑	❑
103.	❑	❑	❑	❑
104.	❑	❑	❑	❑

23

Cardiology

1. The semilunar valves include the _____ valves.

   a. pulmonic and aortic
   b. pulmonic and mitral
   c. mitral and tricuspid
   d. tricuspid and aortic

2. When one or more valves become narrowed because of congenital damage, the valve is said to be:

   a. stenotic.
   b. murmured.
   c. regurgitant
   d. intrinsic.

3. The coronary sinus, a portion of the coronary circulation, is a large vein that opens into the:

   a. aorta.
   b. right atrium.
   c. vena cava.
   d. left ventricle.

4. While assessing a 65-year-old female with atrial fibrillation, you discover her radial pulse is less than her apical pulse. This finding is called pulsus:

   a. paradoxus.
   b. alternans.
   c. deficit.
   d. differential.

5. You are assessing the pulse rate and quality on a 23-year-old male experiencing an asthma attack. You find that the pulse is strong, regular and tachy; however, the pulse decreases considerably during inspiration. This phenomenon is called pulsus:

   a. paradoxus.
   b. alternans.
   c. deficit.
   d. differential.

6. The normal heart sound S1 is caused by vibrations caused by the sudden closure of the _____ valves at the start of ventricular systole.

   a. pulmonic and aortic
   b. pulmonic and mitral
   c. mitral and tricuspid
   d. tricuspid and aortic

7. The abnormal heart sound S3, though sometimes present in healthy young persons, most commonly is associated with moderate to severe:

   a. asthma.
   b. pulmonary embolism.
   c. stroke.
   d. heart failure.

8. The abnormal heart sound that occurs when inflammation is present in the parietal and visceral pericardium is a(an):

   a. murmur.
   b. pericardial friction rub.
   c. S4.
   d. S3.

9. The layer of the heart that lines the chambers of the heart and is continuous with the intima is the:

   a. epicardium.
   b. myocardium.
   c. endocardium.
   d. visceral pericardium.

10. Following a severe steering wheel chest impact, the pericardial space rapidly accumulates fluids resulting in pericardial tamponade. In the average size adult, tamponade can occur with as little as _____ milliliters of fluid.

    a. 25
    b. 50
    c. 75
    d. 100

11. A potentially fatal bacterial infection commonly affecting heart valves is:

    a. epicarditis.
    b. myocarditis.
    c. endocarditis.
    d. scarlet fever.

12. The majority of coronary artery blood flow and myocardial perfusion occurs during which phase of the cardiac cycle?

    a. systole
    b. diastole
    c. asystole
    d. effusion

13. The relationship between increased stroke volume and increased ventricular end-diastolic volume for a given intrinsic contractility is called:

    a. Beck's triad.
    b. Iowa pressure articulation.
    c. autoregulation.
    d. Starling's law of the heart.

14. When a drug's specific action is a negative chronotropic effect, what effect will it have on the heart?

    a. increase heart rate
    b. decrease heart rate
    c. increase force of muscular contractility
    d. decrease force of muscular contractility

15. When a drug has a positive inotropic effect, the drug will affect the heart in which of the following ways?

    a. increase heart rate
    b. decrease heart rate
    c. increase force of muscular contractility
    d. decrease force of muscular contractility

16. Patients who experience _____ pain, most often will be able to localize the pain to a specific area.

    a. somatic
    b. idiopathic
    c. visceral
    d. neurotic

17. A 25-year-old female is complaining of abdominal pain that she describes as intermittent and cramping. What type of pain is the patient most likely experiencing?

    a. somatic
    b. idiopathic
    c. visceral
    d. neurotic

18. Some diabetic patients experience an altered pain perception from a chronic nerve condition called:

    a. dyspepsia.
    b. neuropathy.
    c. parathesia.
    d. ghost pain.

19. People with the preexisting medical condition _____ are more likely to experience a "silent AMI" than those without it.

    a. hypertension
    b. diabetes
    c. Parkinson's
    d. esophageal reflux

20. When there is inadequate blood flow to an organ, such as the heart, _____ occurs initially.

    a. ischemia
    b. infarction
    c. stroke
    d. embolus

21. Restoring blood flow to an organ with inadequate blood flow may be successful if treatment is begun early. All the following are methods of reperfusion therapy, *except*:

    a. chemical thrombolysis.
    b. balloon angioplasty.
    c. coronary artery bypass.
    d. cardiohydrolysis.

22. Pain that is felt at a site that is different from that of the injured or diseased part of the body is called:

    a. referred pain.
    b. irritation.
    c. inflammation.
    d. musculoskeletal.

23. The three primary components used for diagnosis of an acute MI include: cardiac enzyme analysis, abnormal ECG and/or ECG changes, and:

    a. vital signs.
    b. daily use of aspirin.
    c. history.
    d. prehospital treatment.

24. An atypical form of chest pain caused by vasospasm of otherwise normal coronary arteries is called _____ angina.

   a. stable
   b. unstable
   c. Wicket's
   d. Prinzmetal's

25. The most frequent cause of acute MI is:

   a. coronary thrombosis.
   b. hypertension.
   c. trauma.
   d. use of recreational drugs.

26. All the following are classical symptoms associated with ischemic chest pain, *except*:

   a. weakness.
   b. dyspnea.
   c. diaphoresis.
   d. syncope.

27. The ECG wave form that represents the impulse generated as the ventricles depolarize prior to contraction is the:

   a. PR interval.
   b. QRS complex.
   c. J point.
   d. QT interval.

28. Which of the following patients is not a likely candidate for immediate ECG analysis?

   a. 40-year-old female who experienced a near syncopal event.
   b. 2-year-old male having an asthma attack.
   c. 25-year-old male, that received a strong electric shock.
   d. 64-year-old female with severe dehydration and shortness of breath.

29. ST elevation is usually a sign of severe myocardial injury. However, other common causes of ST elevation that may be confused with AMI are:

   a. myocarditis and gout.
   b. syncope and pluerisy.
   c. acute pericarditis and Prinzmetal's angina.
   d. CHF and pulmonary effusion.

30. Patients with right ventricular infarcts often have problems with hypotension and decreased cardiac output, and are very sensitive to drugs that reduce preload such as:

   a. nitroglycerine.
   b. aspirin.
   c. dopamine.
   d. morphine.

31. Twelve lead ECG analyses can help to identify the size and location of the infarct that occurs during an AMI, thus helping to guide treatment. A patient experiencing an inferior wall MI of the left ventricle may have abnormalities in which leads?

   a. V_1 and V_2
   b. V_3 and V_4
   c. II, III and aVF
   d. I, aVL, V_5 and V_6

32. A patient experiencing an acute anterior wall AMI of the left ventricle may have abnormalities in which leads?

   a. V_1 and V_2
   b. V_3 and V_4
   c. II, III and aVF
   d. I, aVL, V_5 and V_6

33. A patient experiencing a septal wall AMI may have abnormalities in which leads?

   a. V_1 and V_2
   b. V_3 and V_4
   c. II, III and aVF
   d. I, aVL, V_5 and V_6

34. The use of drugs, electrolyte imbalances, electrical shock, and trauma are all mechanisms that can produce which of the following conditions?

   a. hypoglycemia
   b. cardiac dysrhythmias
   c. hypertension
   d. Wolff-Parkinson-White syndrome

35. You are interviewing a 74-year-old woman who had a syncopal event while at the market with her daughter. Both the patient and daughter confirm that the patient has a history of periodic loss of consciousness caused by a heart block. They cannot remember what this condition is called, but you suspect which of the following conditions?

   a. unstable syncope
   b. unstable angina
   c. Wolff-Parkinson-White syndrome
   d. Adams-Stokes syndrome

36. Synchronized cardioversion is a timed shock delivered to the heart to convert abnormal rhythms to a normal rhythm. Synchronization is preferred over defibrillation in patients with a pulse because synchronization reduces the energy required to convert and:

    a. reduces the chance of post-shock dysrhythmias.
    b. increases the period of an extra-conduction pathway.
    c. reduces the possibility of pre-excitation syndrome.
    d. increases the stimulation of the relative refractory phase.

37. When injury to the myocardium affects the automaticity and the heart is no longer able to produce the normal pace or rhythm, the treatment of choice in the prehospital setting is:

    a. atropine.
    b. isoproterenol.
    c. external pacing.
    d. defibrillation.

38. Kussmaul's sign may be present during a right ventricular infarction, pericarditis or massive pulmonary embolism and is characterized by:

    a. ascites and shortness of breath.
    b. paradoxical filling of the neck veins during inspiration.
    c. sacral edema and shortness of breath.
    d. pulmonary edema and JVD.

39. You are performing a focused history and physical examination for possible AMI on a 55-year-old patient complaining of substernal chest pain and exertional dyspnea. Which of the following pieces of information from the patient's past medical history will rule out this patient as a candidate for reperfusion therapy?

    a. stable angina
    b. kidney disease
    c. mild hypertension
    d. appendectomy 18 months ago

40. Cardiac muscle tissue has the ability to contract without neural stimulation. This property is called:

    a. self-excitation.
    b. automaticity.
    c. syncytium.
    d. depolarization.

41. Cardiac muscle tissue has the ability to conduct impulses much quicker than regular muscle cells, a property called:

    a. self-excitation.
    b. automaticity.
    c. syncytium.
    d. repolarization.

42. Many patients that take diuretics such as lasix also take potassium to prevent _____ which is an excessive loss of potassium that occurs with diuresis.

    a. hypokalemia
    b. hyperkalemia
    c. hyponatremia
    d. hypercalcemia

43. When cardiac muscle tissue gets an altered amount of potassium, the effect on the heart is a(an):

    a. increased force of contraction.
    b. decreased force of contraction.
    c. slow heart rate.
    d. fast heart rate.

44. Cardiac muscle tissue uses three primary cations to effect depolarization and repolarization of the heart. These three include potassium, sodium and:

    a. phosphate.
    b. gluconate.
    c. caitrate.
    d. calcium.

45. While working as part of a medic team standing by at a marathon, you are treating a runner who is exhausted. The patient's vital signs are R/R 16, B/P 102/50 and H/R 42. After obtaining a focused history from the patient which of the following is the most likely cause of the slow heart rate?

    a. Use of supplemental salt tablets.
    b. Dehydration from over exertion.
    c. Heat stroke.
    d. Hypoglycemia.

46. The pacemaker cells in the _____ of the heart normally initiate the electrical impulses that start the sequence of excitation and conduction through the heart.

    a. SA node
    b. AV node
    c. Bundle branches
    d. Purkinje fibers

47. Backup cardiac pacemaker cells are often called _____, meaning that if the normal pacemaker fails, the next one automatically below it will take over stimulation of the entire sequence.

    a. action potential
    b. PVCs
    c. escape foci
    d. discharges

48. Acetylcholine, a neurotransmitter released by parasympathetic motor neurons, has which of the following effects on the heart?

    a. regulates normal contractions
    b. lowers stroke volume
    c. increases heart rate
    d. enhances automaticity

49. The catacholamine _____, released by the adrenal medulla and sympathetic neurons during sympathetic stimulation, increases stroke volume.

    a. dopamine
    b. norepinephrine
    c. epinephrine
    d. adenosine

50. Sympathetic nerves are located throughout the heart. The parasympathetic nerves are located primarily in the:

    a. bundle of His.
    b. Purkinje fibers.
    c. bundle branches.
    d. SA and AV nodes.

51. An irregular connection between the atria and the ventricles that bypasses the AV node is called a/an:

    a. reentry.
    b. aberration.
    c. accessory pathway.
    d. PVC.

52. When conduction of electrical impulses in the heart experience an alteration of the repolarization wave from its normal direction, which is blocked, to another direction which is not blocked, this is known as:

    a. reentry.
    b. an aberration.
    c. accessory pathway.
    d. a PVC.

53. A pathologic state in which an action potential does not result in systole is:

    a. ECG.
    b. EMD.
    c. PAC.
    d. PSVT.

54. Hypertension is a devastating disease that places an increased work load on the heart. Specifically the extra work load causes the left ventricle to:

    a. dystrophy.
    b. myotrophy.
    c. atrophy.
    d. hypertrophy.

55. The primary types of damage that occur with chronic hypertension are aneurysm, stroke and:

    a. nausea.
    b. deep vein thrombosis.
    c. headache.
    d. renal failure.

56. The treatment plan for hypertensive crisis is to reduce the patient's blood pressure within one or two hours to avoid:

    a. an acute MI.
    b. permanent organ damage.
    c. sudden death.
    d. atherosclerosis.

57. A normal defense mechanism designed to maintain cerebral perfusion after an insult such as a stroke or head injury is called:

    a. cerebral autoregulation.
    b. Beck's triad.
    c. hypotension.
    d. hyptertension.

58. A normal property of the brain that maintains cerebral perfusion within a fairly wide range of mean arterial blood pressures is known as:

    a. cerebral autoregulation.
    b. Beck's triad.
    c. Frank-Starling law.
    d. homeostasis.

59. An inflammation of a vein causing pain in the affected part of the body that is accompanied by stiffness and edema is called:

   a. phlebitis.
   b. ascites.
   c. thrombosis.
   d. angio-edema.

60. A patient affected with Marfan's syndrome may experience sudden death at an early age, usually from which of the following mechanisms?

   a. congestive heart failure
   b. spontaneous papillary rupture
   c. spontaneous pnuemothorax
   d. spontaneous rupture of the aorta

61. You are called to transport a 65-year-old male for evaluation of severe pain in the left calf. The patient tells you the pain began suddenly while he was taking his daily walk, but now that he is sitting, the pain is subsiding. Which of the following conditions do you suspect?

   a. edema
   b. ascites
   c. claudication
   d. muscle cramp

62. In a cardiac contraction, the degree of stretch of the contraction muscle is called the:

   a. atrial pressure point.
   b. ventricular pressure point.
   c. preload.
   d. afterload.

63. The major problems that occur with heart failure are that cardiac output decreases and _____ develop(s).

   a. venous congestion
   b. vaso-spasms
   c. bradycardia
   d. autoregulation

64. In the early stages of heart failure the body senses the decrease in cardiac output and attempts to compensate through stimulation of the:

   a. vagus nerve.
   b. sympathetic nervous system.
   c. Renal buffer system.
   d. MOA system.

65. Left heart failure is more common than right heart failure because the left ventricle is more often affected by:

   a. smoking.
   b. diabetes.
   c. obesity.
   d. chronic hypertension.

66. Prehospital management of cardiogenic shock begins with treating the patient for:

   a. respiratory arrest.
   b. shock.
   c. sepsis infection.
   d. severe dehydration.

67. Chronic right heart failure may present with signs and symptoms of tachycardia, peripheral edema and:

   a. ascites.
   b. syncope.
   c. back pain.
   d. leg pain.

68. Possible definitive treatment choices for cardiogenic shock may include CABG or catheterization of the blocked coronary artery and:

   a. the use of fibrynolitics.
   b. administration of a lasix drip.
   c. non-invasive overdrive pacing.
   d. invasive dialysis.

69. A 57-year-old male who is experiencing an AMI and has no past medical history may present with all the following signs and symptoms, *except*:

   a. shortness of breath.
   b. tachycardia.
   c. sacral edema.
   d. pulmonary edema.

70. The goal in the treatment of CHF is to improve oxygenation and ventilation by:

   a. increasing afterload.
   b. decreasing preload.
   c. administering IV fluid therapy.
   d. stopping the possible infarction.

71. When a patient progresses to a state of severe pulmonary edema, more aggressive treatment such as _____ is required to manage the patient.

   a. external pacing
   b. fluid replacement
   c. ventilatory support
   d. obtaining a 12 lead ECG

72. The most severe form of heart failure, resulting in inadequate cardiac output caused by left ventricular malfunction, is called:

    a. cardiogenic shock.
    b. ischemic shock.
    c. sudden death.
    d. cardiomyopathy.

73. To help differentiate between CHF and APE the paramedic should look for:

    a. shortness of breath.
    b. wet lung sounds.
    c. ECG changes.
    d. past medical history of heart disease.

74. Which of the following is a life-threatening condition with a pathology of an accumulation of fluids into the pericardial sac?

    a. pericarditis
    b. cardiac tamponade
    c. pnuemopericardium
    d. myocarditis

75. You are assessing a 59-year-old female with a chief complaint of dyspnea. Your initial assessment findings reveal a R/R of 34 and labored, crackles in the bases of the lungs, SpO_2 of 90%, P/R of 112 and B/P of 140/100 and she is afebrile. PMHx includes HTN and COPD. Your first differential diagnosis is:

    a. CHF versus APE.
    b. pneumonia versus URI
    c. CHF versus pneumonia
    d. APE versus URI

76. The initial signs and symptoms of cardiogenic shock are the same as seen with:

    a. neurogenic shock.
    b. AMI.
    c. APE.
    d. CVA

77. Peripheral edema is more likely to be present with _____ because it takes several hours to develop.

    a. chronic CHF
    b. pneumonia
    c. acute myocardial infarction
    d. bronchitis

78. When treating a patient with CHF which of the following is paramount to improve oxygenation and ventilation?

    a. Positioning the patient supine.
    b. Positioning the patient upright.
    c. Starting an IV.
    d. Intubating the patient.

79. You have been called to manage a 72-year-old female that awoke suddenly from sleep with shortness of breath and diaphoresis. She tells you that she has a history of heart failure. You suspect that she is presenting with:

    a. anxiety.
    b. exacerbation of COPD.
    c. bronchitis.
    d. paroxysmal nocturnal dyspnea.

80. In right heart failure, blood is not pumped adequately from the _____ into the lungs.

    a. pulmonic circulation
    b. left ventricle
    c. right ventricle
    d. cerebral circulation

81. Right heart failure is more often _____ than _____, and is usually not an emergency unless it is accompanied by left heart failure and pulmonary edema.

    a. life-threatening: not
    b. acute: chronic
    c. chonic: acute
    d. *de novo:* with warning

82. When cardiac pumping is insufficient to meet the circulatory demand of the body, it is called:

    a. mitral valve prolapse.
    b. heart failure.
    c. AMI.
    d. systemic failure.

83. The load against which the heart exerts its contractile force is the:

    a. preload.
    b. afterload.
    c. frontload.
    d. overload.

84. Aneurysms often go unrecognized until the bulging of the sac grows so large that the pressure it exerts on other structures causes symptoms such as:

a. pain.
b. hypotension.
c. hypertension.
d. syncope.

85. If an abdominal aortic aneurysm goes unrecognized or untreated it may grow and burst, usually resulting in:

a. AMI.
b. CVA.
c. paralysis.
d. sudden death.

86. Prehospital management of AAA is limited to recognition of the condition, supportive care and:

a. rapid transport.
b. stabilization prior to transport.
c. definitive treatment.
d. localized treatment.

87. Clinical features associated with hypertensive crisis include:

a. headache, backache and dizziness.
b. headache, vision disturbance and confusion.
c. vision disturbance, nausea and shortness of breath.
d. chest pain, confusion and vomiting.

88. Hypertensive emergencies are related to other emergencies such as intracranial hemorrhage, pulmonary edema, AMI and aortic dissection. When hypertension is associated with these conditions treatment should be directed at the:

a. hypertension.
b. pulmonary edema.
c. AMI.
d. primary problem.

89. You are taking care of an elderly female who you have discovered has accidentally taken an overdose of her potassium medication. Knowing that potassium has important effects on cardiac function what clinical finding would you expect to be present in this patient?

a. bradycardia
b. tachycardia
c. PVCs
d. PACs

90. Unlike other muscle tissue, cardiac muscle tissue has the ability to contract without neural stimulation, a property called:

a. polarization.
b. automaticity.
c. conductivity.
d. enhanced feedback.

91. Aspirin is given to patients with acute chest pain to thin the blood in an effort to:

a. relieve chest pain.
b. restore perfusion.
c. increase myocardial workload.
d. differentiate angina from AMI.

92. _____ sign is a paradoxical filling of the neck veins during inspiration and suggests a right ventricular infarction, massive pulmonary embolism or pericarditis.

a. Beck's
b. Kussmaul's
c. Cushing's
d. Levine's

93. There are several types of pacemakers available for patients with irreversible heart damage. The type of pacemaker a patient receives depends on the:

a. size of the heart.
b. sex of the patient.
c. age of the patient.
d. location of the damage.

94. While interviewing a patient she tells you that she has an implanted pacemaker. During your physical examination of the patient where would you expect to see a scar for the site of the implantation?

a. left upper back
b. right lower abdomen
c. left chest area
d. right thigh

95. When heart muscle becomes hypoxic, the myocardium becomes irritable and may cause:

a. systemic ischemia.
b. blood loss.
c. AMI.
d. dysrhythmias.

96. The clinical manifestation of low arterial pressure, high venous pressure and quiet heart sounds is referred to as:

    a. Beck's triad.
    b. Cushing's triad.
    c. Trousseau's sign.
    d. Cushing's sign.

97. The definitive treatment of cardiac tamponade is to:

    a. place a chest tube.
    b. relieve cardiac compression.
    c. decompress the chest.
    d. administer IV antibiotic therapy.

98. All the following are terms for irregular conduction of electrical pathways in the heart, *except*:

    a. reentry.
    b. aberration.
    c. intrinsic.
    d. accessory.

99. An irregular connection between the atria and ventricles that bypasses the AV node is called a/an _____ pathway.

    a. reentry
    b. aberration
    c. intrinsic
    d. accessory

Test #23 Answer Form

	A	B	C	D			A	B	C	D
1.	❏	❏	❏	❏		27.	❏	❏	❏	❏
2.	❏	❏	❏	❏		28.	❏	❏	❏	❏
3.	❏	❏	❏	❏		29.	❏	❏	❏	❏
4.	❏	❏	❏	❏		30.	❏	❏	❏	❏
5.	❏	❏	❏	❏		31.	❏	❏	❏	❏
6.	❏	❏	❏	❏		32.	❏	❏	❏	❏
7.	❏	❏	❏	❏		33.	❏	❏	❏	❏
8.	❏	❏	❏	❏		34.	❏	❏	❏	❏
9.	❏	❏	❏	❏		35.	❏	❏	❏	❏
10.	❏	❏	❏	❏		36.	❏	❏	❏	❏
11.	❏	❏	❏	❏		37.	❏	❏	❏	❏
12.	❏	❏	❏	❏		38.	❏	❏	❏	❏
13.	❏	❏	❏	❏		39.	❏	❏	❏	❏
14.	❏	❏	❏	❏		40.	❏	❏	❏	❏
15.	❏	❏	❏	❏		41.	❏	❏	❏	❏
16.	❏	❏	❏	❏		42.	❏	❏	❏	❏
17.	❏	❏	❏	❏		43.	❏	❏	❏	❏
18.	❏	❏	❏	❏		44.	❏	❏	❏	❏
19.	❏	❏	❏	❏		45.	❏	❏	❏	❏
20.	❏	❏	❏	❏		46.	❏	❏	❏	❏
21.	❏	❏	❏	❏		47.	❏	❏	❏	❏
22.	❏	❏	❏	❏		48.	❏	❏	❏	❏
23.	❏	❏	❏	❏		49.	❏	❏	❏	❏
24.	❏	❏	❏	❏		50.	❏	❏	❏	❏
25.	❏	❏	❏	❏		51.	❏	❏	❏	❏
26.	❏	❏	❏	❏		52.	❏	❏	❏	❏

	A	B	C	D			A	B	C	D
53.	❏	❏	❏	❏		77.	❏	❏	❏	❏
54.	❏	❏	❏	❏		78.	❏	❏	❏	❏
55.	❏	❏	❏	❏		79.	❏	❏	❏	❏
56.	❏	❏	❏	❏		80.	❏	❏	❏	❏
57.	❏	❏	❏	❏		81.	❏	❏	❏	❏
58.	❏	❏	❏	❏		82.	❏	❏	❏	❏
59.	❏	❏	❏	❏		83.	❏	❏	❏	❏
60.	❏	❏	❏	❏		84.	❏	❏	❏	❏
61.	❏	❏	❏	❏		85.	❏	❏	❏	❏
62.	❏	❏	❏	❏		86.	❏	❏	❏	❏
63.	❏	❏	❏	❏		87.	❏	❏	❏	❏
64.	❏	❏	❏	❏		88.	❏	❏	❏	❏
65.	❏	❏	❏	❏		89.	❏	❏	❏	❏
66.	❏	❏	❏	❏		90.	❏	❏	❏	❏
67.	❏	❏	❏	❏		91.	❏	❏	❏	❏
68.	❏	❏	❏	❏		92.	❏	❏	❏	❏
69.	❏	❏	❏	❏		93.	❏	❏	❏	❏
70.	❏	❏	❏	❏		94.	❏	❏	❏	❏
71.	❏	❏	❏	❏		95.	❏	❏	❏	❏
72.	❏	❏	❏	❏		96.	❏	❏	❏	❏
73.	❏	❏	❏	❏		97.	❏	❏	❏	❏
74.	❏	❏	❏	❏		98.	❏	❏	❏	❏
75.	❏	❏	❏	❏		99.	❏	❏	❏	❏
76.	❏	❏	❏	❏						

24
Neurology

1. A function of the nervous system is to:

   a. monitor internal changes of the body.
   b. circulate nutrients to all body cells.
   c. regulate the neurons.
   d. provide support for the body structures.

2. The largest part of the brain is divided into right and left hemisperes and is called the:

   a. cerebellum.
   b. cerebrum.
   c. diencephalon.
   d. brainstem.

3. The _____ is the location in the brain of higher cognitive functions such as learning and language.

   a. corpus callosum
   b. telencephalon
   c. diencephalon
   d. thalamus

4. Blood enters the brain from the two internal carotid arteries and the:

   a. jugular artery.
   b. iliac artery.
   c. basilar artery.
   d. subclavian artery.

5. The structure which forms a circle around the stalk of the pituitary gland and works as a backup mechanism for complications with cerebral blood flow is called:

   a. foramen magnum.
   b. arch of atlas.
   c. circle of Willis.
   d. cerebral spinal canal.

6. The brainstem contains all the following structures, *except*:

   a. lowbrain.
   b. pons.
   c. medulla.
   d. oblongata.

7. The _____ regulates the biologic clock of the body.

   a. pineal body
   b. medulla
   c. thalamus
   d. optic chiasma

8. The section of the brain responsible for maintaining posture, balance and voluntary coordination of skilled movements is the:

   a. midbrain.
   b. diencephalon.
   c. cerebellum.
   d. brainstem.

9. Cerebrospinal fluid (CSF) is present in the spinal cord, cavities and canals of the brain, as well as the:

   a. temporal gap.
   b. parietal shelf.
   c. epidural space.
   d. subarachnoid space.

10. Which of the following is not a function of CSF?

    a. protection of the brain and spinal cord
    b. supports the brain and spinal cord with nutrients
    c. monitors CO_2 levels in the CSF
    d. oxygenation of tissues

11. _____ is an increase in the amount of CSF, from either a blockage or decrease in normal reabsorption.

    a. Cerebrosis
    b. Hydrocephalus
    c. Cerebroma
    d. Cephalophoma

12. Which of the meninges is the highly vascular covering of the brain and spinal cord?

    a. Dura mater
    b. Pia mater
    c. Arachnoid membrane
    d. Falx cerebelli

13. Meningitis is a potentially life-threatening infection of both the _____ and meninges.

    a. spinal cord
    b. white matter
    c. CSF
    d. gray matter

14. The major difference between gray matter and white matter is that gray matter is:

    a. not covered with myelinated fibers.
    b. covered with myelinated fibers.
    c. ashened colored because of anaerobic metabolism.
    d. there really is no major difference.

15. The fundamental component of the nervous system is the:

    a. myelin.
    b. neuron.
    c. spinal cord.
    d. nerve impulse.

16. All the following are components of the nerve cell body, *except* the:

    a. soma.
    b. dendrite.
    c. axon.
    d. myelin.

17. Nervous tissue requires a tremendous amount of metabolic energy. For this to occur it is essential that there be a constant supply of oxygen and:

    a. potassium.
    b. sodium.
    c. glucose.
    d. carbon dioxide.

18. A disease process that destroys the myelin sheath and infects the nerve fibers, impairing nerve function is called:

    a. multiple sclerosis.
    b. Parkinson's disease.
    c. epilepsy.
    d. Lou Gehrig's disease.

19. Nerve cells communicate with each other primarily through the:

    a. peripheral system.
    b. flowing of acetylcholine
    c. the limbic system.
    d. synapses.

20. High in the brainstem is the _____, which is responsible for maintaining consciousness.

    a. reticular activating system
    b. limbic system
    c. ANS
    d. CNS

21. The twelve pair of cranial nerves are a component of which part of the nervous system?

    a. autonomic
    b. peripheral
    c. structural
    d. functional

22. _____ is a disorder of the CNS, named after the famous baseball player Lou Gehrig. It has a rapidly progressive deterioration leading to atrophy of all body muscles and death.

    a. Bell's palsy
    b. ALS
    c. Cerebral palsy
    d. Parkinson's disease

23. A term for a chronic, progressive disease of the CNS characterized by exacerbation and remission of assorted multiple neurologic symptoms is:

    a. Epilepsy.
    b. Bell's palsy.
    c. Multiple sclerosis.
    d. Parkinson's disease.

24. All the following are infectious diseases of the nervous system, *except*:

    a. hydrocephalus.
    b. encephalitis.
    c. tetanus.
    d. poliomyelitis.

25. You are assessing a 28-year-old male complaining of a severe headache. Just before losing consciousness in front of you he tells you that it came on very suddenly after he experienced a loud sound like a bang in his head. Which of the following conditions do you suspect was the cause of this event?

    a. CVA
    b. TIA
    c. Ruptured aneurysm
    d. Meningitis

26. All the following are common causes of dementia, *except*:

    a. Alzheimer's disease.
    b. tumor.
    c. head trauma
    d. amnesia

27. Ischemia, ICP, cerebral edema and brain herniation are all _____ injuries from traumatic brain injury.

    a. primary
    b. secondary
    c. tertiary
    d. irreversible

28. A mild closed head injury that results in a transient loss of brain function with or without a loss of consciousness is called:

    a. amnesia.
    b. contusion.
    c. concussion.
    d. contra-coup.

29. All the following are significant factors in reduction in morbidity and mortality of brain injury patients, *except*:

    a. hyperventilation.
    b. maintenance of ABCs.
    c. rapid transport to a trauma center.
    d. CT scanning.

30. Which of the following is not a common emergent neurologic condition?

    a. TIA
    b. CVA
    c. Syncope
    d. Parkinson's

31. The major difference between a stroke and a TIA is that:

    a. a TIA always precedes a stroke.
    b. a stroke always precedes a TIA.
    c. the TIA has no lasting effect.
    d. the stroke is considered a warning sign.

32. An undiagnosed TIA is a very high risk factor for:

    a. hypertension.
    b. a major stroke.
    c. new onset diabetes.
    d. heart disasese

33. A sudden temporary change in behavior, sensory, or motor activity caused by an excessive or chaotic electrical discharge of one or more groups of neurons in the brain is known as a:

    a. TIA.
    b. CVA
    c. seizure.
    d. palsy.

34. Which of the following is not a phase of a seizure?

    a. preictal
    b. atonic
    c. ictal
    d. postictal

35. A seizure characterized by impairment of consciousness, including an aura is a _____ seizure.

    a. simple partial
    b. complex partial
    c. absence
    d. complete motor

36. Prolonged or repeated seizures are true emergencies because:

    a. brain damage can occur.
    b. the patient can swallow the tongue.
    c. the patient forgets to breathe.
    d. the acid in the blood decreases.

37. Non-cardiac syncope often occurs in patients with no underlying disease, usually from a stressor such as pain, emotion or:

    a. heat.
    b. cold.
    c. medication.
    d. strobe lights.

38. How is a patient's mental status best assessed?

    a. by speaking with the patient
    b. by assessing the cranial nerves
    c. by checking for symmetry of motor response
    d. by checking for deficits in coordination and reflexes

39. What is the most significant aspect of a neurologic assessment?

    a. performing serial assessment
    b. a positive Babinski sign
    c. absence of seizure activity
    d. medication compliance

40. First developed in 1974, the _____ is an objective measure of the patient's level of consciousness.

    a. GCS
    b. AVPU
    c. Babinski sign
    d. CT scan

41. A respiratory pattern in which an extended inspiratory effort or gasping with a brief expiration, caused by pressure, damage or surgical removal of the pons in the area of CN IV is called:

    a. ataxic.
    b. Biot's respiration.
    c. cluster breathing.
    d. apneusis.

42. While assessing an unconscious, head-injured victim of a MVC, you observe the patient's respiratory effort as a pattern of cycles of apnea and hyperventilation. You recognize this pattern as:

    a. autisms.
    b. Kussmaul's breathing.
    c. Cheyne-Stokes respirations.
    d. apneusis.

43. Involuntary neurologic activities such as yawning, hic-cupping, coughing and vomiting are called:

    a. ataxics.
    b. autisms.
    c. clusters.
    d. central neurologic initiations.

44. _____ breathing often precedes agonal breathing and apnea and has no pattern or rhythm with depth or rate.

    a. Biot's
    b. Kussmaul's
    c. Ataxic
    d. Cluster

45. The term for normal visual function of the eyes which depends on the ability of both eyes to fix on the same subject is:

    a. diplopia.
    b. binocular vision.
    c. medial gaze.
    d. vergence reflex.

46. The term _____ refers to the adjustment of the eyes to variations in distance.

    a. accommodation
    b. acuity
    c. conjugate gaze
    d. divergence

47. An involuntary movement of the eyes that can be in any direction, but more often is either verticle or horizontal, is:

    a. doll's eyes.
    b. dysconjugate gaze.
    c. nystagmus.
    d. diplopia.

48. An abnormal constriction of the pupils, caused by certain types of infection and some types of drug overdose is called:

    a. anisocoria.
    b. glaucoma.
    c. dystonia.
    d. miosis.

49. Nearly ten percent of the population has a congenital inequality of their pupil sizes. The term for this condition is:

    a. anisocoria.
    b. glaucoma.
    c. akinesia.
    d. miosis

50. A brief involuntary movement of distal extremities and facial muscles, which often occurs in Huntington's disease, Parkinson's disease and thyrotoxosis, is:

    a. chorea.
    b. ballism.
    c. myclonus.
    d. tics.

51. The condition of slow and irregular involuntary winding movements of the extremities, as seen in cerebral palsy, encephalitis and some drug side effects, is:

    a. akinesia.
    b. athetosis.
    c. dystonia.
    d. dyskinesia.

52. A disorder with characteristics of lack of muscle coordination, involuntary muscle movement, tics, incoherent grunts, barks and cursing is called:

    a. tremors.
    b. Creutzfeldt-Jakobs disease.
    c. Tourette syndrome.
    d. Wernicke syndrome.

53. Assessing extraocular movements (EOMs) is the best single method for measuring brainstem integrity. Which of the following is a test for checking EOMs?

   a. assess for palmar drift
   b. assess the patient's gait
   c. assess the six cardinal positions of gaze
   d. assess discriminative touch, dull versus sharp

54. While assessing a patient presenting with new stroke symptoms such as: dysphasia, difficulty swallowing and chewing, which cranial nerve do you suspect is being affected?

   a. X
   b. VIII
   c. VI
   d. V

55. _____ is an abnormal gait characterized by unsteady, uncoordinated, wide at the base step, as seen with drunkenness, heavily medicated persons or certain medical conditions.

   a. Steppage
   b. Ataxia
   c. Festination
   d. Spastic hemiparesis

56. The loss of sensory and motor function below certain levels of the spine defines a/an:

   a. spinal cord injury.
   b. frontal lobe lesion.
   c. injury to Broca's area.
   d. precursor to ICP.

57. Patients experiencing cerebral vascular accidents including stroke, intracerebral or subarachnoid hemorrhage can present with typical signs of _____, which can make diagnosis of the underlying problem difficult.

   a. hypothermia
   b. heat stroke
   c. hyperglycemia
   d. memory loss

58. The most common signs of brain dysfunction are AMS and:

   a. hyperglycemia.
   b. loss of motor control.
   c. speech deficits.
   d. behavioral changes.

59. You have been called to care for an unconscious patient with a known brain tumor. The patient presents with the jaws clenched, arms and legs extended. You suspect the lesion is located in the diencephalon, midbrain or:

   a. pons.
   b. medulla.
   c. thalamus.
   d. insula.

60. _____ posturing, also referred to as flexion, is associated with a lesion at or above the upper brainstem.

   a. Broca's
   b. Wernicke's
   c. Decorticate
   d. Decerebrate

61. Cushing's triad is a(an) _____ sign of rising ICP.

   a. early
   b. late
   c. unreliable
   d. not

62. Babinski's reflex is a test to assess for spinal cord dysfunction, specifically in the _____ portion of the motor control system.

   a. pyramidal
   b. extrapyramidal
   c. ipsilateral
   d. lateral

63. Both sides of the brain communicate via _____ to carry out many complex functions.

   a. the corpus callosum
   b. Broca's area
   c. Wernicke's area
   d. the island of Reil

64. The _____ lobe of the brain receives and translates somatic sensations of pain, touch, pressure, heat and cold, and body position.

   a. frontal
   b. parietal
   c. occipital
   d. temporal

65. The _____ links the nervous and endocrine systems, as well as the mind (psyche) and body.

   a. thalamus
   b. insula
   c. pineal body
   d. hypothalamus

66. CSF is produced in the _____ and is completely re-placed several times each day.

   a. spine
   b. epidural space
   c. ventricles of the brain
   d. arachnoid space

67. The dura mater has three significant inner extentions, the falx cerebelli, falx cerebri and the:

   a. stalk.
   b. soma.
   c. cortex.
   d. tentorium.

68. What type of bleeding occurs in a subdural hematoma?

   a. venous
   b. arterial
   c. systemic
   d. metabolic

69. Of the three types of structural neurons, only the _____ are located only in the brain and spinal cord.

   a. intraneurons
   b. afferent
   c. efferent
   d. interneurons

70. _____ are extensions of the nerve cell body with branches that conduct impulses to the cell body, relaying information to the neuron.

   a. Axons
   b. Dendrites
   c. DNA
   d. RNA

71. The layer or coating around the axon that protects the axon process and increases the conduction of nerve impulses is the:

   a. myelin.
   b. stratum.
   c. swathe.
   d. jacket.

72. A collection of the blood caused by a ruptured blood vessel that is enclosed in an organ, tissue or body space is a/an:

   a. aneurysm.
   b. abscess.
   c. stroke.
   d. hematoma.

73. The most common developmental defect of the CNS occurring while in utero is:

   a. hydrocephalus.
   b. shingles.
   c. spina bifida.
   d. polio.

74. _____ is a viral infection causing inflammation of the gray matter of the spinal cord that may temporarily or permanently affect neurologic functions.

   a. Poliomyelitis
   b. Abscess
   c. Spina bifida
   d. Meningitis

75. Which of the following conditions may be seen with a head CT scan?

   a. concussion
   b. contusion
   c. amnesia
   d. aphasia

76. _____ is the type of amnesia that affects the ability to recall memories from the past.

   a. Aphasic
   b. Non-phasic
   c. Anterograde
   d. Retrograde

77. All the following are causes of neurologic emergencies, *except*:

   a. metabolic derangements.
   b. cerebrovascular disease.
   c. AMI.
   d. neoplasms.

78. _____ stroke is the most common and is caused by a clot that blocks an artery.

   a. Ischemic
   b. Nocturnal
   c. Hemorrhagic
   d. Embolic

79. You are using a thrombolytic checklist on a patient presenting with stroke symptoms. Which of the following is an exclusion critierion for the use of fibryolitics?

   a. alert mental status
   b. able to give consent
   c. uncontrolled hypertension
   d. onset of symptoms <three hours

80. Which of the following medications is made from a plant called belladonna, a drug which causes the pupils to dilate?

    a. Atropine
    b. Bretylium
    c. Dopamine
    d. Atrovent

81. The _____ test is used in comatose patients to assess for brainstem or oculomotor injury, after neck injury has been ruled out.

    a. accomodation
    b. dolls-head maneuver
    c. drop-foot
    d. pronator drift

82. The difference of _____ millimeter(s) or more in the size of the pupils is abnormal.

    a. one
    b. two
    c. three
    d. four

83. _____ is the loss of ability to speak because of a defect in or loss of language function.

    a. Ataxia
    b. Aphasia
    c. Dysarthria
    d. Dysphonia

84. All the following are terms used to describe a patient's muscle tone, *except*:

    a. normal.
    b. rigid.
    c. spastic.
    d. neural.

85. When describing the patient's mental status, avoid terms such as stupor, lethargic and obtunded because they:

    a. all mean the same thing.
    b. mean different things to different people.
    c. are difficult to spell.
    d. are not real medical terms.

86. To assess the unconscious patient for neurologic deficits, which of the following would not be reliable?

    a. an irregular breathing pattern
    b. withdrawing from painful stimulus
    c. Babinski's reflex
    d. vision disturbances

87. Loss of lateral eye movement is an early sign of:

    a. vision loss.
    b. rising ICP.
    c. decreasing ICP.
    d. an orbital fracture.

88. You are assessing the driver of an automobile that was rear-ended at a moderate speed. The patient is complaining of severe pain in the left leg immediately after the collision, but there is no apparent trauma to the leg. Which of the following do you suspect?

    a. herniated disc
    b. spinal fracture
    c. muscle cramp
    d. faking

89. A functional disorder of the CNS, characterized by unilateral faical paralysis caused by compression of cranial nerve VII (facial nerve), is called:

    a. a brain abscess.
    b. a neoplasm.
    c. Bell's palsy.
    d. ALS.

90. What part of day do thrombotic strokes typically occur?

    a. late morning
    b. early afternoon
    c. early evening
    d. during sleep

91. The most common causes of seizures in infants includes all the following, *except*:

    a. epilepsy.
    b. trauma from childbirth.
    c. electrolyte abnormalities.
    d. infection.

92. The phase of a seizure characterized by a loss of consciousness with muscle contraction is called:

    a. preictal.
    b. aura.
    c. tonic.
    d. clonic.

93. A _____ event is a transient loss of consciousness caused by a decreased blood supply to the brain.

   a. TIA
   b. CVA
   c. syncopal
   d. seizure

94. The term _____ means new growth and is used synonymously with tumor.

   a. abscess
   b. migraine
   c. neoplasm
   d. foci

95. All the following conditions are examples of neurologic disorders, *except*:

   a. Parkinson's disease.
   b. Alzheimer's disease.
   c. shingles.
   d. hypertension.

96. Tic douloureux is pain in one or more of the three branches of the _____ cranial nerve that runs along the face.

   a. III
   b. V
   c. VIII
   d. XII

97. Glaucoma can occur as a congenital defect, a result of another eye disorder, and is associated with:

   a. heredity.
   b. trauma.
   c. hyperthyroidism.
   d. female gender.

98. When a patient's Babinski sign is affected, what type of disorder would the patient most likely have?

   a. ballism
   b. pyramidal
   c. extrapyramidal
   d. myoclonus

99. Which part of the neurologic examination is the least exact and informative except in the case of spinal cord injury?

   a. mental status
   b. reflexes
   c. motor function
   d. sensory function

100. The primary motor cortex located in the _____ is connected with the association motor cortex in the basal ganglia and cerebellum.

   a. frontal lobe
   b. occipital lobe
   c. midbrain
   d. parietal lobe

Test #24 Answer Form

	A	B	C	D			A	B	C	D
1.	❏	❏	❏	❏		27.	❏	❏	❏	❏
2.	❏	❏	❏	❏		28.	❏	❏	❏	❏
3.	❏	❏	❏	❏		29.	❏	❏	❏	❏
4.	❏	❏	❏	❏		30.	❏	❏	❏	❏
5.	❏	❏	❏	❏		31.	❏	❏	❏	❏
6.	❏	❏	❏	❏		32.	❏	❏	❏	❏
7.	❏	❏	❏	❏		33.	❏	❏	❏	❏
8.	❏	❏	❏	❏		34.	❏	❏	❏	❏
9.	❏	❏	❏	❏		35.	❏	❏	❏	❏
10.	❏	❏	❏	❏		36.	❏	❏	❏	❏
11.	❏	❏	❏	❏		37.	❏	❏	❏	❏
12.	❏	❏	❏	❏		38.	❏	❏	❏	❏
13.	❏	❏	❏	❏		39.	❏	❏	❏	❏
14.	❏	❏	❏	❏		40.	❏	❏	❏	❏
15.	❏	❏	❏	❏		41.	❏	❏	❏	❏
16.	❏	❏	❏	❏		42.	❏	❏	❏	❏
17.	❏	❏	❏	❏		43.	❏	❏	❏	❏
18.	❏	❏	❏	❏		44.	❏	❏	❏	❏
19.	❏	❏	❏	❏		45.	❏	❏	❏	❏
20.	❏	❏	❏	❏		46.	❏	❏	❏	❏
21.	❏	❏	❏	❏		47.	❏	❏	❏	❏
22.	❏	❏	❏	❏		48.	❏	❏	❏	❏
23.	❏	❏	❏	❏		49.	❏	❏	❏	❏
24.	❏	❏	❏	❏		50.	❏	❏	❏	❏
25.	❏	❏	❏	❏		51.	❏	❏	❏	❏
26.	❏	❏	❏	❏		52.	❏	❏	❏	❏

	A	B	C	D		A	B	C	D
53.	❑	❑	❑	❑	77.	❑	❑	❑	❑
54.	❑	❑	❑	❑	78.	❑	❑	❑	❑
55.	❑	❑	❑	❑	79.	❑	❑	❑	❑
56.	❑	❑	❑	❑	80.	❑	❑	❑	❑
57.	❑	❑	❑	❑	81.	❑	❑	❑	❑
58.	❑	❑	❑	❑	82.	❑	❑	❑	❑
59.	❑	❑	❑	❑	83.	❑	❑	❑	❑
60.	❑	❑	❑	❑	84.	❑	❑	❑	❑
61.	❑	❑	❑	❑	85.	❑	❑	❑	❑
62.	❑	❑	❑	❑	86.	❑	❑	❑	❑
63.	❑	❑	❑	❑	87.	❑	❑	❑	❑
64.	❑	❑	❑	❑	88.	❑	❑	❑	❑
65.	❑	❑	❑	❑	89.	❑	❑	❑	❑
66.	❑	❑	❑	❑	90.	❑	❑	❑	❑
67.	❑	❑	❑	❑	91.	❑	❑	❑	❑
68.	❑	❑	❑	❑	92.	❑	❑	❑	❑
69.	❑	❑	❑	❑	93.	❑	❑	❑	❑
70.	❑	❑	❑	❑	94.	❑	❑	❑	❑
71.	❑	❑	❑	❑	95.	❑	❑	❑	❑
72.	❑	❑	❑	❑	96.	❑	❑	❑	❑
73.	❑	❑	❑	❑	97.	❑	❑	❑	❑
74.	❑	❑	❑	❑	98.	❑	❑	❑	❑
75.	❑	❑	❑	❑	99.	❑	❑	❑	❑
76.	❑	❑	❑	❑	100.	❑	❑	❑	❑

25

Endocrinology

1. The most common of the endocrine emergencies is _____, which occurs more frequently than all the rest combined.

   a. fluid imbalance
   b. altered mental status
   c. diabetic problems
   d. respiratory problems

2. Which of the following is not a risk factor predisposing to endocrine disease?

   a. Hyperlipidemia
   b. Heredity
   c. Hypothyroidism
   d. Hypopituitarism

3. Diabetes is the leading cause of all the following conditions, *except*:

   a. adult blindness.
   b. death.
   c. nontraumatic lower extremity amputations.
   d. end-stage kidney failure.

4. The endocrine system is an integrated _____ and co-ordination system enabling reproduction, growth and development, and regulation of energy.

   a. chemical
   b. fluid
   c. muscle
   d. nerve

5. The endocrine system, together with the _____ system, maintains internal homeostasis of the body and coordinates responses to environmental changes and stress.

   a. GI
   b. integumentary
   c. biofeedback
   d. nervous

6. _____ regulate many body functions, such as growth, reproduction, temperature, metabolism and blood pressure.

   a. Antigens
   b. Hormones
   c. Receptors
   d. Emotions

7. Endocrines are called "ductless glands" because they secret their chemical hormones directly into the:

   a. brain.
   b. heart.
   c. lungs.
   d. blood.

8. Which of the following is not a major gland of the endocrine system?

   a. Hypothalamus
   b. Pituitary
   c. Thyroid
   d. Pancreas

9. The _____ gland, sometimes known as the "master gland" is located at the base of the brain in the cranial cavity.

   a. parathyroid
   b. adrenal
   c. pituitary
   d. gonad

10. Which of the following endocrine glands is responsible for maintaining normal levels of calcium in the blood?

    a. Parathyroid
    b. Adrenal
    c. Pituitary
    d. Ovaries

11. The _____ is considered an organ of both the digestive and the endocrine systems.

    a. thyroid
    b. parathyroid
    c. pancreas
    d. testes

12. The _____ gland(s) is/are responsible for secretion of the hormones vital in maintaining the body's water and salt balance.

   a. pancreas
   b. insulin
   c. pituitary
   d. adrenal

13. Though the specific pathophysiology varies for each disease, endocrine emergencies typically arise from any of the following, *except*:

   a. excessive hormone production.
   b. excessive sympathetic stimulation.
   c. failure of normal hormone production.
   d. failure of feedback inhibition systems.

14. In the body's normal regulation of the blood sugar level, insulin is released from the pancreas together with:

   a. epinephrine and glucagon.
   b. glucagon.
   c. amino acids.
   d. fatty acids.

15. Insulin moves sugar molecules from the blood into the cell, where they are:

   a. stored.
   b. bathed.
   c. reconstituted.
   d. broken down.

16. _____ occurs as a result of a viral infection of the pancreas leading to the formation of antibodies to pancreatic beta-cells that produce insulin.

   a. Type I diabetes
   b. Type II diabetes
   c. Obesity
   d. Insulin receptor resistance

17. Diabetic patients do not always have the classic symptoms of myocardial ischemia such as crushing substernal chest pain because:

   a. glucose is the sole source of oxidative metabolism for the CNS.
   b. insulin numbs the pain.
   c. many diabetics have some form of neuropathy.
   d. elevated blood lipid levels alter sensation.

18. Hypoglycemia of more than 20–30 minutes duration results in the production of toxic compounds in the brain that cause:

   a. cardiac arrest.
   b. excessive levels of heat production.
   c. a decrease in the thyroid function.
   d. permanent neuronal damage.

19. Many patients with hyperglycemia are significantly _____, therefore _____ is/are part of the primary treatment.

   a. hyperthermic: cooling
   b. hypothermic: heat
   c. dehydrated: fluids
   d. altered in mental status: insulin

20. Diabetic patients lack the normal effects of insulin, therefore sugar and other substances such as _____ fail to enter the cells properly.

   a. amino acids
   b. glycogen
   c. proteins
   d. triglycerides

21. Diabetic ketoacidosis (DKA) is a metabolic condition consisting of hyperglycemia, dehydration and the accumulation of _____ in the body.

   a. ketones and ketoacids
   b. free fatty acids
   c. amino acids
   d. uric acid

22. The effects of osmotic diuresis in diabetic patients cause frequent urination. At times this can lead to dehydration. Depending on the severity of their condition, the patient may also be deficient in:

   a. ketones and ketoacids.
   b. neurons.
   c. calcium.
   d. total body potassium.

23. The most common reason a diabetic patient develops DKA is because of:

   a. excess glucagon.
   b. infection.
   c. too much insulin.
   d. too little insulin.

24. Which of the following statements about DKA is incorrect?

    a. Not all patients with hyperglycemia will have DKA.
    b. Distinguishing between hyperglycemia and DKA in the field is easy.
    c. Many patients with hypoglycemia are in coma, but not shock.
    d. Many patients with DKA are not in a coma.

25. During periods of insulin deficiency, _____ is/are broken down to provide energy.

    a. ketones
    b. glucagon
    c. stored fats
    d. epinephrine

26. Ketoacidosis develops when the level of ketones in the _____ is too _____.

    a. blood: high.
    b. pancreas: high.
    c. blood: low.
    d. pancreas: low.

27. The diabetic emergency that occurs from a relative insulin deficiency that leads to marked hyperglycemia, but with the absence of ketones and acidosis, is called:

    a. hypoosmolar hyperglycemic nonketotic coma.
    b. hyperosmolar hyperglycemic nonketotic coma.
    c. nonketotic mellitis.
    d. nonketotic osmolitis.

28. Many long-standing diabetic patients remain asymptomatic until their sugar level drops low enough to result in loss of consciousness. This occurs because:

    a. early warning signs from the counter-regulatory hormones fail.
    b. they have aquired dysfunction of the peripheral nervous system.
    c. they develop a tolerance to symptoms.
    d. early warning signs from the beta-cells are inactivated.

29. Which of the following substances can increase a person's sensitivity to hypoglycemia, which may result in a person feeling hypoglycemic symptoms at blood sugar levels not usually associated with causing problems?

    a. Poppy seeds
    b. Chocolate
    c. Peanuts
    d. Caffeine

30. The production of glucagons and epinephrine stimulate enzymes that break down glycogen to glucose. This process is called:

    a. homeostasis.
    b. Harada's syndrome.
    c. gluconeogenesis.
    d. glycogenolysis.

31. Hyperglycemia is a common finding in _____ caused by insulin resistance and increased glycogenolysis.

    a. massive head trauma
    b. Cushing's sydrome
    c. thyrotoxicosis
    d. myxedema coma

32. Signs and symptoms of thyrotoxicosis may include any of the following, *except*:

    a. fever and flushing.
    b. CHF.
    c. tachycardia or new onset a-fib.
    d. fruity breath odor.

33. Before the diagnosis of _____ is established, patients often have fatigue, lethargy, and gradual weight gain for years.

    a. hyperthyroidsim
    b. hypothyroidism
    c. myxedema coma
    d. Cushing's syndrome

34. The term myxedema generically refers to any and all symptoms of hypothyroidism and may typically include any of the following, *except*:

    a. cool dry skin and slowed reflexes.
    b. hypertension.
    c. coarse thin hair and brittle nails.
    d. hyperglycemia.

35. Persons with myxedema coma may typically present with any of the following conditions, *except*:

    a. dehydration and potassium imbalance.
    b. respiratory depression.
    c. hemodynamically significant bradydysrhythmias.
    d. hypothermia.

36. _____ is a metabolic syndrome resulting from hyper-secretion of the glucocorticoid hormone, cortisol, which affects carbohydrate, protein, and lipid metabolism.

    a. Cushing's syndrome
    b. Adrenal insufficiency
    c. Addison's disease
    d. Graves' disease

37. All the following are typical signs and symptoms of Cushing's syndrome, *except*:

    a. abnormal pattern of fat distribution.
    b. increased libido.
    c. adult-onset acne.
    d. excess growth of body hair.

38. Which of the following preexisting conditions would a patient's primary acute complaint not be directly related to?

    a. Cushing's syndrome
    b. Thyroid storm
    c. Adrenal insuffiency
    d. Hyperglycemia

39. Autoimmune destruction of the adrenal glands is the most common cause of adrenal insufficiency and is called:

    a. Cushing's syndrome.
    b. thyroid storm.
    c. Addison's disease.
    d. Graves' disease.

40. Adrenal insufficiency is inadequate production of adrenal hormones, primarily _____, for any of a number of reasons.

    a. adrenocortical
    b. cortisol and aldosterone
    c. follicle-stimulating hormone (FSH)
    d. parathyroid hormone (PTH)

41. The pathophysiology of adrenal insufficiency is that the normal feedback loop between the hypothalamus, pitiuitary gland and adrenal glands are suppressed because of:

    a. the use of oral or inhaled steroids.
    b. daily injections of insulin.
    c. the use of oral hypoglycemic agents.
    d. daily estrogen use.

42. Signs any symptoms of chronic adrenalin sufficiency may include any of the following, *except*:

    a. anorexia and weight loss.
    b. muscle and joint pain.
    c. salt craving and abdominal pain.
    d. decreased pigmentation.

43. Acute adrenal insufficiency, sometimes called an Addisonian crisis, presents as hypotension, hypoglycemia and severe:

    a. hypovolemia.
    b. hypercarbia.
    c. weight loss.
    d. muscle and joint pain.

44. Protrusion of the eyeballs (exophthalmus) is a common physical finding in patients with:

    a. hyperthyroidism.
    b. hypothyroidism.
    c. myxedema coma.
    d. Cushing's syndrome.

45. Which of the following is not an oral hypoglycemic agent?

    a. Glucotrol®
    b. Glyburide®
    c. Rezulin®
    d. Ogen®

46. The onset of action is faster and duration is shorter with _____ insulin preparations.

    a. beef
    b. pork
    c. human
    d. chicken

47. In addition to $D_{50}W$, thiamine is also considered to be of value in the management of the hypoglycemic diabetic patient who is an alcoholic or:

    a. hypothermic.
    b. malnourished.
    c. hypokalemic.
    d. hypotensive.

48. Your patient has a nontraumatic altered mental status. His vital signs are H/R 110, B/P 74/44, R/R 20, and his skin is warm and moist. His spouse tells you that he is not diabetic, but he does have asthma and takes steriod inhalers daily. You check his glucose level, and it is 40 mg/dl. After assuring that his airway and breathing are adequate, what would be the next appropriate step in care?

    a. Administer glucagon
    b. Give fluids boluses
    c. Administer $D_{50}W$
    d. Administer thiamine

49. As hypoglycemia alone, does not typically result in hypotension, which of the following conditions is the patient discussed in question 48 most likely experiencing?

    a. Acute adrenal insufficiency
    b. Cushing's syndrome
    c. Myxedema
    d. Thyrotoxicosis

50. Cushing's syndrome is caused by the hypersecretion of glucocorticoids by the _____ gland(s).

    a. adrenal
    b. thymus
    c. reproductive
    d. pancreas

51. You are assessing a 22-year-old male with insulin dependent diabetes mellitus (IDDM), who is having a diabetic event. His girlfriend called because she could not get him up this morning, and says he has been sick with a bad cold for several days. The patient's eyes are open, but he cannot verbalize a response. His breathing is deep and rapid, his skin is warm and dry, and he looks dehydrated. Vital signs are R/R 40, B/P 84/50, P/R 118. While you are checking his glucose level, which diabetic emergency do you suspect?

    a. Hypoglycemia
    b. Hyperglycemia
    c. HHNC
    d. None of the above

52. What is the significance about the respirations of the patient described in question 51?

    a. He is hyperventilating because of dehydration.
    b. This is the body's response to hypo-osmolarity and high pH.
    c. Deep respirations are a response to increased acid levels from ketones.
    d. The deep and rapid breathing is caused by the congestion from his cold.

53. For which of the following conditions is the patient described in question 51 at risk without intervention?

    a. permanent brain damage
    b. septic shock
    c. cardiac arrest
    d. all of the above

54. Which of the following treatment plans would be the most appropriate for the patient described in question 51?

    a. High flow oxygen, IV fluid boluses and glucagon.
    b. High flow oxygen, IV fluid boluses.
    c. IV, $D_{50}W$ and thiamine.
    d. IV, $D_{50}W$ and IV antibiotics in the hospital.

55. You have responded to a suburban residence for a 60-year-old male with an altered mental status. A neighbor called EMS because the patient is having stroke symptoms and is unable to get out of bed today. The patient is conscious, but very confused. His responses are slow and he feels week. He denies any pain or history of diabetes, and his vital signs are R/R 20, B/P 100/50, P/R 62, and his skin is warm and dry. Which of the following conditions do you suspect first?

    a. CVA
    b. diabetic emergency
    c. AMI
    d. all of the above

56. Further evaluation of the patient described in question 55 reveals that his medications include beta-blocker and antihypertensive meds. His SpO_2 is 99% with oxygen. Before you begin transport, which of the following would be of most value to make a differential diagnosis?

    a. 12 lead ECG
    b. glucose reading
    c. neurologic examination
    d. medication changes

57. What is the significance of the medications for the patient described in question 55?

    a. Beta-blockers will conceal compensatory signs of shock.
    b. Antihypertensives may precipitate hypoglycemia.
    c. Antihypertensives may conceal hyperglycemia.
    d. Beta-blockers may precipitate a stroke.

58. Put in order from quickest to slowest, the treatment response to a hypoglycemic event when IV access is unobtainable.

    a. Oral glucose, glucagon, orange juice
    b. Glucagon, Glucophage®, oral glucose
    c. Orange juice, Glucophage®, glucagon
    d. Glucophage®, glucagon, oral glucose

59. Which of the following hormones produced in the pancreas, stimulates an increase in blood sugar?

    a. Insulin
    b. Glucagon
    c. Beta-cell
    d. Cortisone

60. Complaints of abdominal pain are associated with which endocrine emergency?

    a. adrenal gland disorders
    b. hypoglycemia
    c. DKA
    d. all of the above

61. You respond to a call for a patient who fell and cannot get up. You find a 47-year-old female who fell while getting out of bed. She has no specific pain, but is c/o increased weakness over the last week. You immediately recognize that she has one of the classic physical findings, the _____ that is associated with Cushing's syndrome.

    a. moon face
    b. bulging eyes
    c. extreme peripheral edema
    d. fruity breath odor

62. You assist the patient described in question 61 to a chair, and she allows you to assess her and take her vital signs. You find that her arms and legs appear to be wasting, compared to the rest of her body. She also has unusual stretch marks on her skin. You attribute these findings to be _____ with Cushing's disease.

    a. typical findings
    b. non-compliance of medications associated
    c. side effects of medications associated
    d. none of the findings associated

63. Which of the following conditions is characterized by the body breaking down fat rather than glucose as its energy source?

    a. Hypoglycemia
    b. DKA
    c. Pancreatitis
    d. Insulin shock

64. Which of the following gland(s) is the only one(s) with both endocrine and exocrine functions?

    a. Thyroid
    b. Parathyroids
    c. Pancreas
    d. Adrenals

65. Which of the following gland(s) is responsible for the secretion of antidiuretic hormone?

    a. Ovaries
    b. Testes
    c. Thymus
    d. Pituitary

Test #25 Answer Form

	A	B	C	D			A	B	C	D
1.	❏	❏	❏	❏		27.	❏	❏	❏	❏
2.	❏	❏	❏	❏		28.	❏	❏	❏	❏
3.	❏	❏	❏	❏		29.	❏	❏	❏	❏
4.	❏	❏	❏	❏		30.	❏	❏	❏	❏
5.	❏	❏	❏	❏		31.	❏	❏	❏	❏
6.	❏	❏	❏	❏		32.	❏	❏	❏	❏
7.	❏	❏	❏	❏		33.	❏	❏	❏	❏
8.	❏	❏	❏	❏		34.	❏	❏	❏	❏
9.	❏	❏	❏	❏		35.	❏	❏	❏	❏
10.	❏	❏	❏	❏		36.	❏	❏	❏	❏
11.	❏	❏	❏	❏		37.	❏	❏	❏	❏
12.	❏	❏	❏	❏		38.	❏	❏	❏	❏
13.	❏	❏	❏	❏		39.	❏	❏	❏	❏
14.	❏	❏	❏	❏		40.	❏	❏	❏	❏
15.	❏	❏	❏	❏		41.	❏	❏	❏	❏
16.	❏	❏	❏	❏		42.	❏	❏	❏	❏
17.	❏	❏	❏	❏		43.	❏	❏	❏	❏
18.	❏	❏	❏	❏		44.	❏	❏	❏	❏
19.	❏	❏	❏	❏		45.	❏	❏	❏	❏
20.	❏	❏	❏	❏		46.	❏	❏	❏	❏
21.	❏	❏	❏	❏		47.	❏	❏	❏	❏
22.	❏	❏	❏	❏		48.	❏	❏	❏	❏
23.	❏	❏	❏	❏		49.	❏	❏	❏	❏
24.	❏	❏	❏	❏		50.	❏	❏	❏	❏
25.	❏	❏	❏	❏		51.	❏	❏	❏	❏
26.	❏	❏	❏	❏		52.	❏	❏	❏	❏

	A	B	C	D			A	B	C	D
53.	❏	❏	❏	❏		60.	❏	❏	❏	❏
54.	❏	❏	❏	❏		61.	❏	❏	❏	❏
55.	❏	❏	❏	❏		62.	❏	❏	❏	❏
56.	❏	❏	❏	❏		63.	❏	❏	❏	❏
57.	❏	❏	❏	❏		64.	❏	❏	❏	❏
58.	❏	❏	❏	❏		65.	❏	❏	❏	❏
59.	❏	❏	❏	❏						

26
Allergies and Anaphylaxis

1. When protective cells are able to recognize infections as they enter the body and destroy them prior to causing harm, this is called a/an:

    a. antigen.
    b. antibody.
    c. immune response.
    d. immunity.

2. An _____ is an overreaction by the body's immune response to normally harmless foreign substances, which causes damage to body tissues.

    a. antigen
    b. antibody
    c. allergic reaction
    d. allergy

3. When an antigen and the IgE antibody react, the combination leads to release of mediators from:

    a. basophils and mast cells.
    b. histamines.
    c. leukotrienes.
    d. antibodies.

4. Swelling of the skin caused by leakage of fluid from the blood vessels into the interstitial and subcutaneous tissues is called:

    a. urticaria.
    b. angioneurotic edema.
    c. angiocerebral edema.
    d. perisacral edema.

5. The most common causes of anaphylaxis include all the following, *except*:

    a. drugs.
    b. insect stings.
    c. blood products.
    d. IV fluids.

6. Which of the vital signs findings is not usually associated with an allergic reaction?

    a. Tachycardia
    b. Bradycardia
    c. Tachypnea
    d. Hypotension

7. As anaphylaxis develops, mast cells located in the skin, respiratory tract, and _____ release mediators that are apparent as physical signs and symptoms.

    a. GI tract
    b. nervous system
    c. cardiovascular system
    d. renal system

8. The epinephrine auto-injector contains _____ mg for adults and _____ mg for children.

    a. 0.5; 0:25
    b. 0.5; 0:05
    c. 0.3; 0.33
    d. 0.3; 0.15

9. Besides epinephrine, what other medication classification does the paramedic administer to a patient in anaphylaxis?

    a. Beta-blocker
    b. Antihistamine
    c. Antidiuretic
    d. ACE inhibitor

10. Which of the following medications is not administered by a paramedic to a patient in anaphylaxis?

    a. Bronchodilator
    b. Histamine
    c. Steroid
    d. Vassopressor

11. When is epinephrine appropriate for IV use over SQ for the patient in anaphylaxis?

    a. When the patient's auto-injector is empty.
    b. When the patient has an AMS.
    c. When the paramedic has taken PO Benadryl® prior to EMS arriving.
    d. When peripheral circulation is so poor SQ injections will be ineffective.

12. Which of the following would be the most helpful for the paramedic to determine what type of snake or spider bite a patient has sustained?

    a. The size of the bite.
    b. The shape of the bite.
    c. Markings of the animal.
    d. Time of the bite.

13. _____ is a natural sap from the rubber tree used to make natural rubber products.

    a. Gum
    b. Latex
    c. Lidocaine
    d. Powder

14. Patients in anaphylaxis may be given corticosteriods which:

    a. slow histamine release.
    b. have a fast acting effect.
    c. help to produce immunity.
    d. stimulate the antigen effect.

15. The histamine released during anaphylaxis may produce any of the following effects, except:

    a. decreased arterial pressure.
    b. increased arterial pressure.
    c. increased capillary permeability.
    d. spasms of the bronchioles.

16. Immunity may be acquired in any of the following manners, *except*:

    a. rendered.
    b. natural.
    c. active.
    d. passive.

17. Benedryl® is given to patients for allergic reactions because it:

    a. increases heart rate and strength of contractions.
    b. will mediate IgE.
    c. competes with histamine at the receptor sites blocking the effects of histamine.
    d. stimulates the antigen effect.

18. Which of the following is not a CNS response to anaphylaxis?

    a. Headache
    b. Tearing
    c. Dizziness
    d. Bronchoconstriction

19. Beta agonists help to reverse some of the _____ associated with anaphylaxis.

    a. edema
    b. bronchospasm
    c. nausea
    d. vasodilation

20. When the body releases histamine in response to exposure to an antigen, the body is trying to:

    a. vasoconstrict bronchial muscles.
    b. increase dilation of the capillaries.
    c. decrease permeability of the arterioles.
    d. minimize exposure to the antigen.

21. Your patient is a 6-year-old male who is having an allergic reaction to a known substance (nuts). The exposure occurred 30 minutes ago and he now has hives on his torso. His parents gave him 25 mg of Benadryl® PO just before calling EMS. Your primary concern for this patient is:

    a. the airway.
    b. histamine release.
    c. vasodilation.
    d. IV access.

22. Your management of the patient described in question 21 includes a calm approach with oxygen and:

    a. IV epinephrine 0.1 mg/kg (1:10,000).
    b. IM epinephrine 1.0 mg/kg (1:1,000).
    c. SC epinephrine 0.01 mg/kg (1:1,000).
    d. SC epinephrine 0.1 mg/kg (1:1,000).

23. Which of the following corticosteriods is not used in anaphylaxis by the paramedic to slow histamine release and capillary leakage?

    a. Aminophylline
    b. Solu-Medrol®
    c. Hydrocortisone
    d. Nortriptyline

24. The speed of an anaphylactic reaction depends on the route of exposure and the:

    a. degree of sensitivity.
    b. level of consciousness.
    c. patient's age.
    d. preexisting medical conditions.

25. The type of reaction an individual experiences depends on the speed of the reaction and the:

    a. route of exposure.
    b. target organ.
    c. patient's age.
    d. preexisting medical conditions.

26. The patient you are treating for an anaphylactic reaction is wheezing, hypotensive, and tachycardic five minutes after you have administered epinephrine. Which of the following should the patient receive next?

    a. Albuterol
    b. Repeat epi and give fluid boluses
    c. Benedryl®
    d. Dopamine

27. The patient described in question 26 continues to be hypotensive and tachycardic despite the efforts of your previous treatment. How would you manage the patient enroute to the hospital?

    a. Apply MAST/PASG and initiate a rapid transport.
    b. Start administration of a vassopressor.
    c. Prepare for a difficult intubation.
    d. Repeat epi and fluid boluses.

28. Urticaria or hives occur as a result of the fluid shift that happens when:

    a. blood vessels dilate and become permeable.
    b. the interstitial spaces overflow into the capillaries.
    c. the intracellular spaces constrict.
    d. antihistamines are no longer effective.

29. What is the mechanism by which Benadryl® helps to clear up hives?

    a. Antihistamines stimulate histamines to withdraw into mast cells.
    b. Antihistamines block H_2 receptors in the skin.
    c. Histamines are destroyed when antihistamines block H_1 receptor sites.
    d. Antihistamines block H_1 receptors in blood vessels.

30. Which of the following effects from the medication dopamine is not desired in anaphylaxis?

    a. increased cardiac contractibility
    b. increased peripheral vasoconstriction
    c. renal and mesentery artery vasodilation
    d. maintenance of systolic pressure

Test #26 Answer Form

	A	B	C	D
1.	❏	❏	❏	❏
2.	❏	❏	❏	❏
3.	❏	❏	❏	❏
4.	❏	❏	❏	❏
5.	❏	❏	❏	❏
6.	❏	❏	❏	❏
7.	❏	❏	❏	❏
8.	❏	❏	❏	❏
9.	❏	❏	❏	❏
10.	❏	❏	❏	❏
11.	❏	❏	❏	❏
12.	❏	❏	❏	❏
13.	❏	❏	❏	❏
14.	❏	❏	❏	❏
15.	❏	❏	❏	❏

	A	B	C	D
16.	❏	❏	❏	❏
17.	❏	❏	❏	❏
18.	❏	❏	❏	❏
19.	❏	❏	❏	❏
20.	❏	❏	❏	❏
21.	❏	❏	❏	❏
22.	❏	❏	❏	❏
23.	❏	❏	❏	❏
24.	❏	❏	❏	❏
25.	❏	❏	❏	❏
26.	❏	❏	❏	❏
27.	❏	❏	❏	❏
28.	❏	❏	❏	❏
29.	❏	❏	❏	❏
30.	❏	❏	❏	❏

27

Gastroenterology and Urology

1. There are three major types of acute abdominal pain: visceral, somatic, and:

    a. involuntary.
    b. voluntary.
    c. referred.
    d. diffuse.

2. _____ pain is caused by stimulation of nerve fibers in the parietal peritoneum by chemical or bacterial inflammation.

    a. Visceral
    b. Somatic
    c. Biliary
    d. Radiating

3. _____ pain is caused by sudden stretching or distention of a hollow organ.

    a. Visceral
    b. Somatic
    c. Biliary
    d. Radiating

4. You are assessing a 28-year-old male complaining of acute abdominal pain radiating around the right side to the back and angle of the scapula. Which of the following is most likely the cause of the pain?

    a. pancreas
    b. gallbladder
    c. kidney stone
    d. duodenal ulcer

5. Possible conditions associated with left lower quadrant pain of the abdomen include:

    a. PID, diverticulitis, and ovarian cyst.
    b. AMI, appendicitis, pancreatitis.
    c. Cholecystitis, duodenal ulcer, and bowel obstruction.
    d. Gallbladder, lesion, pyelonephritis.

6. A 65-year-old male with cardiac disease is complaining of a sudden onset of pain in his upper thighs and lumbosacral area. You suspect the cause of the pain to be a/an:

    a. AMI.
    b. pulled muscle.
    c. ruptured aneurysm.
    d. appendicitis.

7. The most common cause of "false alarm" in GI bleeding calls is:

    a. bowel obstruction.
    b. ectopic pregnancy.
    c. swallowed blood from a nosebleed.
    d. Mallory-Weiss tear.

8. Common causes for upper GI bleeding include all the following, *except*:

    a. peptic ulcer disease.
    b. diverticulosis.
    c. acute gastritis.
    d. esophagitis.

9. All the following are common causes for lower GI bleeding, *except*:

    a. esophageal varices.
    b. tumors.
    c. polyps.
    d. fissures.

10. You are assessing a 30-year-old male who is in tears and complaining of acute non-traumatic abdominal pain that radiates into the groin and external genitalia. You suspect the cause of the pain to be:

    a. STD.
    b. renal colic.
    c. appendicitis.
    d. bowel obstruction.

11. While preparing to transport a nursing home resident to the ED for evaluation, the staff reports that the patient has had a melena BM today. What was unusual about the stool?

    a. It appeared tarry and black.
    b. It smelled of vomitus.
    c. Bright red blood was present.
    d. It was yellowish in color.

12. Initial treatment of any patient with GI bleeding, regardless of the location, begins with the administration of high flow oxygen and:

    a. rapid transport to the ED.
    b. treatment for shock.
    c. treatment for pain control.
    d. nasogastric tube placement.

13. _____ is an acute inflammation of the gallbladder, usually caused by gallstones.

    a. Colitis
    b. Cholecystitis
    c. Crohn's disease
    d. Diverticulitis

14. Your partner is assessing a 35-year-old male with symptoms of malaise, nausea, vomiting, and tenderness on palpation of the upper-right quadrant of the abdomen. After moving the patient to the ambulance you notice the patient's sclera look yellow. What do you suspect is the patient's problem?

    a. Reflux esophagitis
    b. Diverticulitis
    c. Gastroenteritis
    d. Acute hepatitis

15. Orthostasis usually occurs with a _____ percent loss of circulating volume.

    a. 5–10
    b. 15–20
    c. 25–30
    d. >35

16. Which of the following causes of abdominal pain is not an immediate life threat?

    a. Acute MI
    b. Ruptured ectopic pregnancy
    c. Ruptured viscus
    d. Reflux esophagitis

17. The _____ is the most important part of the diagnosis in acute abdominal pain.

    a. blood pressure
    b. history
    c. patient's age
    d. type of pain

18. A slow onset of abdominal pain is more commonly associated with which of the following conditions?

    a. appendicitis
    b. ectopic pregnancy
    c. renal infarction
    d. splenic infarction

19. During the interview with a 38-year-old female complaining of GI distress, she tells you the pain began shortly after eating lunch. The lunch consisted of fatty food from a fast-food take-out place. Which of the following conditions do you suspect is the cause of the abdominal pain?

    a. Cholecystitis
    b. Pancreatitis
    c. Gastroenteritis
    d. Obstruction

20. A 40-year-old male with severe abdominal pain that began the day before and has progressively worsened, is lying completely still. The patient is very distressed when any attempt is made to move him. What do you suspect is the nature of his distress?

    a. muscle spasms
    b. colic
    c. peritoneal inflammation
    d. obstruction

21. Which of the following characteristics of bowel sounds is the most significant in the field?

    a. decreased sounds
    b. increased sounds
    c. absence of sounds
    d. abnormal sounds

22. The presence of rebound tenderness in the abdomen during the physical examination indicates:

    a. colic.
    b. obstruction.
    c. shock.
    d. peritoneal irritation.

23. In which of the following age groups is a positive tilt test an unreliable finding?

   a. < 13
   b. 20–30
   c. 30–50
   d. > 65

24. Probably the most common GI abnormality, which includes symptoms of bloating, pain, and often violent diarrhea, is:

   a. acute gastroenteritis.
   b. acute cholecystitis.
   c. lactose intolerance.
   d. bowel obstruction.

25. A condition that is most frequently found in young adults and is characterized by recurrent abdominal pain, usually crampy in nature, and diarrhea, alternating with periods of constipation, is known as:

   a. acute gastroenteritis.
   b. lactose intolerance.
   c. renal colic.
   d. irritable bowel syndrome.

26. The fluid wave test is performed on the abdomen to assess for the presence of:

   a. tenderness.
   b. ascites.
   c. masses.
   d. edema.

27. Patients that are being treated for acute GI emergencies get nothing by mouth (NPO) because they may need an empty stomach for emergency surgery and:

   a. a full stomach impedes diagnostic testing.
   b. the release of digestive enzymes often worsens the condition.
   c. pain management is contraindicated on a full stomach.
   d. their medication only works on an empty stomach.

28. _____ is a general term for a method, involving a semipermeable membrane, used to separate smaller particles from larger ones in a liquid mixture.

   a. Sifting
   b. DPL
   c. Osmosis
   d. Dialysis

29. The common causes of urologic emergencies include all the following, *except*:

   a. kidney stones.
   b. UTIs.
   c. bowel torsion.
   d. acute urinary retention.

30. Complications associated with hemodialysis may include all the following, *except*:

   a. vascular access problems.
   b. hypotension.
   c. chest pain.
   d. hypoglycemia.

31. Special considerations for care of the dialysis patient with an acute problem includes:

   a. avoiding taking a BP in any extremity with a fistula.
   b. only taking a BP in the extremity with a graft.
   c. accessing Medical Control for orders to start an IV.
   d. never asking advice from the dialysis technician.

32. You are transporting a nursing home resident to the hospital for evaluation of dysuria, frequency, urgency, and suprapubic pain. The patient has had the symptoms for two days. What do you suspect is the problem?

   a. kidney stone
   b. UTI
   c. bowel obstruction
   d. bladder obstruction

33. A 20-year-old female is complaining of abdominal pain and acute urinary retention. Which of the following conditions must be ruled out first?

   a. UTI
   b. ectopic pregnancy
   c. kidney stone
   d. pyelonephritis

34. You are called to a local high school for a male complaining of acute abdominal pain. Upon arrival and initial assessment, you have found that the patient was playing basketball when suddenly he felt severe pain in his left testicle. He denies having abdominal pain, but feels nausea. You suspect which of the following?

   a. torsion of the testicle
   b. kidney stone
   c. renal infection
   d. UTI

35. Based on the scenario above, which of the following treatments may be helpful?

    a. ice
    b. oxygen
    c. Trendelenburg's position
    d. aspirin

36. One of the functions of the urinary system is:

    a. maintaining proper balance between water and salts in the blood.
    b. to produce aldosterone.
    c. to excrete potassium to solidify waste products.
    d. helping the body eliminate sugar.

37. You are treating a 56-year-old male patient with a complaint of exertional chest pain. Your thorough history taking has revealed that the patient took Viagra® last night. Which of the following treatments would be most appropriate for the relief of this patient's chest pain?

    a. oxygen only
    b. oxygen and nitroglycerin
    c. oxygen and morphine
    d. morphine only

38. The most common STDs in both genders are gonorrhea, syphilis, and:

    a. hepatitis B.
    b. chlamydia.
    c. HIV.
    d. herpes.

39. During your assessment of a 30-year-old male complaining of acute severe abdominal pain that radiates into the right flank area, you discover that the patient has a history of kidney stones. The patient tells you this pain is just like when he had a kidney stone before. After attention to the ABCs, your management plan for this patient includes:

    a. rapid transport.
    b. pain management.
    c. supportive care only.
    d. treating for shock.

40. Conditions that result in abdominal pain, but do not originate in the abdomen, include all the following, *except*:

    a. pneumonia.
    b. black widow spider bite.
    c. herpes zoster.
    d. food poisoning.

41. Which of the following groups do not commonly present with atypical signs during a GI emergency?

    a. trauma
    b. children
    c. elderly
    d. pregnant women

42. _____ pain is pain from one area that is being sensed in another because of embryologic nerve distribution patterns.

    a. Referred
    b. Acute
    c. Guarded
    d. Reflex

43. A/an _____ GI bleed is bleeding proximal to the duodenojejunal junction.

    a. upper
    b. lower
    c. acute
    d. non-traumatic

44. Which of the following is a definition for the term "hematochezia"?

    a. Vomiting bright red blood
    b. Bright red blood in the stool
    c. Tarry, sticky black stool
    d. Vomiting "coffee grounds" old blood

45. Estimating the amount of blood lost from reports of stool and vomitus volume are likely to be:

    a. accurate if reported by a paramedic.
    b. candid as reported by the patient.
    c. reliable when reported by a home health aide.
    d. unreliable.

46. Appendicitis is inflammation of the appendix caused by occlusion of the lumen by a:

    a. small tumor.
    b. small piece of stool.
    c. blood clot.
    d. large lesion.

47. Cholecystitis is an acute inflammation of the gall bladder that blocks the lumen, interfering with:

    a. blood flow.
    b. bile flow.
    c. insulin production.
    d. urine production.

48. _____ is a general term indicating inflammation of the colon for any of a number of reasons.

    a. Diverticulitis
    b. Diverticulosis
    c. Colitis
    d. Gastritis

49. Dilations of the veins of the esophagus secondary to increased portal vein pressures result in:

    a. cirrhosis.
    b. peptic ulcer.
    c. gastric ulcer.
    d. varices.

50. Dilations of the veins in the lower portion of the colon result in:

    a. tumors.
    b. hemorrhoids.
    c. colitis.
    d. varices.

Test #27 Answer Form

	A	B	C	D			A	B	C	D
1.	❏	❏	❏	❏		26.	❏	❏	❏	❏
2.	❏	❏	❏	❏		27.	❏	❏	❏	❏
3.	❏	❏	❏	❏		28.	❏	❏	❏	❏
4.	❏	❏	❏	❏		29.	❏	❏	❏	❏
5.	❏	❏	❏	❏		30.	❏	❏	❏	❏
6.	❏	❏	❏	❏		31.	❏	❏	❏	❏
7.	❏	❏	❏	❏		32.	❏	❏	❏	❏
8.	❏	❏	❏	❏		33.	❏	❏	❏	❏
9.	❏	❏	❏	❏		34.	❏	❏	❏	❏
10.	❏	❏	❏	❏		35.	❏	❏	❏	❏
11.	❏	❏	❏	❏		36.	❏	❏	❏	❏
12.	❏	❏	❏	❏		37.	❏	❏	❏	❏
13.	❏	❏	❏	❏		38.	❏	❏	❏	❏
14.	❏	❏	❏	❏		39.	❏	❏	❏	❏
15.	❏	❏	❏	❏		40.	❏	❏	❏	❏
16.	❏	❏	❏	❏		41.	❏	❏	❏	❏
17.	❏	❏	❏	❏		42.	❏	❏	❏	❏
18.	❏	❏	❏	❏		43.	❏	❏	❏	❏
19.	❏	❏	❏	❏		44.	❏	❏	❏	❏
20.	❏	❏	❏	❏		45.	❏	❏	❏	❏
21.	❏	❏	❏	❏		46.	❏	❏	❏	❏
22.	❏	❏	❏	❏		47.	❏	❏	❏	❏
23.	❏	❏	❏	❏		48.	❏	❏	❏	❏
24.	❏	❏	❏	❏		49.	❏	❏	❏	❏
25.	❏	❏	❏	❏		50.	❏	❏	❏	❏

28

Toxicology

1. The majority of the reported poisoning exposures occur in:

   a. the patient's home.
   b. a workplace.
   c. recreational facilities.
   d. on the highway.

2. The largest number of poisoning deaths occur in which age group?

   a. 1 to 8
   b. 9 to 19
   c. 20 to 49
   d. 50 to 70

3. Of the following, which is not a predisposing risk factor for a toxic emergency?

   a. pediatric ingestions
   b. adult ingestions
   c. suicide attempts
   d. occupational exposures

4. An example of a toxic effect on the respiratory system includes:

   a. the inability of the cells to manufacture ATP.
   b. a slowing of the transmission of nerve impulses.
   c. the development of pulmonary edema.
   d. the paralysis of the muscles.

5. Of the following, which is not one of the four routes by which toxic substances enter the body?

   a. injection
   b. exhaustion
   c. inhalation
   d. ingestion

6. A substance may pass through the skin and enter the body. This is known as:

   a. ingestion.
   b. inhalation.
   c. absorption.
   d. exhaustion.

7. When a toxic substance enters the body through an insect's stinger this is by the _____ route.

   a. absorption
   b. injection
   c. inhalation
   d. ingestion

8. An example of a creature with a toxic substance that is particular to the South, especially Florida, is:

   a. rattlesnakes.
   b. brown recluse spiders.
   c. coral snakes.
   d. Jellyfish.

9. General signs and symptoms that are suggestive of a poisoning include:

   a. burning and tearing of the eyes.
   b. decreased sweating and salivation.
   c. headache, syncopy, and low blood sugar.
   d. cold body temperature.

10. Sometimes the vital signs are an indication of the poisoning agent. Tachycardia suggests:

    a. pesticide poisoning.
    b. stimulant ingestion.
    c. aspirin toxicity.
    d. narcotic injection.

11. The poisoned patient who took a large quantity of _____ may be hyperthermic.

    a. alcohol
    b. a narcotic
    c. a sedative
    d. aspirin

12. The blood pressure is often elevated with an overdose of:

    a. depressants.
    b. aspirin.
    c. cocaine.
    d. pesticides.

13. Several groups of drugs that present with similar clinical patterns of toxicology are called a:

    a. syndrome.
    b. toxidrome.
    c. paradyme.
    d. prognosis.

14. A narcotic poisoning may result in _____ pupils.

    a. unequal
    b. dilated
    c. constricted
    d. fixed

15. Each of the following are examples of toxidromes, *except*:

    a. infectious agents.
    b. cholinergics.
    c. hallucinogens.
    d. sympathomimetics.

16. Common agents that fall into the toxidrome referred to as anticholinergics include:

    a. pesticides and nerve agents.
    b. LSD, PCP, and mescaline.
    c. tricyclic antidepressants and mushrooms.
    d. diet pills, caffeine, and cocaine.

17. Euphoria, hypotension and respiratory depression are most commonly found with which toxidrome?

    a. sympathomimetics
    b. narcotics
    c. anticholinergics
    d. hallucinogens

18. Tachycardia, diaphoresis, chest pain, and stroke are most commonly caused by which toxidrome?

    a. sympathomimetics
    b. anticholinergics
    c. cholinergics
    d. narcotics

19. What is the most common route of poisoning?

    a. absorption
    b. inhalation
    c. ingestion
    d. injection

20. The first cardinal principle of management for all EMS providers when dealing with a toxicologic emergency is to:

    a. consider specific antidotes.
    b. consider decontamination of the patient.
    c. ensure your own safety first.
    d. maintain an open airway and breathing.

21. The difference between a poisoning and an overdose is:

    a. poisoning involves exposure to a substance that is generally harmful and has no beneficial effects.
    b. overdose suggests an excessive exposure to a substance that is not normally used to treat humans.
    c. there is no difference between the two terms and they are used interchangeably.
    d. all of the above are correct.

22. The induction of vomiting should not be done for patients who are suspected to have taken any of the following, *except*:

    a. acid.
    b. lye.
    c. asprin.
    d. petroleum products.

23. Vomiting should not be induced if the patient:

    a. has taken pills.
    b. is over 50 years old.
    c. has a decreased mental status.
    d. is a known drug abuser.

24. The paramedic should not induce vomiting if the patient has ingested all the following, *except*:

    a. corrosives, such as strong acids or alkali.
    b. petroleum products.
    c. an overdose of amphetamines.
    d. iodine, silver nitrate or strychnine.

25. Gastric dialysis is a mechanism of poison removal aided by the administration of:

    a. activated charcoal.
    b. ipecac syrup.
    c. tincture of benzene.
    d. milk or mild soap.

26. When treating a 27-year-old male patient who has a history of depression you determine the patient may have taken 10 to 20 tricyclic antidepressants. His vitals are within normal range, and he is alert at this time. What treatment should be considered?

    a. administer 2 mg Narcan
    b. transport to the poison control center
    c. consider administering activated charcoal
    d. quickly restrain the patient

27. Exposure to systemic toxins, such as carbon monoxide, often result in:

    a. hypoxia.
    b. vertigo.
    c. diaphoresis.
    d. edema.

28. In all patients taken out of a fire the paramedic should suspect:

    a. food poisoning.
    b. drug overdose.
    c. chlorine inhalation.
    d. carbon monoxide exposure.

29. When substances pass through the skin into the blood stream this is called:

    a. ingestion.
    b. inhalation.
    c. absorption.
    d. injection.

30. A chemical that _____ in the fat of the skin is likely to cause poisoning by absorption.

    a. slowly dissolves
    b. does not dissolve
    c. dissolves easily
    d. traps large particles

31. Symptoms of general toxicity include all the following, *except*:

    a. paralysis.
    b. headache.
    c. AMS.
    d. vomiting.

32. Patients presenting with muscle fasciculation and paralysis may be suffering from:

    a. cholinergic overdose.
    b. CNS toxicity.
    c. aspirin overdose.
    d. narcotic overdose.

33. Your patient is a 22-year-old female who is 7 months pregnant. Apparently she took an overdose of over-the-counter medication designed to relieve abdominal cramping. She is alert and oriented and her vital signs are within normal range. What is your best course of treatment?

    a. induce vomiting with syrup of ipecac
    b. restrain her as she may become violent
    c. monitor her ABCs and administer oxygen
    d. administer activated charcoal and rush her to the ED

34. What does the pathophysiology of poisoning by inhalation involve?

    a. The substance is absorbed into the bloodstream in the intestines.
    b. The substance is absorbed at the alveolar level leading to systemic toxicity.
    c. The material is absorbed through the skin into the muscles.
    d. The material moves across the blood-brain barrier into the venous system.

35. What desired effect is most helpful to the patient when the paramedic administers Narcan?

    a. immediate withdrawal symptoms from the overdose
    b. reversal of the hypertension
    c. reversal of the respiratory depression
    d. a heightened sensitivity to the surrounding environment

36. Of the following, which substance is not usually absorbed through the skin?

    a. pesticides
    b. nitro
    c. wax
    d. insecticide

37. If your patient was exposed to a herbicide, which antidote may prove useful if authorized by Medical Control to administer?

    a. narcan
    b. atropine
    c. solu-medrol
    d. nitrous oxide

38. Your patient is a 52-year-old male who was working in the fields of his farm all day. His wife called the ambulance because he has been acting crazy and very shaky and drooling at the dinner table. What could be wrong with him?

    a. He has taken an overdose of painkillers.
    b. He is diabetic and missed a lunch.
    c. He had an excessive exposure to insecticides.
    d. He is having a stroke.

39. An acquired resistance to the therapeutic effects of usual doses of a drug is referred to as:

    a. addiction.
    b. tolerance.
    c. dependence.
    d. drug abuse.

40. A psychologic craving for or reliance on a chemical agent is referred to as a/an:

    a. addiction.
    b. tolerance.
    c. dependence.
    d. drug abuse.

41. What is the source of most illegal drugs in the United States?

    a. smuggling from Columbia
    b. stolen shipments to hospital pharmacies
    c. artificially manufactured in college labs
    d. they are grown in rural areas

42. A substance which is often abused and called blow or candy on the street is called:

    a. marijuana.
    b. sedative-hypnotics.
    c. cocaine.
    d. opiates.

43. Medications that are often abused, yet are medically prescribed for bedwetting, seizures and Tourette's syndrome, include:

    a. narcotics.
    b. tricyclic antidepressants.
    c. cyanide.
    d. sedative-hypnotics.

44. A drug that is frequently abused, which decreases inhibitory synapses in the brain, then excitatory synapses causing euphoria followed by depression, is called a/an:

    a. opiate.
    b. alcohol.
    c. barbiturates.
    d. mushroom.

45. The symptoms of _____ syndrome include agitation, anxiety, ataxia, coma, and confusion.

    a. hydrocarbon
    b. serotonin
    c. postural
    d. anerobic

46. Use of hydrocarbons causing CNS alteration, cardiac dysfunction and liver dysfunction is often referred to as:

    a. huffing.
    b. freebasing.
    c. snorting.
    d. none of the above.

47. The early signs of carbon monoxide poisoning include all the following, *except*:

    a. coma.
    b. headache.
    c. nausea.
    d. vomiting.

48. When a patient is thought to have sustained carbon monoxide poisoning, his/her management should include high concentration oxygen and consideration for:

    a. activated charcoal.
    b. syrup of ipecac.
    c. a hyperbaric chamber.
    d. a large dose of atropine.

49. The management of an aspirin overdose may include all the following, *except*:

    a. activated charcoal.
    b. glucose administration.
    c. antiseizure medication.
    d. spirits of amnonia.

50. You have been called to a housing project where three preschoolers play in the hallways and basement. The building is old, decaying, and sorely in need of repair. The parent of one child states that her son is complaining of a diffuse crampy abdominal pain and has diarrhea. He has been acting uncoordinated, irritable and has memory lapses. What could be the cause of this sickness?

    a. Carbon monoxide poisoning from a faulty heating unit.
    b. Lead poisoning from eating paint chips.
    c. Hydrocarbon poisoning from inhaling glue fumes.
    d. An overdose of cocaine from a needle found in the basement.

Test #28 Answer Form

	A	B	C	D			A	B	C	D
1.	❏	❏	❏	❏		26.	❏	❏	❏	❏
2.	❏	❏	❏	❏		27.	❏	❏	❏	❏
3.	❏	❏	❏	❏		28.	❏	❏	❏	❏
4.	❏	❏	❏	❏		29.	❏	❏	❏	❏
5.	❏	❏	❏	❏		30.	❏	❏	❏	❏
6.	❏	❏	❏	❏		31.	❏	❏	❏	❏
7.	❏	❏	❏	❏		32.	❏	❏	❏	❏
8.	❏	❏	❏	❏		33.	❏	❏	❏	❏
9.	❏	❏	❏	❏		34.	❏	❏	❏	❏
10.	❏	❏	❏	❏		35.	❏	❏	❏	❏
11.	❏	❏	❏	❏		36.	❏	❏	❏	❏
12.	❏	❏	❏	❏		37.	❏	❏	❏	❏
13.	❏	❏	❏	❏		38.	❏	❏	❏	❏
14.	❏	❏	❏	❏		39.	❏	❏	❏	❏
15.	❏	❏	❏	❏		40.	❏	❏	❏	❏
16.	❏	❏	❏	❏		41.	❏	❏	❏	❏
17.	❏	❏	❏	❏		42.	❏	❏	❏	❏
18.	❏	❏	❏	❏		43.	❏	❏	❏	❏
19.	❏	❏	❏	❏		44.	❏	❏	❏	❏
20.	❏	❏	❏	❏		45.	❏	❏	❏	❏
21.	❏	❏	❏	❏		46.	❏	❏	❏	❏
22.	❏	❏	❏	❏		47.	❏	❏	❏	❏
23.	❏	❏	❏	❏		48.	❏	❏	❏	❏
24.	❏	❏	❏	❏		49.	❏	❏	❏	❏
25.	❏	❏	❏	❏		50.	❏	❏	❏	❏

29

Environmental Conditions

1. Examples of an environmental emergency include all the following, *except*:

   a. atmospheric pressure.
   b. heat stoke.
   c. hypothermia.
   d. frostbite.

2. Which of the following age groups are at greater risk for environmental emergencies than others?

   a. teens and geriatrics
   b. middle age and geriatrics
   c. small children and geriatrics
   d. early adult and geriatrics

3. Which of the following general health issues makes a person more susceptible to environmental influences?

   a. Obesity
   b. Smoking
   c. Cancer
   d. Hypertension

4. Predisposing medical conditions that are particularly risky conditions making a person more susceptible to environmental conditions include all the following, *except*:

   a. diabetes.
   b. CHF.
   c. thyroid disease.
   d. hypertension.

5. Which of the following medications results in an impaired ability to sweat and dissipate heat?

   a. Tricyclic antidepressants
   b. Antidiabetics
   c. Aspirin
   d. Diuretics

6. An example of an environmental challenge that involves atmospheric pressure is a _____ accident.

   a. freefalling
   b. diving
   c. caving
   d. skiing

7. Of the following, which is not a principal type of environmental illness?

   a. High altitude sickness
   b. Heat cramps
   c. Radiation burns
   d. Cold diuresis

8. Which of the following is not a major component of the body's thermoregulatory mechanism?

   a. Hypothalamus
   b. Metabolic rate
   c. Central blood vessels
   d. Skin

9. Body heat is generated as a side effect of normal _____ processes.

   a. systemic
   b. cell-mediated
   c. metabolic
   d. neural

10. _____ refers to normal body means of heat loss and gain.

    a. Thermoregulation
    b. Radiation
    c. Conduction
    d. Homeostasis

11. Body heat is gained or dissipated by which of the following mechanisms?

    a. Convection
    b. Homeostasis
    c. Metabolysis
    d. Electrolyte balance

12. When a person lays on a cold surface such as a cold floor, heat is lost from the body by means of:

    a. radiation.
    b. conduction.
    c. convection.
    d. evaporation.

13. When the body is exposed to very high temperatures _____ becomes the only effective method of heat dissipation.

   a. radiation
   b. conduction
   c. convection
   d. evaporation

14. In heat cramps and heat exhaustion, the underlying problem involves:

   a. dehydration.
   b. exposure.
   c. localized injury.
   d. inadequate thermogenesis.

15. Signs of thermolysis include:

   a. shivering and loss of coordination.
   b. diaphoresis and flushing.
   c. tachypnea and chest pain.
   d. slurred speech and ataxia.

16. A person who is properly acclimatized to warm temperatures is less likely to:

   a. sweat.
   b. disrupt sodium concentrations.
   c. vasodilate.
   d. maintain adequate fluid intake.

17. The primary causes of hypothermia are cold water immersion, cold weather exposure and _____ hypothermia.

   a. urban
   b. acute
   c. subacute
   d. chronic

18. You are evaluating a 55-year-old female who was outside watching her grandson play ball. She has a c/c of dizziness when she stands up and a headache. Her clothing is wet with perspiration, but her skin temperature feels normal. Which of the following heat syndromes do you suspect she is experiencing?

   a. Cramps
   b. Exhaustion
   c. Stroke
   d. Exertional heat stroke

19. Your management plan for the patient described in question 18, is to cool her off in your ambulance and:

   a. treat for dehydration.
   b. provide high flow oxygen.
   c. apply ice or ice packs.
   d. administer salt tablets.

20. Severe infection (sepsis) may actually result in _____ when the body's fever-production centers are overwhelmed.

   a. heat exhaustion
   b. heat stroke
   c. hypothermia
   d. exposure

21. There is a high incident of heat exhaustion in individuals with all the following circumstances, *except*:

   a. mall walkers.
   b. people taking water pills.
   c. prolonged bouts of diarrhea.
   d. young children.

22. Medications that can predispose a patient to hypothermia include all the following, *except*:

   a. narcotics.
   b. antiseizure medications.
   c. antihistamines.
   d. antidiabetics.

23. Fever is a normal response to the release of chemicals called _____ and usually results from an infection.

   a. pyrogens
   b. pyrexia
   c. pylorus
   d. purines

24. _____ is a normal response to an intact thermoregulatory system, while _____ develops when the thermoregulatory system has failed.

   a. Shivering: hypothermia
   b. Fever: heat stroke
   c. Diaphoresis: heat exhaustion
   d. AMS: heat cramps

25. With the exception of _____, wet clothing loses approximately 90% of its insulating value.

   a. wool
   b. polyester
   c. denim
   d. cotton

26. Conditions that may contribute to hypothermia include all the following, *except*:

   a. hypothyroidism.
   b. brain dysfunction.
   c. hypoglycemia.
   d. hyperglycemia.

27. Which of the following conditions is not usually a predisposing factor for hypothermia?

   a. Acute stroke
   b. Intoxication
   c. Shock
   d. AMI

28. The severity of hypothermia is determined by the core body temperature (CBT) and the presence of:

   a. frostbite.
   b. signs and symptoms.
   c. frost nip.
   d. cold diuresis

29. A CBT of less than _____ is suggestive of severe hypothermia.

   a. 95°F
   b. 90°F
   c. 85°F
   d. 80°F

30. A person who has been hiking for several hours in the winter would most likely be at risk for _____ hypothermia.

   a. acute
   b. subacute
   c. chronic
   d. urban

31. An elderly stroke victim who has fallen, and is unable to move off a tile floor would most likely be at risk for _____ hypothermia.

   a. acute
   b. subacute
   c. chronic
   d. urban

32. Sometimes hypothermia is a sign of another disease such as:

   a. stroke.
   b. hypoglycemia.
   c. hyperthyroidism.
   d. hyperplasia.

33. Which of the following cardiac dysrhythmias/disturbances is more common during the rewarming phase rather than the development of hypothermia?

   a. Atrial fibrillation
   b. Ventricular fibrillation
   c. J waves
   d. Long Q-T

34. Which of the following considerations is most accurate regarding the treatment of severe hypothermia patients?

   a. Cold may affect the potency of first-line cardiac drugs.
   b. The risk of v-fib increases with orotracheal intubation.
   c. The risk of v-fib increases with nasotracheal intubation.
   d. The hypothermic heart is never resistant to defibrillation.

35. The most common dysrhythmias in hypothermia-associated cardiac arrest are:

   a. bradycardia and heart blocks.
   b. V-fib and asystole.
   c. V-tach and a-fib.
   d. bradycardia and asystole.

36. The American Heart Association recommends that _____ in v-fib hypothermia-cardiac arrest.

   a. defibrillation be attempted as soon as possible
   b. lidocaine be administered in double the normal dose
   c. bretylium be administered in one-half the normal dose
   d. defibrillation be withheld until the patient can be rewarmed

37. During the management of the near-drowning patient, the paramedic should assume that the patient is _____ until proven otherwise.

   a. brain dead
   b. hypothermic
   c. in v-fib
   d. experiencing laryngospasm

38. For the paramedic managing the hypothermic patient, the first priority after airway, breathing and circulation is to:

   a. administer a prophylactic antidysrhythmic.
   b. dress and protect frostbitten extremities.
   c. start an IV lifeline.
   d. stop ongoing heat loss.

39. Frostbite is the formation of _____ within the tissues affected.

   a. hematomas
   b. blood clots
   c. ice crystals
   d. cellulitis

40. The paramedic can differentiate superficial frostbite and deep frostbite by:

    a. deep frostbitten skin has a white, waxy appearance.
    b. superficial frostbite feels hard to palpation.
    c. superficial frostbite only affects small children and the elderly.
    d. deep frostbite has a temporary decreased loss of sensation.

41. Often when a frostbitten area is rewarmed, the patient complains of the area feeling numb. This feeling is caused by:

    a. the formation of acute cellulitis.
    b. lack of oxygen.
    c. the presence of small hematomas.
    d. the formation of blisters.

42. When treating a drowning victim the paramedic should consider the single most important factor in adult drowning, which is:

    a. the use of alcohol and mind-altering drugs.
    b. associated hypothermia.
    c. an acute medical problem may have precipitated the drowning.
    d. suicide attempt may have been the cause.

43. Signs and symptoms of near drowning may include any of the following, *except*:

    a. progressive dyspnea.
    b. wheezing.
    c. respiratory arrest.
    d. hiccups.

44. Aspiration of either seawater or freshwater decreases pulmonary compliance and results in:

    a. tension pneumothorax.
    b. hypoxia.
    c. pneumonia.
    d. upper respiratory infection.

45. The endpoints in near drowning, no matter what type of water involved, include all the following, *except*:

    a. metabolic acidosis.
    b. pulmonary edema.
    c. respiratory arrest.
    d. aspiration injuries.

46. The three types of drowning include dry, wet and:

    a. primary.
    b. secondary.
    c. tertiary.
    d. central.

47. Several complications can occur following near drowning incidents, and include all the following, *except*:

    a. persistent laryngeal spasms.
    b. persistent hypoxemia.
    c. infection.
    d. persistent neurologic deficit.

48. The best predictor of the severity of neurologic deficit following a near drowning is the:

    a. type of water the patient aspirated.
    b. time to the first spontaneous gasp following removal from the water.
    c. presence of preexisting medical conditions.
    d. temperature of the water.

49. _____ drowning is defined as the recurrence of respiratory distress after successful recovery from the initial drowning incident and can occur within a few minutes or up to four days later.

    a. Wet
    b. Primary
    c. Secondary
    d. Central

50. SCUBA is an acronym for:

    a. sealed and condensed underwater breathing apparatus.
    b. self-compressed underwater breathing aperture.
    c. self-contained underwater breathing apparatus.
    d. solid-compact underwater breathing aperture.

51. Which of the following is not a law of gas that applies to diving emergencies?

    a. Boyle's law
    b. Henry's law
    c. Dalton's law
    d. George's law

52. _____ law states that the volume of a gas varies inversely with the absolute pressure or as the pressure increases, the gas volume decreases.

    a. Boyle's
    b. Henry's
    c. Dalton's
    d. George's

53. When a diver ascends, but forgets to exhale on the way up, the pressure will _____ with ascent and the volume of gas trapped in the lungs will _____:

   a. decrease: expand.
   b. decrease: shrink.
   c. increase: expand.
   d. increase: shrink.

54. Which of the following injuries will the diver in question 53 most likely experience if the condition persists?

   a. Stroke
   b. Pericardial tamponade
   c. Pneumothorax
   d. Loss of consciousness

55. Decompression sickness is an illness during or after ascent secondary to rapid release of _____ in the blood.

   a. an air embolus
   b. nitrogen bubbles
   c. hydrogen bubbles
   d. subcutaneous air

56. A patient with decompression sickness is c/o pain in the legs and shoulders two days after a dive. These symptoms are associated with the:

   a. bends.
   b. staggers.
   c. chokes.
   d. itches.

57. Divers can experience *nitrogen narcosis* at various depths because of the narcotic effect of dissolved nitrogen in the body. The effect is analogous to excessive ethanol levels and the cause is attributed to _____ law.

   a. Boyle's
   b. Henry's
   c. Dalton's
   d. George's

58. Preexisting conditions that can predispose some divers to the possibility of air embolism during or after a dive include all the following, *except*:

   a. smoker.
   b. asthma.
   c. COPD.
   d. sinus infection.

59. Your patient is a 33-year-old male diver who is lying on the pier. He is experiencing stroke-like symptoms immediately after surfacing from an 80-foot dive. He has left-sided motor deficit and is c/o of left-sided numbness and vertigo. Which of the following conditions do you suspect?

   a. Air embolism
   b. Decompression sickness
   c. Nitrogen narcosis
   d. ARDS

60. After managing and supporting the ABCs, how would you manage the patient described in question 59?

   a. Complete a thrombolic checklist.
   b. Consider pain management therapy.
   c. Consider decompression therapy.
   d. Treat for stroke only.

61. When obtaining information about a patient who is experiencing an emergency related to diving, which of the following is not a significant factor?

   a. The number of dives today.
   b. The depths of today's dives.
   c. The type of gas mixture used.
   d. Did the patient fly in an airplane more than 24 hours ago?

62. Hyperbaric oxygen is beneficial in both _____ and decompression sickness.

   a. pneumothorax
   b. tamponade
   c. DVT
   d. air embolism

63. Long delays are common for the treatment of decompression sickness in the lay diving populations because of:

   a. lack of recognition of symptoms.
   b. the distance to hyperbaric treatment areas.
   c. all diving sites are in foreign countries.
   d. the dive boats rarely have radios.

64. During the predive surface phase of a dive, any of the following potential problems may occur, *except*:

   a. air embolism.
   b. motion sickness.
   c. hyperventilation.
   d. near drowning.

65. During which phase of a dive do squeeze syndromes, involving the ears, most commonly occur?

    a. Predive surface
    b. Descent
    c. Bottom
    d. Postdive surface

66. The most common altitude syndromes include all the following, *except*:

    a. acute mountain sickness (AMS).
    b. high altitude pulmonary edema (HAPE).
    c. high altitude cerebral edema (HACE).
    d. acute flying sickness (AFS).

67. High altitude illness occurs as a result of decreased atmospheric pressure, resulting in:

    a. hypercarbia.
    b. hypoxia.
    c. vertigo.
    d. dehydration.

68. Causes of high altitude illness include all the following, *except*:

    a. mountain climbing.
    b. flying in an unpressurized aircraft.
    c. skydiving.
    d. SCUBA diving at high altitudes.

69. Your patient is a mountain climber who has been sick for two days following an ascent of a mountain in excess of 8,000 feet. He is c/o dizziness, headache, irritability and exertional SOB. Which of the following conditions do you suspect he has?

    a. AMS
    b. HAPE
    c. HACE
    d. AFS

70. The most important treatment the paramedic can provide for the patient described in question 69 is to:

    a. administer high flow oxygen.
    b. administer a diuretic.
    c. transport to a hyperbaric therapy center.
    d. administer Nifedipine®.

71. You are treating a patient who has suffered first-degree burns that cover 35% of the BSA. You are cooling her with normal saline during the transport. Which of the following mechanisms of heat loss is the patient experiencing?

    a. Conduction
    b. Radiation
    c. Evaporation
    d. All of the above

72. The patient you are evaluating has frostnip on her fingers and face. While obtaining the focused history on this patient, which of the following are factors that may increase her susceptibility to frostbite?

    a. Diabetes and smoker.
    b. Headache and sinus infection.
    c. Allergy to PNC.
    d. Hearing deficit.

73. A diver has experienced *squeeze* during his last dive. Which body areas can be affected by squeeze?

    a. Thighs and calves
    b. Feet and mouth
    c. Ears and sinuses
    d. Hands and shoulders

74. For the last two hours, a rescue crew has been carrying a hiker out of the woods. The hiker lost his footing on ice and fractured his femur. The patient is very cold and within the last 10 minutes has stopped shivering. Why has his shivering stopped?

    a. He has gone into shock.
    b. His core temperature has reached 92°F.
    c. His glucose stores are depleted.
    d. He has acute mountain sickness.

75. A diver is experiencing nitrogen narcosis. What is the primary danger for this diver?

    a. impaired thinking
    b. barotrauma
    c. air embolism
    d. hypoxia

76. When working in high humidity climates, it is important to recall that sweating becomes ineffective if the relative humidity exceeds _____ percent.

    a. 15
    b. 35
    c. 55
    d. 75

77. A patient who has generalized hypothermia has been removed from the cold environment. If he has an open airway and no nausea he should be allowed to:

   a. refuse medical attention.
   b. drink warm fluids.
   c. walk around to help warm the body.
   d. smoke a cigarette.

78. On the scene at a private residence, you arrive to the backyard to find a small crowd standing around two people doing CPR. The patient is a teenage male who was pulled from the pool. A witness saw the male dive into the pool and then float to the surface face down. Considering the MOI what injury(s) has the patient most likely sustained?

   a. Head trauma
   b. SCI
   c. Barotraumas
   d. Decompression sickness

79. You and your crew take over CPR and continue resuscitative efforts for the patient described in question 78. Initially the patient was easy to ventilate, but now lung compliance is getting hard to bag. What do you suspect is the cause of the increased resistance in ventilation?

   a. Gastric distention
   b. Rising ICP
   c. Pneumothorax
   d. Hypercarbia

80. To correct the problem of increased resistance in ventilation of the patient described in question 78 the paramedic would:

   a. decompress the stomach.
   b. hyperventilate the patient.
   c. decompress the chest.
   d. intubate the patient.

Test #29 Answer Form

	A	B	C	D		A	B	C	D
1.	❑	❑	❑	❑	27.	❑	❑	❑	❑
2.	❑	❑	❑	❑	28.	❑	❑	❑	❑
3.	❑	❑	❑	❑	29.	❑	❑	❑	❑
4.	❑	❑	❑	❑	30.	❑	❑	❑	❑
5.	❑	❑	❑	❑	31.	❑	❑	❑	❑
6.	❑	❑	❑	❑	32.	❑	❑	❑	❑
7.	❑	❑	❑	❑	33.	❑	❑	❑	❑
8.	❑	❑	❑	❑	34.	❑	❑	❑	❑
9.	❑	❑	❑	❑	35.	❑	❑	❑	❑
10.	❑	❑	❑	❑	36.	❑	❑	❑	❑
11.	❑	❑	❑	❑	37.	❑	❑	❑	❑
12.	❑	❑	❑	❑	38.	❑	❑	❑	❑
13.	❑	❑	❑	❑	39.	❑	❑	❑	❑
14.	❑	❑	❑	❑	40.	❑	❑	❑	❑
15.	❑	❑	❑	❑	41.	❑	❑	❑	❑
16.	❑	❑	❑	❑	42.	❑	❑	❑	❑
17.	❑	❑	❑	❑	43.	❑	❑	❑	❑
18.	❑	❑	❑	❑	44.	❑	❑	❑	❑
19.	❑	❑	❑	❑	45.	❑	❑	❑	❑
20.	❑	❑	❑	❑	46.	❑	❑	❑	❑
21.	❑	❑	❑	❑	47.	❑	❑	❑	❑
22.	❑	❑	❑	❑	48.	❑	❑	❑	❑
23.	❑	❑	❑	❑	49.	❑	❑	❑	❑
24.	❑	❑	❑	❑	50.	❑	❑	❑	❑
25.	❑	❑	❑	❑	51.	❑	❑	❑	❑
26.	❑	❑	❑	❑	52.	❑	❑	❑	❑

	A	B	C	D		A	B	C	D
53.	❏	❏	❏	❏	67.	❏	❏	❏	❏
54.	❏	❏	❏	❏	68.	❏	❏	❏	❏
55.	❏	❏	❏	❏	69.	❏	❏	❏	❏
56.	❏	❏	❏	❏	70.	❏	❏	❏	❏
57.	❏	❏	❏	❏	71.	❏	❏	❏	❏
58.	❏	❏	❏	❏	72.	❏	❏	❏	❏
59.	❏	❏	❏	❏	73.	❏	❏	❏	❏
60.	❏	❏	❏	❏	74.	❏	❏	❏	❏
61.	❏	❏	❏	❏	75.	❏	❏	❏	❏
62.	❏	❏	❏	❏	76.	❏	❏	❏	❏
63.	❏	❏	❏	❏	77.	❏	❏	❏	❏
64.	❏	❏	❏	❏	78.	❏	❏	❏	❏
65.	❏	❏	❏	❏	79.	❏	❏	❏	❏
66.	❏	❏	❏	❏	80.	❏	❏	❏	❏

30

Infectious and Communicable Diseases

1. A microorganism capable of causing disease is a/an:

    a. host.
    b. pathogen.
    c. parasite.
    d. infectious agent.

2. Nonpathogenic bacteria that live on the human skin, in the GI tract and in mucous membranes are called:

    a. normal flora.
    b. protozoa.
    c. fungi
    d. virus.

3. A single cell microscopic parasitic organism that causes infection is a/an:

    a. normal flora.
    b. protozoa.
    c. fungus.
    d. virus.

4. A parasitic organism that can only live within a cell of a living animal or plant is a/an:

    a. helminth.
    b. host.
    c. fungi.
    d. virus.

5. Bacterial infections cause:

    a. nausea.
    b. malnourishment.
    c. headache.
    d. fever.

6. All the following can influence an individual's susceptibility to infection, *except*:

    a. age.
    b. gender.
    c. nutrition.
    d. latency period.

7. Which of the following is an example of an external barrier found on the human body?

    a. hair
    b. teeth
    c. skin
    d. ear wax

8. The period after an exposure has occurred to a host when the infection cannot be transmitted to someone else is the _____ period.

    a. refractory
    b. latency
    c. communicable
    d. disease

9. The duration of time between exposure to a host and the development of signs and symptoms of the disease is the _____ period.

    a. communicable
    b. incubation
    c. immune
    d. inflammatory

10. The duration of time from onset of symptoms to resolution of symptoms or death is called the _____ period.

    a. refractory
    b. resolution
    c. distribution
    d. disease

11. The _____ is responsible for reporting to the County Health Department communicable diseases seen by prehospital health care providers.

    a. paramedic
    b. hospital
    c. patient's personal physician
    d. nursing home

12. The Ryan-White Act of 1990 requires that exposure notification to emergency responders must be made within _____ hours.

    a. 12
    b. 24
    c. 48
    d. 72

13. OSHA is an example of a _____ level agency involved in disease outbreak.

    a. Federal
    b. State
    c. Local
    d. Private sector

14. CDC recommends all the following immunizations for EMS providers, *except*:

    a. HCV
    b. HBV
    c. Polio
    d. MMR

15. Which of the following infections can be caused by needle stick?

    a. HBV, HCV, & HIV
    b. HBV, HIV & pneumonia
    c. HIV, UTI & URI
    d. HIV, TB & pneumonia

16. The single most important task a health care provider can do to reduce the transmission of communicable disease is:

    a. not recap needles.
    b. dispose of all needles into sharps containers.
    c. place biohazards in red bags.
    d. wash hands.

17. All the following are examples of a significant exposure, *except*:

    a. needle stick
    b. blood contact with broken skin.
    c. inhaling air droplets.
    d. fecal contact to hands.

18. Which of the following clinical findings would lead you to suspect a patient is infectious?

    a. shortness of breath
    b. hypertensive teenager
    c. hypothermic geriatric
    d. hypothermic pediatric

19. What is the most common serious infectious disease in the United States?

    a. HIV
    b. AIDS
    c. Hepatitis
    d. TB

20. How many types of hepatitis are there?

    a. 5
    b. 6
    c. 7
    d. 8

21. A person started the series of three hepatitis B vaccinations, but failed to receive the last shot. Now, two years later, he wants to complete the vaccination. How should he complete the series?

    a. restart the entire series
    b. repeat only the second dose
    c. complete only the third dose
    d. completion is no longer recommended

22. Primary contraction of HCV is through direct contact with blood, such as a needle stick and:

    a. sexual contact.
    b. airborne droplet.
    c. indirect contact with urine.
    d. indirect contact with feces.

23. Which of the following infectious diseases does not have a known vaccine?

    a. HBV
    b. HCV
    c. Chickenpox
    d. Pneumococcal disease

24. What is the primary mode of transmission for HAV?

    a. needle stick
    b. oral–fecal
    c. airborne droplet
    d. direct contact with blood

25. What is the most common symptom of active TB?

    a. productive cough
    b. shortness of breath
    c. fever
    d. weakness

26. Which, of the following, does not pose a risk for transmission of HBV and HCV?

a. needle stick
b. open sore contact
c. sexual contact
d. contact with saliva

27. Which, of the following, is the cause of most stomach ulcers?

a. stress
b. spicy foods
c. stomach acid
d. bacteria

28. An acute viral infectious disease of the CNS that causes painful muscle spasms in the throat and interferes with swallowing, leading to dehydration and death is:

a. salmonella.
b. rabies.
c. AIDS.
d. arbovirus.

29. _____ is usually transmitted to humans by eating foods contaminated with animal feces.

a. Salmonella
b. Rabies
c. Lyme disease
d. Arbovirus

30. A person infected with _____ can pass on the disease by touching food after using the toilet and not washing his/her hands.

a. salmonella
b. varicella
c. Lyme disease
d. arbovirus

31. Lyme disease is transmitted by a tick bite. The infection does not occur until an infected tick has been attached for _____ hours.

a. 6–12
b. 12–24
c. 24–36
d. 36–48

32. Signs and symptoms of _____ include flu-like symptoms, muscle ache, joint pain with or without a rash.

a. chickenpox
b. rabies
c. Lyme disease
d. pneumonia

33. All the following are examples of infectious agents, *except*:

a. bacteria.
b. helminths.
c. protozoa.
d. gram stain.

34. An example of a human internal barrier that protects against infectious diseases is:

a. normal flora.
b. an inflammatory response.
c. Cushing's response.
d. endorphins.

35. The liaison that makes notification between the hospital and an exposed emergency responder is the EMS agency's:

a. medical director.
b. designated officer.
c. chief supervisor.
d. dispatcher.

36. _____ is an example of a national level agency involved in disease outbreak.

a. CDC
b. NIOSH
c. U.S. Fire Protection Administration
d. HMO

37. _____ is included in the top ten recommended vaccinations for children.

a. HAV
b. Varicella
c. Influenza
d. HPV

38. _____ is an approach to infection control, which is based on the assumption that all blood and body fluids are potentially infectious.

a. BSI
b. PPE
c. Hand washing
d. Biohazard labeling

39. The most commonly spread illnesses passed on by touching droplets from sneezing and coughing are influenza, the common cold and:

a. TB
b. HPV
c. pneumonia
d. staph

40. Biohazardous wastes are placed in _____ bags that are labeled accordingly for disposal.

   a. clear
   b. yellow
   c. red
   d. green

41. All needles and sharps must be discarded in _____ that are properly labeled.

   a. red bags
   b. puncture proof containers
   c. red containers
   d. unbreakable glass containers

42. All the following are clinical features of an infectious or communicable disease, *except*:

   a. coughing.
   b. nuchal rigidity.
   c. a bleeding laceration.
   d. hepatomegaly.

43. A _____ is a test using a sample of blood to measure the amount of antibody against a particular antigen in that blood.

   a. gloucomene
   b. titer
   c. ram stain
   d. hemacult

44. After a paramedic is exposed to HBV while on the job, the _____ must assure and pay for proper medical follow-up.

   a. patient
   b. paramedic
   c. employer
   d. hospital

45. In the United States, TB is most prevalent in nursing homes, homeless shelters, prisons, and:

   a. shopping malls.
   b. migrant farm camps.
   c. hospitals.
   d. community housing developments.

46. _____ is often called the stomach flu. It is incorrectly used to describe many types of infections and irritations of the digestive tract.

   a. Ulcers.
   b. Esophageal reflux
   c. Gastroenteritis
   d. *Helicobacteria pylori*

47. Diseases caused by _____ include the West Nile virus, encephalitis, yellow fever and dengue.

   a. the Lyme tick
   b. arbovirus
   c. meningitis
   d. the plague

48. Advanced clinical features of _____ include AMS, paralyseis, parethesia, stiff neck, sensitivity to light, arrhythmias and chest pain.

   a. varicella
   b. salmonella
   c. Lyme disease
   d. HBV

49. The principal forms of plague are bubonic, septicemic and:

   a. pneumonic.
   b. pulmonic.
   c. cardiogenic.
   d. enteric.

50. In recent times the most cases of plague in the United States have been reported in New Mexico, Arizona, California and:

   a. Alaska.
   b. Colorado.
   c. New York.
   d. Florida.

Test #30 Answer Form

	A	B	C	D			A	B	C	D
1.	❏	❏	❏	❏		26.	❏	❏	❏	❏
2.	❏	❏	❏	❏		27.	❏	❏	❏	❏
3.	❏	❏	❏	❏		28.	❏	❏	❏	❏
4.	❏	❏	❏	❏		29.	❏	❏	❏	❏
5.	❏	❏	❏	❏		30.	❏	❏	❏	❏
6.	❏	❏	❏	❏		31.	❏	❏	❏	❏
7.	❏	❏	❏	❏		32.	❏	❏	❏	❏
8.	❏	❏	❏	❏		33.	❏	❏	❏	❏
9.	❏	❏	❏	❏		34.	❏	❏	❏	❏
10.	❏	❏	❏	❏		35.	❏	❏	❏	❏
11.	❏	❏	❏	❏		36.	❏	❏	❏	❏
12.	❏	❏	❏	❏		37.	❏	❏	❏	❏
13.	❏	❏	❏	❏		38.	❏	❏	❏	❏
14.	❏	❏	❏	❏		39.	❏	❏	❏	❏
15.	❏	❏	❏	❏		40.	❏	❏	❏	❏
16.	❏	❏	❏	❏		41.	❏	❏	❏	❏
17.	❏	❏	❏	❏		42.	❏	❏	❏	❏
18.	❏	❏	❏	❏		43.	❏	❏	❏	❏
19.	❏	❏	❏	❏		44.	❏	❏	❏	❏
20.	❏	❏	❏	❏		45.	❏	❏	❏	❏
21.	❏	❏	❏	❏		46.	❏	❏	❏	❏
22.	❏	❏	❏	❏		47.	❏	❏	❏	❏
23.	❏	❏	❏	❏		48.	❏	❏	❏	❏
24.	❏	❏	❏	❏		49.	❏	❏	❏	❏
25.	❏	❏	❏	❏		50.	❏	❏	❏	❏

31

Behavioral and Psychiatric Disorders

1. A/an _____ is a strong feeling, often accompanied by physical signs such as tachycardia and diaphoresis.

   a. disorder
   b. emotion
   c. nightmare
   d. daydream

2. Any disturbance of emotional balance, manifested by maladaptive behavior and impaired function, is called:

   a. insanity.
   b. mental disorder.
   c. normalcy.
   d. malfunction.

3. Which of the following statements about mental illness is true?

   a. In the United States, behavioral and psychiatric disorders incapacitate more people than all other health problems combined.
   b. Mental disorders are most often incurable.
   c. Studies have shown that most mentally disabled patients are unstable and dangerous.
   d. Abnormal behavior is always bizarre.

4. Which of the following statements about mental illness is false?

   a. In many cases psychiatric illness has an organic basis.
   b. Many patients with mental illness are calm and never present a danger.
   c. Having a mental disorder is cause for embarrassment and shame.
   d. Modern medical and psycho-therapeutic techniques can provide stabilized treatment for most mental disorders.

5. All the following are types of classifications of psychiatric disorders, *except*:

   a. anxiety.
   b. mood.
   c. adolescence.
   d. substance-related.

6. Delirium and dementia are examples of _____ disorders.

   a. cognitive
   b. psychotic
   c. mood
   d. somatoform

7. _____ is a type of disorder that involves gross distortions of reality.

   a. Anxiety
   b. Schizophrenia
   c. Substance-related
   d. Somatoform

8. A mood disorder consisting of alternating periods of depression and mania is called:

   a. dementia.
   b. psychosis.
   c. hallucinations.
   d. bipolar.

9. Panic disorders, phobias, and post-traumatic syndromes are all examples of _____ disorders.

   a. insanity
   b. mood
   c. anxiety
   d. paranoia

10. Dependence is a _____ craving for a chemical agent, resulting from abuse or addiction.

    a. psychologic
    b. physical
    c. neural
    d. spiritual

11. _____ disorders are a group of neurotic disorders with symptoms suggesting physical disease, but with no demonstrable organic causes.

    a. Dissociative
    b. Somatoform
    c. Eating
    d. Factitious

12. A type of neurosis in which emotions are so repressed that a split occurs in the personality is what type of disorder?

    a. dissociative
    b. somatoform
    c. insanity
    d. factitious

13. _____ disorders are a large category of mental disorders characterized by inflexible and maladaptive behavior that impairs a person's ability to function in society.

    a. Dissociative
    b. Impulsive
    c. Personality
    d. Schizophrenic

14. All the following factors can alter the behavior of an ill or injured individual, *except*:

    a. the patient's perception of the health care provider.
    b. the patient's perceived degree of pain or severity of illness.
    c. a history of previous emotional illness.
    d. future experiences of the actual degree of pain or severity of illness.

15. With respect to medical legal concerns, the paramedic should be aware of local facilities and procedures for:

    a. alcohol ingestion.
    b. registration of sexual predators.
    c. crisis intervention.
    d. definitive care.

16. The paramedic is responsible for knowing both local protocols and _____ regarding treatment of persons with mental illnesses.

    a. family wishes
    b. state laws
    c. advanced directives
    d. federal briefs

17. Many mental illnesses have been shown to occur from chemical alteration in the brain. These chemicals are called:

    a. neurons.
    b. antidepressants.
    c. neurotransmitters.
    d. neuters.

18. Just because a person is on a "psych" drug does not mean that he/she has an emotional illness, as several of these agents are useful in other conditions such as:

    a. diabetes.
    b. toothaches.
    c. acne.
    d. migraine headaches.

19. When a paramedic is assessing a patient displaying abnormal motor activity, he/she should always consider the possibility of hypoxia, drug intoxification, blood sugar abnormality, and:

    a. pain.
    b. abnormal thought content.
    c. stimulated intellectual function.
    d. mood disorders.

20. During the assessment of a patient, the paramedic should be alert for examples of overt behaviors associated with behavioral and psychiatric disorders such as:

    a. poor hygiene.
    b. hypoglycemia.
    c. a lack of family support.
    d. multiple pets.

21. _____ are irrational, intense, and obsessive fears of specific things such as an object or a physical situation.

    a. Hysterias
    b. Impulses
    c. Anxieties
    d. Phobias

22. Which of the following is an example of when the paramedic may need to transport a patient against his or her will?

    a. when the patient has no available transportation
    b. when the patient exhibits a danger to others
    c. when dental care is needed
    d. after the patient falls and needs assistance getting up

23. Most people have fears and concerns. However, these fears become _____ when they significantly interfere with normal daily activities.

    a. phobias
    b. addictions
    c. impulses
    d. nightmares

24. The state of incoherent excitement, confused speech, restlessness, and sometimes hallucinations often caused by acute illness or drug intoxication is referred to as:

    a. depression.
    b. delirium.
    c. dementia.
    d. paranoia.

25. As a rule, most experts believe that the paramedic will be able to provide better care to a person with a behavioral emergency when _____ are not present.

    a. police
    b. relatives
    c. EMS supervisors
    d. pets

26. A _____ is something done by a person intending to ask for help, rather than die.

    a. homicide attempt
    b. homicide gesture
    c. suicide attempt
    d. suicide gesture

27. A behavioral emergency only occurs when a person is:

    a. insane.
    b. neurotic.
    c. unable to cope.
    d. experiencing a loss.

28. _____ is when a patient has no conception whatsoever of reality.

    a. Psychosis
    b. Neurosis
    c. Anxiety
    d. Phobia

29. The best way to deal with a patient experiencing hallucinations is:

    a. to use a chemical restraint.
    b. the "talk-down" technique.
    c. to use physical restraint.
    d. to shout at the patient.

30. All the following are signs or symptoms that a person is depressed, *except*:

    a. paranoia.
    b. significant weight gain.
    c. sleep disturbances.
    d. decreased appetite.

31. Organic causes of apparent emotional and psychiatric illness in older patients include all the following, *except*:

    a. prescribed medications.
    b. polypharmacy.
    c. climate changes.
    d. severe infections.

32. Mania or excessive hyperactivity is an example of a(an) _____ disorder.

    a. impulsive control
    b. eating
    c. personality
    d. mood

33. _____ is a condition characterized by an overwhelming desire to continue taking a drug on which one has become "hooked" through repeated consumption.

    a. Dependence
    b. Intoxication
    c. Addiction
    d. Abuse

34. _____ relates to acute effects of taking a substance and may or may not be related to dependence.

    a. Alcoholism
    b. Intoxication
    c. Addiction
    d. Abuse

35. True _____ is both a psychologic and physical event, whereby the patient has both a physical and psychologic craving for the drug, as well as the effect.

   a. dependence
   b. intoxication
   c. addiction
   d. neurosis

36. As a rule, if a person has a psychiatric disorder and then develops a drug addiction or alcoholism, the underlying psychiatric condition:

   a. improves.
   b. worsens.
   c. is cured.
   d. shows no change.

37. With respect to emotional illness, the term for assuming a certain body–language position suggestive of a particular emotion is:

   a. affect.
   b. fear.
   c. mental status.
   d. posture.

38. The term _____ refers to a state of mind in which one is uncertain of the present time, place, or self-identity.

   a. anger
   b. delirium
   c. confusion
   d. bipolar

39. The term _____ refers to the emotional tone behind an expressed emotion or behavior.

   a. fear
   b. anxiety
   c. affect
   d. mental status

40. While interviewing an emotionally disturbed patient, which of the following is a therapeutic interview technique the paramedic might use?

   a. look directly into the patient's eyes
   b. promptly interrupt the patient when he/she becomes too talkative
   c. avoid asking questions about the immediate problem
   d. engage in active listening

41. Management of behavioral emergencies begins with maintaining scene and personal safety and then the paramedic should:

   a. begin the physical exam.
   b. build a good rapport with the patient.
   c. wait until the crisis team arrives before beginning care.
   d. have the police stand over the patient.

42. If a situation escalates and you become trapped by the patient, what should you do until help arrives?

   a. scream for help
   b. do not say anything
   c. keep talking to the patient
   d. threaten the patient with bodily harm

43. All the following are factors that increase the risk that a person is suicidal, except:

   a. no prior history of suicide attempts.
   b. male gender.
   c. excessive alcohol or drug use.
   d. a person who is divorced.

44. Studies report that the risk of suicide in men is double that of women after experiencing a divorce or marital separation primarily because:

   a. men are mentally weaker than women.
   b. women have better support systems.
   c. men lack certain female hormones.
   d. women tend to remarry more quickly than men.

45. The term _____ refers specifically to physical problems brought about by underlying emotional problems.

   a. somatogenesis
   b. pseudopsychosis
   c. psychosomatic illness
   d. psychogenic disease

46. Clues that a patient may develop violent behavior include all the following, except:

   a. pacing back and forth.
   b. bragging about being a tough guy.
   c. domestic violence situation.
   d. attempted suicide.

47. Which of the following statements about neurotic fear is true:

   a. A person with neurosis is probably insane.
   b. People with neurosis are not crazy.
   c. Most people with neurosis cannot cope with their fears.
   d. Neurosis is a normal anxiety reaction to a perceived fear.

48. Elderly persons commonly appear to have organic illnesses such as cardiac conditions when, in reality, they are:

   a. severely depressed.
   b. lonely.
   c. over-medicated.
   d. under-medicated.

49. Which of the following statements best describes how phobias can be unhealthy?

   a. Phobias can cause AMS.
   b. People with phobias are prone to AMI.
   c. Phobias are not unhealthy.
   d. Phobias can interfere with daily living activities.

50. Which of the following statements about "open-ended" questions is not true?

   a. They are used to encourage better patient responses.
   b. They tend to lead the patient to a specific answer.
   c. They are less likely to provoke an untoward patient response.
   d. They give the patient an opportunity to vent.

Test #31 Answer Form

	A	B	C	D		A	B	C	D
1.	❏	❏	❏	❏	26.	❏	❏	❏	❏
2.	❏	❏	❏	❏	27.	❏	❏	❏	❏
3.	❏	❏	❏	❏	28.	❏	❏	❏	❏
4.	❏	❏	❏	❏	29.	❏	❏	❏	❏
5.	❏	❏	❏	❏	30.	❏	❏	❏	❏
6.	❏	❏	❏	❏	31.	❏	❏	❏	❏
7.	❏	❏	❏	❏	32.	❏	❏	❏	❏
8.	❏	❏	❏	❏	33.	❏	❏	❏	❏
9.	❏	❏	❏	❏	34.	❏	❏	❏	❏
10.	❏	❏	❏	❏	35.	❏	❏	❏	❏
11.	❏	❏	❏	❏	36.	❏	❏	❏	❏
12.	❏	❏	❏	❏	37.	❏	❏	❏	❏
13.	❏	❏	❏	❏	38.	❏	❏	❏	❏
14.	❏	❏	❏	❏	39.	❏	❏	❏	❏
15.	❏	❏	❏	❏	40.	❏	❏	❏	❏
16.	❏	❏	❏	❏	41.	❏	❏	❏	❏
17.	❏	❏	❏	❏	42.	❏	❏	❏	❏
18.	❏	❏	❏	❏	43.	❏	❏	❏	❏
19.	❏	❏	❏	❏	44.	❏	❏	❏	❏
20.	❏	❏	❏	❏	45.	❏	❏	❏	❏
21.	❏	❏	❏	❏	46.	❏	❏	❏	❏
22.	❏	❏	❏	❏	47.	❏	❏	❏	❏
23.	❏	❏	❏	❏	48.	❏	❏	❏	❏
24.	❏	❏	❏	❏	49.	❏	❏	❏	❏
25.	❏	❏	❏	❏	50.	❏	❏	❏	❏

32

Hematology

1. What is the name of the body system that produces blood cells?

   a. Hepatic
   b. Hemophilic
   c. Hematopoietic
   d. Uremic

2. The key components of the body system described in question 1, include the liver, spleen and:

   a. kidneys.
   b. bone marrow.
   c. gray matter.
   d. CFS.

3. The majority of the blood cells are formed in the:

   a. spleen.
   b. liver.
   c. lungs.
   d. bone marrow.

4. The average pH of the blood is:

   a. 7.30
   b. 7.35
   c. 7.40
   d. 7.45

5. Men have approximately _____ cc of blood per kg of body weight.

   a. 60
   b. 70
   c. 80
   d. 90

6. During fetal development, red blood cells are produced in the:

   a. lungs.
   b. kidneys.
   c. umbilical cord.
   d. spleen.

7. All the elements in the red cells, white cells and platelets are derived from the:

   a. leukocytes.
   b. stem cell.
   c. monocytes.
   d. erythrocytes.

8. How many days do mature red blood cells normally circulate in the blood?

   a. 30
   b. 60
   c. 120
   d. 240

9. Hemoglobin byproducts are excreted by the body in the form of:

   a. bilirubin.
   b. hemotoxins.
   c. urine.
   d. cytokines.

10. The measure of the number of red blood cells per unit of blood volume is called the:

    a. pulse oximetry.
    b. end tidal CO_2.
    c. hematocrit.
    d. hematacult.

11. When a patient has a low number of red blood cells, this chronic condition is called:

    a. hematuria.
    b. polycythemia.
    c. hypocythemia.
    d. anemia.

12. The normal range of hematocrit for women is:

    a. 36–46.
    b. 44–49.
    c. 50–54.
    d. 55–60.

13. The normal range of hematocrit for men is:

    a. 36–42.
    b. 40–45.
    c. 41–53.
    d. 50–55.

14. Neutrophils, eosinophils and basophils are different types of:

    a. platelets.
    b. granulocytes.
    c. leucocytes.
    d. hemoglobins.

15. Cells without intracellular granules are called:

    a. neutrophils.
    b. monocytes.
    c. exudates.
    d. hemocells.

16. The main function of a leukocyte is to:

    a. carry oxygen to body cells.
    b. provide the color for the blood.
    c. maintain host defenses against infection.
    d. keep the blood clean of byproducts.

17. Another name for pus is:

    a. anemic discharge.
    b. purulent exudate.
    c. productive sputum.
    d. polycythemia.

18. Antibody-mediated immunity is also called:

    a. humoral immunity.
    b. anemia.
    c. cellular immunity.
    d. leukemia.

19. When a patient has a low number of WBCs this is called:

    a. leukopenia.
    b. leukocytosis.
    c. leukemia.
    d. anemia.

20. Platelets circulate in the blood for an average of _____ days before being removed by the spleen.

    a. 2–5
    b. 7–10
    c. 20–28
    d. 30–45

21. The aggregation of platelets may be decreased by:

    a. high cholesterol in foods.
    b. polycythemia.
    c. anti-inflammatory drugs.
    d. chronic anemia.

22. Immediately after vascular injury, which of the following occurs?

    a. The vessel contracts in the vicinity of injury.
    b. Platelets bind to the exposed binding sites.
    c. Bound platelets release granules that recruit further platelets.
    d. All of the above.

23. The substance that is the final "glue" that completes the blood clot is:

    a. hemoglobin.
    b. epithelium.
    c. fibrin.
    d. elastin.

24. Human blood groups are determined by the presence or absence of two antigens, A and B, on the surface of _____cells.

    a. platelet
    b. red blood
    c. white blood
    d. stem

25. The universal blood recipients with type _____ blood have no antibodies.

    a. A
    b. B
    c. AB
    d. O

26. People with type _____ have no antigens and are considered universal donors.

    a. A
    b. B
    c. AB
    d. O

27. Which of the following hematologic conditions is associated with shortness of breath and severe abdominal pain?

    a. Anemia
    b. Sickle cell crisis
    c. Leukemia
    d. Myeloma

28. The hematologic condition which rarely affects females but is sex-linked by transmission from a mother to a son and is characterized by excessive bleeding after minor wounds is:

    a. amemia.
    b. sickle cell disease.
    c. hemophilia.
    d. leukemia.

29. _____ results from a malignant tumor of blood-forming tissues, and is characterized by abnormalities of the bone marrow, spleen, lymph nodes and liver.

    a. Polycythemia
    b. Sickle cell disease
    c. Hemophilia
    d. Leukemia

30. Which of the following drugs or herbs does not decrease the aggregation of platelets?

    a. Thyme
    b. Aspirin
    c. Ibuprofen
    d. Ginseng

31. _____ is the body's natural and normal way of preventing excess blood clot formation.

    a. Fibrinolysis
    b. Electrolysis
    c. Plasminolysis
    d. Neutrolysis

32. The main function of leukocytes is to maintain host defenses against infection, particularly _____ infection.

    a. viral
    b. bacterial
    c. fungal
    d. protozoa

33. Which of the following granulocytes in the blood are important in fighting allergic reactions?

    a. Neutrophils and eosinophils
    b. Neutrophils and basophils
    c. Eosinophils and basophils
    d. None of the above.

34. When a clinician refers to a patient's H & H, they are referring to the patient's hematocrit and:

    a. hypoxia.
    b. hemoglobin.
    c. hematology.
    d. hematuria.

35. Which of the following conditions when severe, is characterized by fatigue, dyspnea, chest pain or syncopy?

    a. Anemia
    b. Leukemia
    c. Lymphomas
    d. Hemophilia

Test #32 Answer Form

	A	B	C	D			A	B	C	D
1.	❑	❑	❑	❑		19.	❑	❑	❑	❑
2.	❑	❑	❑	❑		20.	❑	❑	❑	❑
3.	❑	❑	❑	❑		21.	❑	❑	❑	❑
4.	❑	❑	❑	❑		22.	❑	❑	❑	❑
5.	❑	❑	❑	❑		23.	❑	❑	❑	❑
6.	❑	❑	❑	❑		24.	❑	❑	❑	❑
7.	❑	❑	❑	❑		25.	❑	❑	❑	❑
8.	❑	❑	❑	❑		26.	❑	❑	❑	❑
9.	❑	❑	❑	❑		27.	❑	❑	❑	❑
10.	❑	❑	❑	❑		28.	❑	❑	❑	❑
11.	❑	❑	❑	❑		29.	❑	❑	❑	❑
12.	❑	❑	❑	❑		30.	❑	❑	❑	❑
13.	❑	❑	❑	❑		31.	❑	❑	❑	❑
14.	❑	❑	❑	❑		32.	❑	❑	❑	❑
15.	❑	❑	❑	❑		33.	❑	❑	❑	❑
16.	❑	❑	❑	❑		34.	❑	❑	❑	❑
17.	❑	❑	❑	❑		35.	❑	❑	❑	❑
18.	❑	❑	❑	❑						

Gynecology and Obstetrics

1. Which of the following structures does not form the female external genitalia?

   a. mons pubis
   b. urethra
   c. perineum
   d. urinary meatus

2. Which of the following structures of the female genitalia is responsible for sexual hormone secretion?

   a. ovaries
   b. fallopian tubes
   c. myometrium
   d. fimbriae

3. Which of the following statements is incorrect in reference to the fallopian tubes?

   a. Ova take 3 to 4 days to travel through the fallopian tubes.
   b. The fimbriae at the ends of the tubes are connected to the ovaries.
   c. Fallopian tubes extend out laterally from the top of the uterus.
   d. Fallopian tubes are also known as oviducts.

4. The base of the uterus is called the:

   a. fundus.
   b. cervix.
   c. uterine cavity.
   d. endometrium.

5. A developing child in utero under eights weeks gestation is called the:

   a. fetus.
   b. embryo.
   c. ova.
   d. oocyte.

6. The umbilical vein is responsibility for:

   a. the production of amniotic fluid.
   b. carrying fetal blood to the placenta.
   c. returning oxygenated blood from the fetus to the placenta.
   d. returning oxygenated blood from the placenta to the fetus.

7. Amniocentesis is a procedure that removes a sample of amniotic fluid for the purpose of evaluation of all the following, *except*:

   a. gender of the child.
   b. genetic disorders.
   c. biochemical disorders.
   d. multiple fetuses.

8. The normal menstrual cycle is 28 days and can be divided into three phases: menses, the proliferative phase and:

   a. the secretory phase.
   b. the sloughing phase.
   c. PMS.
   d. post-capillary washout.

9. All the following are true about premenstrual dysphoric disorder, *except* the:

   a. condition involves physical symptoms.
   b. condition involves emotional symptoms.
   c. cause of the condition is hormonal.
   d. treatment of the condition is aimed at relieving the symptoms.

10. Abnormal amenorrhea can occur with all the following, *except*:

    a. extreme and prolonged exercise.
    b. malnutrition.
    c. syphilis.
    d. pregnancy.

11. The hormone _____ is responsible for stimulating bone and muscle growth.

    a. estrogen
    b. progesterone
    c. actin
    d. testosterone

12. The hormone responsible for restoring and preparing the uterus for pregnancy after menses is:

    a. estrogen.
    b. progesterone.
    c. oxytocin.
    d. pitocin.

13. Fertilization is the union of the egg and sperm which forms the:

    a. zygote.
    b. ovum.
    c. fetus.
    d. corpus luteum.

14. Common signs and symptoms associated with pelvic inflammatory disease (PID) include all the following, *except*:

    a. nausea and vomiting.
    b. acute abdominal pain.
    c. headache.
    d. abnormal discharge.

15. _____ is the leading cause of female infertility and ectopic pregnancy.

    a. peritonitis
    b. genital warts
    c. vaginal yeast infections
    d. PID

16. What is the most common bacterial STD?

    a. Syphilis
    b. Gonorrhea
    c. Pubic lice
    d. Chlamydia

17. Besides menstruation, other causes of vaginal bleeding include all the following, *except*:

    a. labor.
    b. sexual abuse.
    c. PID.
    d. UTI.

18. Cystitis is a _____ infection, which often occurs secondary to a urinary tract infection (UTI).

    a. kidney
    b. bladder
    c. urethra
    d. ovarian

19. You are assessing a 26-year-old female who is 24 weeks pregnant. She is complaining of acute abdominal pain that is constant and severe. The pregnancy has been normal and she has prenatal care. She feels the baby moving. However, she is having a small amount of bloody discharge that just began. You suspect which of the following?

    a. ectopic pregnancy.
    b. abruptio placenta.
    c. placenta previa.
    d. spontaneous abortion.

20. How do you manage the patient described in question 19?

    a. Administer high flow oxygen and begin transport.
    b. Treat for shock and begin transport.
    c. Have the patient call her gynecologist because delivery is imminent.
    d. Prepare the patient mentally for a spontaneous abortion.

21. Pregnant women with a negative Rh factor may become sensitized if the fetus has a positive Rh factor. If a fetus in any subsequent pregnancies has a positive Rh factor, Rh antibodies may cross the placenta and:

    a. suppress the immune response.
    b. destroy fetal cells.
    c. cause gestational diabetes.
    d. precipitate preclampsia.

22. You are dispatched to a call of respiratory distress. Upon arrival you find a 36-year-old female who is 38 weeks pregnant. She is having severe difficulty breathing that began one hour ago and is getting progressively worse. She has no history of asthma, COPD or cardiac problems and her pregnancy has been normal with regular prenatal care. What do you suspect is the problem?

    a. Heart attack
    b. Hyperventilation
    c. Pulmonary embolism
    d. Pneumothrorax

23. Your management plan for the patient in question 22 includes:

    a. IV fluid replacement.
    b. nebulized albuterol treatment.
    c. assisted breathing and chest decompression.
    d. rapid transport for a life-threatening condition.

24. Normal changes that occur during pregnancy include all the following, *except*:

    a. increased heart rate.
    b. decreased B/P during second trimester.
    c. increased peripheral edema.
    d. increased cardiac output.

25. Women in third trimester pregnancy are at increased risk of vomiting during injury and illness because of:

    a. a decreased tidal volume.
    b. slowed peristalsis.
    c. increased appetite.
    d. nausea from morning sickness.

26. Palpation of the fundus during active labor is performed to determine all the following, *except*:

    a. size of the baby's head.
    b. length of contraction.
    c. measure height of fundus to estimate gestational age.
    d. strength of contraction.

27. Back labor is back pain caused by the fetus pressing against the _____ during labor.

    a. spine
    b. kidneys
    c. bladder
    d. vena cava

28. The hormone _____ secreted by the pituitary gland stimulates the uterus to produce stronger contractions.

    a. estrogen
    b. progesterone
    c. oxytocin
    d. epinephrine

29. In which of the following cases would it be appropriate not to start an IV on a woman in active labor?

    a. contractions are abnormal
    b. labor is two weeks early, but the mother is mentally competent and refuses
    c. postpartem hemorrhage began before delivery of the placenta
    d. the mother is full term with twins

30. While assisting the mother during delivery, the paramedic prepares to prevent an explosive delivery by:

    a. coaching the mother to breathe deeply.
    b. coaching the mother to pant during contractions.
    c. having the mother raise her hips when the head delivers.
    d. holding one hand on the baby's head while the mother is pushing.

31. Once the baby's head delivers the paramedic should:

    a. inspect the head for trauma.
    b. inspect for a nuchal cord.
    c. perform the first APGAR score.
    d. dry the head and face.

32. Once the baby's head is out, the natural progression is for the baby's face to turn:

    a. laterally.
    b. superiorly.
    c. purple.
    d. inferiorly.

33. The APGAR score is a well-accepted assessment score chart for evaluating infants by rating the muscle tone, heart rate, respirations and:

    a. reflex and color.
    b. color and weight.
    c. B/P and reflex.
    d. B/P and color.

34. In the field the primary reason to cut the cord soon after the birth is that:

    a. the baby will suckle quicker.
    b. stage III of labor will progress quicker.
    c. the baby will be easier to manage and assess.
    d. the mother will not tear the cord.

35. When the cord is not cut immediately, the infant should be placed _____ to prevent placental transfusion.

    a. at a higher level than the placenta
    b. at a lower level than the placenta
    c. in an incubator
    d. in an infant swaddler

36. When access for medication is needed in the newborn, which of the following is preferred?

    a. IO
    b. ET
    c. umbilical vein cannulation
    d. umbilical artery cannulation

37. You have arrived at the scene of a serious MVC and find an unconscious young women, who is obviously pregnant, behind the wheel. She is breathing agonal respirations as you approach. You assist her ventilations while your crew quickly extricates her from the vehicle. You advise your crew to position her on a long board with:

    a. her legs elevated.
    b. her head elevated.
    c. right side of the board elevated slightly.
    d. left side of the board elevated slightly.

38. You continue to aggressively treat the patient in the previous question by intubating her, while your crew obtains vital signs. Her pulse is 110 and B/P is 80/40. Your management plan enroute includes:

    a. aggressive fluid replacement.
    b. the application of MAST/PASG.
    c. the use of vasopressors.
    d. rapid transport to the nearest ED

39. Listening for fetal heart tones is the standard of care:

    a. for distressed fetuses in the prehospital setting.
    b. only when a Doppler is available.
    c. only in third trimester pregnancies.
    d. in the clinical setting and not in the field.

40. All the following are correct about Braxton Hicks contractions, *except* they:

    a. are relatively short-lived and benign.
    b. are practice contractions to prepare the uterus.
    c. can be relieved by drinking milk.
    d. are often relieved with mild exercise.

41. The primary impact on the fetus from a state of shock in the mother includes:

    a. increased risk of hypothermia.
    b. hypoglycemic environment for the fetus.
    c. decreased liver function for the fetus.
    d. shunting of blood from the fetus.

42. Which of the following is a secondary injury from a sexual assault?

    a. lacerations to the external genitalia
    b. STDs
    c. bruising on the mons pubis
    d. rectal tears

43. Preserving evidence from the crime scene by the paramedic includes all the following, *except*:

    a. bringing the victims clothing to the ED.
    b. bagging each item separately.
    c. using plastic bags to bag saved items.
    d. asking the victim not to bathe.

44. After assessing and addressing any life-threatening conditions, the management of the victim of a sexual assault is focused on:

    a. preserving evidence of the crime.
    b. providing emotional support.
    c. cleaning superficial wounds.
    d. reporting the crime to the appropriate person.

45. Sexual assault is a crime of violence and can occur in any age group. It is estimated that _____ females are raped during her lifetime.

    a. 1 in 3
    b. 1 in 5
    c. 1 in 10
    d. 1 in 20

46. _____ is the cessation of ovarian function and menstrual activity.

    a. Menarche
    b. Menopause
    c. Amenorrhea
    d. Mittleschmerz

47. All the following are examples of gynecologic emergencies, *except*:

    a. gall stones.
    b. ruptured ovarian cyst.
    c. ectopic pregnancy.
    d. sexual assault.

48. _____ is characterized by lower abdominal pain experienced by some women at the time of ovulation.

    a. Menarche
    b. Menopause
    c. Amenorrhea
    d. Mittleschmerz

49. _____ is an acute or chronic inflammation of the endometrium caused by bacterial infection.

    a. Endometriosis
    b. Endomeritis
    c. Cystitis
    d. Oophritis

50. The complications of vaginal bleeding include:

    a. infection.
    b. tissue scarring.
    c. shock and death.
    d. infertility.

51. You have been called to a multiparous woman who is having contractions and is at 34 weeks gestation. She tells you that the baby has not yet moved into a head down position. Her labor is very active and she feels like the baby is coming. You move the patient to your stretcher and prepare for transport. What is your management plan for this patient?

    a. Begin rapid transport to the hospital.
    b. Prepare for imminent delivery.
    c. Administer Pitocin®, as the fetus is premature.
    d. Position the mother in Trendelenburg's position.

52. How would you assess the woman in question 51 for signs of imminent delivery?

    a. Measure the height of her fundus.
    b. Count her contractions.
    c. Observe the birth canal for crowning.
    d. Palpate the fundus for strength of contractions.

53. Next how would you continue to manage the patient in question 52?

   a. Start an IV and prepare an OB delivery kit.
   b. Monitor, reassess and continue rapid transport.
   c. Titrate the Pitocin® drip until desired affect is obtained.
   d. Call ahead to the ED to advise of cesarean section delivery.

54. As your partner backs into the ED the baby's feet and buttocks present. How would you continue?

   a. Ask the patient to stop pushing.
   b. Quickly move her into the ED before the head delivers.
   c. Allow the cord to deliver and support the body.
   d. Place a gloved hand in the birth canal to hold the fetus.

55. You are dispatched to a residence for postpartum hemorrhage. You arrive and find that a 32-year-old woman has given birth to a healthy baby with the help of a certified midwife. The pregnancy and birth were normal; however, after the delivery of the placenta the patient has had heavy blood loss, despite uterine massage. What is your management plan for this patient?

   a. Assist the midwife with direct pressure on the uterus.
   b. Treat for shock and begin transport.
   c. Encourage the mother to have the baby nurse during transport.
   d. Insert trauma dressings in the birth canal, apply MAST/PASG and begin transport.

56. Before you began transport, the midwife showed you that the placenta was whole and during your assessment of the patient, you do not observe any peritoneal tears. You suspect the cause of the heavy bleeding may be all the following, *except*:

   a. lack of uterine tone.
   b. a vaginal or cervical tear.
   c. a clotting disorder.
   d. the presence of an undelivered fetus.

57. Despite all your treatment on scene and enroute to the hospital, the patient continues to hemorrhage and is dropping her blood pressure steadily. You call Medical Control and give report. The doctor gives you an order to:

   a. administer an additional fluid bolus of up to two liters.
   b. begin a Pitocin® drip.
   c. stop uterine massage and inflate MAST/PASG.
   d. begin a dopamine drip.

58. In preparation for multiple births, such as with twins, the paramedic should expect all the following, *except*:

   a. delivery is never in the same manner as individual delivery.
   b. the mother may not know she is having twins.
   c. nearly 40% of twin deliveries are premature
   d. a breach presentation of one of the twins is common.

59. It is rare that the paramedic would ever have to place a gloved hand into the birth canal to manage the delivery. These rare occurrences include an umbilical cord presentation and a:

   a. complicated breach delivery.
   b. shoulder dystocia presentation.
   c. nuchal cord presentation.
   d. cephalopelvic disproportion.

60. After assisting with the normal delivery of a healthy baby, the patient suddenly complains of severe lower abdominal pain. She does not deliver the placenta, but begins heavy bleeding and the uterus is presenting from the vagina. You immediately recognize this as uterine inversion. Your management plan for this patient is to:

   a. attempt to deliver the placenta to control the bleeding.
   b. cover the protruding tissue with moist, sterile dressings.
   c. prepare to intubate the patient as she will probably develop a pulmonary embolis.
   d. start an IV, apply MAST/PASG and begin a rapid transport.

Test #33 Answer Form

	A	B	C	D		A	B	C	D
1.	❏	❏	❏	❏	27.	❏	❏	❏	❏
2.	❏	❏	❏	❏	28.	❏	❏	❏	❏
3.	❏	❏	❏	❏	29.	❏	❏	❏	❏
4.	❏	❏	❏	❏	30.	❏	❏	❏	❏
5.	❏	❏	❏	❏	31.	❏	❏	❏	❏
6.	❏	❏	❏	❏	32.	❏	❏	❏	❏
7.	❏	❏	❏	❏	33.	❏	❏	❏	❏
8.	❏	❏	❏	❏	34.	❏	❏	❏	❏
9.	❏	❏	❏	❏	35.	❏	❏	❏	❏
10.	❏	❏	❏	❏	36.	❏	❏	❏	❏
11.	❏	❏	❏	❏	37.	❏	❏	❏	❏
12.	❏	❏	❏	❏	38.	❏	❏	❏	❏
13.	❏	❏	❏	❏	39.	❏	❏	❏	❏
14.	❏	❏	❏	❏	40.	❏	❏	❏	❏
15.	❏	❏	❏	❏	41.	❏	❏	❏	❏
16.	❏	❏	❏	❏	42.	❏	❏	❏	❏
17.	❏	❏	❏	❏	43.	❏	❏	❏	❏
18.	❏	❏	❏	❏	44.	❏	❏	❏	❏
19.	❏	❏	❏	❏	45.	❏	❏	❏	❏
20.	❏	❏	❏	❏	46.	❏	❏	❏	❏
21.	❏	❏	❏	❏	47.	❏	❏	❏	❏
22.	❏	❏	❏	❏	48.	❏	❏	❏	❏
23.	❏	❏	❏	❏	49.	❏	❏	❏	❏
24.	❏	❏	❏	❏	50.	❏	❏	❏	❏
25.	❏	❏	❏	❏	51.	❏	❏	❏	❏
26.	❏	❏	❏	❏	52.	❏	❏	❏	❏

	A	B	C	D		A	B	C	D
53.	❏	❏	❏	❏	57.	❏	❏	❏	❏
54.	❏	❏	❏	❏	58.	❏	❏	❏	❏
55.	❏	❏	❏	❏	59.	❏	❏	❏	❏
56.	❏	❏	❏	❏	60.	❏	❏	❏	❏

34

Trauma Systems and Mechanism of Injury

1. Approximately _____ unexpected trauma deaths occur in the United States each year.

   a. 10,000
   b. 100,000
   c. 150,000
   d. 500,000

2. The top five causes of trauma death include MVCs, falls, poisonings, fire, burns, and:

   a. drowning.
   b. bike accidents.
   c. skiing accidents.
   d. motor cycle accidents.

3. Getting a complete and accurate history of the accident can help to identify as many as 95% of the injuries present, because:

   a. the patient can tell where he/she is injured.
   b. witnesses can tell where the patient is injured.
   c. the police can identify the injuries.
   d. many MOIs have predictable patterns of injuries.

4. What percent of trauma is life-threatening?

   a. > 1%
   b. 5%
   c. 10%
   d. 15%

5. The two major factors for traumatic injury are amount of energy exchanges to the body and:

   a. the patient's age.
   b. anatomic structures that are involved.
   c. PMH.
   d. the use of any safety restraints.

6. The three phases of trauma care include preincident, postincident and:

   a. golden hour.
   b. incident.
   c. platinum ten minutes.
   d. physical therapy.

7. After personal safety and maintenance of the patient's ABCs, _____ is the most important information to obtain in any trauma victim.

   a. MOI
   b. PMH
   c. organ donor status
   d. DNAR status

8. Paramedics can make a big difference in trauma prevention by doing all the following, *except*:

   a. assisting in public education of seat belt use.
   b. setting the example.
   c. promoting legislation to reduce the use of weapons.
   d. filling out an organ donor card.

9. The paramedic can make a significant impact on the life or death of a trauma victim by:

   a. wearing the appropriate PPE.
   b. stabilizing the patient prior to transport.
   c. minimizing scene time when appropriate.
   d. transporting the trauma patient to the nearest facility.

10. The paper, *Accidental Death and Disability: The Neglected Disease of Modern Society* is also known as the:

   a. Ryan-White Act.
   b. Highway Safety Act of 1966.
   c. Trauma Prevention Act.
   d. White Paper.

11. The components of a trauma system include all the following, *except*:

    a. injury prevention programs.
    b. hospice care.
    c. definitive care.
    d. trauma critical care.

12. A trauma _____ is a reporting system designed to collect trauma-related data in an effort to improve the quality and cost-effectiveness of care and to aid in outcomes of research.

    a. registry
    b. chronicle
    c. journal
    d. catalog

13. Which of the following statements about trauma centers is not correct?

    a. Trauma centers must meet strict criteria to be designated a trauma center.
    b. A delineated criterion for a trauma center includes personnel.
    c. A delineated criterion for a trauma center includes use of air–medical transport.
    d. Not all hospitals that care for acutely injured patients are trauma centers.

14. Which of the following is not a criteria for transport to a Level I trauma center?

    a. Multiple system trauma
    b. Trauma cardiac arrest
    c. Severe burns
    d. Pregnant patient

15. Which of the following is not an indication for the use of air–medical transport?

    a. Access to remote areas.
    b. Access to specialty equipment.
    c. Lengthy ground transport.
    d. Morbidly obese patient.

16. Which of the following is not a contraindication or relative contraindication (depending on the aircraft) for the use of air–medical transport?

    a. access to personnel with specialty skills
    b. inclement weather conditions
    c. extremely combative patients
    d. patients with barotraumas

17. _____ means that energy cannot be created or destroyed, only transferred or exchanged.

    a. Kinetic energy
    b. Force
    c. Newton's first law of motion
    d. Conservation of energy

18. An object in motion tends to stay in motion, and an object at rest tends to stay at rest, describes:

    a. kinetic energy.
    b. force.
    c. Newton's first law of motion.
    d. conservation of energy.

19. _____ means that the more speed that is involved, the more energy there is.

    a. Kinetic energy
    b. Force
    c. Newton's first law of motion
    d. Conservation of energy

20. _____ is the creation of a cavity in an object that can be permanent or temporary.

    a. Energy
    b. Force
    c. Cavitation
    d. Puncture

21. Which of the following components of kinetic energy make the greatest impact on a trauma victim?

    a. Mass
    b. Velocity
    c. Acceleration
    d. Deceleration

22. Which of the following are the actual units for kinetic energy?

    a. foot-pounds
    b. mile-grams
    c. meter-liter
    d. inch-ounces

23. When does the Golden Hour for the trauma victim begin?

    a. When the first responder arrives at the patient's side.
    b. When the paramedic arrives on the scene.
    c. Immediately after the injury is sustained.
    d. Immediately upon arriving at the ED.

24. What is meant by the third collision in the MOI of a trauma victim?

    a. Third collision is the internal organs striking against the body.
    b. This is a triad of injuries involving the head, neck and spine.
    c. Third collision refers to multiple injuries.
    d. Third collision pertains to children involved in motor vehicle collisions.

25. Why are some bullets designed to tumble when fired from a gun?

    a. Tumbling bullets are faster.
    b. Tumbling decreases the force of impact.
    c. Penetration is streamlined with tumbling.
    d. Tumbling creates greater tissue damage.

26. Blunt trauma is associated with acceleration and deceleration forces in all the following, *except*:

    a. motor vehicle collisions.
    b. auto pedestrian collisions.
    c. falls.
    d. GSWs.

27. Which of the following MOIs is not usually associated with predictable injury patterns?

    a. Motorcycle collisions
    b. Auto–pedestrian collisions
    c. Falls
    d. GSWs

28. The three phases associated with the blast effect are the primary phase, the secondary phase, and the _____ phase.

    a. late
    b. triage
    c. tertiary
    d. end-stage

29. During the secondary phase of the blast effect, the potential for injury comes from:

    a. the heat wave.
    b. flying articles.
    c. pressure waves.
    d. the patient striking an object.

30. Which of the following penetrating MOIs has the greatest potential for energy exchange?

    a. High power rifle
    b. Knife
    c. Shotgun
    d. Hanging

31. Which of the following will generate the greatest amount of kinetic energy?

    a. 90 kg patient traveling at 30 mph
    b. 80 kg patient traveling at 40 mph
    c. 70 kg patient traveling at 50 mph
    d. 60 kg patient traveling at 60 mph

32. You are assessing a patient that was a victim of a significant blast injury. He has the clinical findings of a closed pneumothorax. Which of the following is the most likely cause of his injury?

    a. Heat wave
    b. Compression
    c. Flying article
    d. Sound wave

33. During the _____ phase of the blast effect, injuries can result from the patient becoming a flying object and striking other objects.

    a. primary
    b. secondary
    c. late
    d. tertiary

34. Your patient is the victim of a motorcycle collision and has bilateral femur fractures. What type of impact did the patient most likely sustain?

    a. Frontal
    b. Rear-end
    c. Side
    d. Rotational

35. Cervical spine injuries are most common with what type of collision?

    a. Frontal
    b. Rear-end
    c. Primary
    d. Secondary

36. Your patient was assisted out of a house fire by a fireman who found him lying on the bedroom floor unconscious? Which of the following pieces of information about the MOI is the most significant for this patient?

    a. Cause of the fire.
    b. When the fire was started.
    c. Smoke condition in the room in which the patient was found.
    d. Presence of a carbon monoxide detector in the house.

37. What is the most likely cause of the unconsciousness in the patient described in question 36?

    a. Airway burns
    b. Super heated air
    c. CO_2 inhalation
    d. Shock

38. The patient you are assessing fell from a tall ladder while at work. Which of the following aspects of the MOI should the paramedic focus on?

    a. Point of impact of the body.
    b. The distance of the fall.
    c. The type of surface of the impact.
    d. All of the above.

39. When a projectile such as a bullet passes through the body, it creates a wave of pressure that can compress organs and tissue causing:

    a. contusion, fracture or rupture.
    b. liquidation.
    c. collapse and disintegration.
    d. spontaneous combustion.

40. Which of the following aspects of a GSW should the paramedic focus on?

    a. The gender of the shooter.
    b. The wind speed at the time of the shooting.
    c. The level of gravity at the time of the shooting.
    d. None of the above.

41. Your patient is the victim of a motorcycle collision where he was T-boned at an intersection by a car? Which of the following injury patterns are most associated with lateral impact motorcycle collisions?

    a. Bilateral femur fractures
    b. Crush injuries
    c. Pelvis dislocation
    d. Pneumothorax

42. Which of the following is an injury associated with third collision MOI?

    a. Brain contusion
    b. Fractured pelvis
    c. Dislocated knee
    d. Neck injury

43. By performing a rapid assessment and life-saving procedures, minimizing scene time to _____ minutes and transporting the patient to an appropriate facility, the paramedic makes the difference between life or death for a trauma patient.

    a. 10
    b. 15
    c. 30
    d. 60

44. As a general rule the entrance wound of a GSW is usually smaller than the exit wound because of:

    a. proximity of the shooter.
    b. positioning of the patient.
    c. cavitation.
    d. dissection.

45. During the primary phase of the blast effect there is a pressure wave that can cause major damage on the:

    a. eyes and skin.
    b. lungs and GI tract.
    c. head and neck.
    d. hearing.

46. The pathologic effects of the pressure wave during the blast effect include:

    a. lacerations and bruising.
    b. rupture of an organ or air embolism.
    c. whiplash and sprains.
    d. shattering.

47. During the third phase of an auto–pedestrian collision the patient can sustain injuries from:

    a. the impact of the vehicle.
    b. the fall on to the hood of the vehicle.
    c. going into the vehicle.
    d. being run over by the vehicle.

48. The victim of a motorcycle collision that does not wear a helmet has a _____ % increased risk of brain injury.

    a. 30
    b. 50
    c. 300
    d. 500

49. Which of the following statements about air bags is *not* correct?

    a. Air bags provide supplemental protection.
    b. Air bags may produce facial and forearm abrasions.
    c. Air bags do not work without the use of seat belts.
    d. The protective covers can explode into the chest of the occupant.

50. Which of the following statements about shoulder restraints is correct?

    a. They prevent hyperflexion of the upper torso.
    b. The do not prevent forward motion of the upper torso in frontal impact collisions.
    c. Neck injuries can still be prevented even without the use of a lap restraint.
    d. Shoulder restraints provide more benefit when the seat is very close to the dashboard.

Test #34 Answer Form

	A	B	C	D			A	B	C	D
1.	❏	❏	❏	❏		26.	❏	❏	❏	❏
2.	❏	❏	❏	❏		27.	❏	❏	❏	❏
3.	❏	❏	❏	❏		28.	❏	❏	❏	❏
4.	❏	❏	❏	❏		29.	❏	❏	❏	❏
5.	❏	❏	❏	❏		30.	❏	❏	❏	❏
6.	❏	❏	❏	❏		31.	❏	❏	❏	❏
7.	❏	❏	❏	❏		32.	❏	❏	❏	❏
8.	❏	❏	❏	❏		33.	❏	❏	❏	❏
9.	❏	❏	❏	❏		34.	❏	❏	❏	❏
10.	❏	❏	❏	❏		35.	❏	❏	❏	❏
11.	❏	❏	❏	❏		36.	❏	❏	❏	❏
12.	❏	❏	❏	❏		37.	❏	❏	❏	❏
13.	❏	❏	❏	❏		38.	❏	❏	❏	❏
14.	❏	❏	❏	❏		39.	❏	❏	❏	❏
15.	❏	❏	❏	❏		40.	❏	❏	❏	❏
16.	❏	❏	❏	❏		41.	❏	❏	❏	❏
17.	❏	❏	❏	❏		42.	❏	❏	❏	❏
18.	❏	❏	❏	❏		43.	❏	❏	❏	❏
19.	❏	❏	❏	❏		44.	❏	❏	❏	❏
20.	❏	❏	❏	❏		45.	❏	❏	❏	❏
21.	❏	❏	❏	❏		46.	❏	❏	❏	❏
22.	❏	❏	❏	❏		47.	❏	❏	❏	❏
23.	❏	❏	❏	❏		48.	❏	❏	❏	❏
24.	❏	❏	❏	❏		49.	❏	❏	❏	❏
25.	❏	❏	❏	❏		50.	❏	❏	❏	❏

35

Hemorrhage and Shock

1. The two general locations of severe hemorrhage are:

    a. head and neck.
    b. extremities and back.
    c. internal and external.
    d. chest and pelvis.

2. When a patient has signs of hypovolemia and there are no external reasons, the paramedic should consider:

    a. esophageal varices.
    b. occult GI bleeding.
    c. dehydration.
    d. head trauma.

3. Bleeding described as spurting bright red is usually from a/an:

    a. vein.
    b. artery.
    c. capillary.
    d. vesicle.

4. A patient was shot in the stomach. Upon arrival, after assuring the police have secured the scene, the paramedic is able to talk directly to the patient who is alert and complaining of severe pain. The paramedic is unable to obtain a radial pulse. What grade/stage of hemorrhage would you suspect the patient is in?

    a. One
    b. Two
    c. Three
    d. Four

5. Based on the scenario above approximately how much blood has the patient lost up to the point of initial assessment by the paramedic?

    a. up to 15%
    b. 15 to 25%
    c. 25 to 35%
    d. greater than 35%

6. What treatment would be appropriate for this patient?

    a. High flow O_2
    b. Two large bore IVs enroute
    c. Trendelenburg's position
    d. All of the above

7. When the systolic BP drops from a hemorrhage, it is referred to as _____ shock.

    a. hypervolemic
    b. decompensated
    c. irreversible
    d. compensated

8. In the formula CO = HR x SV, the SV is usually approximately _____ per heartbeat in an adult.

    a. 25 cc
    b. 50 cc
    c. 70 cc
    d. 120 cc

9. For the short term, to increase the cardiac output it is easiest for the body to:

    a. decrease vascular resistance.
    b. vasodilate.
    c. increase heart rate.
    d. increase stroke volume.

10. What is the objective measure of vasoconstriction during hemorrhage?

    a. increase in systolic pressure
    b. increase in diastolic pressure
    c. decrease in systolic pressure
    d. decrease in diastolic pressure

11. For the long term, how can you increase your SV?

    a. add more volume by an IV infusion
    b. take medication to slow the heart rate
    c. aerobic exercise on a regular basis
    d. lift weight on a regular basis

12. All the following are alpha-1 effects of epinephrine, *except*:

    a. vasoconstriction.
    b. increase in PVR.
    c. decrease in afterload.
    d. increase in afterload.

13. When the patient is hypovolemic, the beta-1 effects of epinephrine include:

    a. positive chronographic effect.
    b. positive inatropic effect.
    c. positive dromotropic effect.
    d. all of the above.

14. The chemical that is released during shock, which starts to act as an antidiuretic, is called:

    a. insulin.
    b. aldosterone.
    c. arginine vasopressin.
    d. glucagon.

15. A potent vasoconstrictor that promotes sodium reabsorption and decreases urine output in shock states is:

    a. insulin.
    b. aldosterone.
    c. arginine vasopressin
    d. angiotensin II.

16. Following injury and volume loss, the patient is often:

    a. hypoglycemic.
    b. hyperglycemic.
    c. flushed and warm.
    d. depleted of urine.

17. When the compensatory mechanisms are overwhelmed, all the following occur, *except*:

    a. preload decreases.
    b. cardiac output decreases.
    c. myocardial blood supply increases.
    d. capillary and cellular changes occur.

18. At the cellular level, during low perfusion states when the postcapillary sphincter relaxes, this is called the _____ phase.

    a. ischemia
    b. washout
    c. stagnation
    d. final

19. During low perfusion states the precapillary sphincters relax in response to lactic acid and:

    a. decreased carbon dioxide.
    b. vasomotor center failure.
    c. hypothermia.
    d. aerobic metabolism.

20. _____ shock is characterized by signs and symptoms of late shock, but is refractory to treatment.

    a. Hypovolemic
    b. Distributive
    c. Irreversible
    d. Obstructive

21. Which one of the following signs or symptoms may differentiate cardiogenic shock from hypovolemic shock?

    a. chief complaint of chest pain
    b. presence of tachycardia
    c. absence of diaphoresis
    d. poor CTC

22. Which of the following signs may differentiate distributed shock from hypovolemic shock?

    a. chief complaint of dyspnea
    b. presence of tachycardia
    c. absence of diaphoresis
    d. flushed skin

23. Which of the following signs may differentiate obstructive shock from hypovolemic shock?

    a. chief complaint of abdominal pain
    b. presence of JVD
    c. presence of tachycardia
    d. poor CTC

24. Intravenous volume expanders that have the same tonicity as plasma are _____ solutions.

    a. isotonic
    b. hypertonic
    c. hypotonic
    d. synthetic

25. When using intravenous volume expanders it is necessary to recall that only about _____ of the fluid infused stays in the intravascular space.

    a. 1/4
    b. 1/3
    c. 1/2
    d. 2/3

26. When a crystalloid IV volume expander such as normal saline is used, the amount that shifts out of the intravascular space moves into the _____ within approximately one hour.

    a. interstitial space
    b. lungs
    c. intracellular compartment
    d. kidneys

27. Which of the following statements is most correct about intravenous volume expanders?

    a. They should only be used enroute to the ED.
    b. Hypertonic solutions are best in the prehospital setting.
    c. Isotonic solutions are not routinely used in or out of the ED.
    d. They do not carry hemoglobin.

28. You are assessing an 18-year-old male who crashed his dirt bike. He has an obvious closed femur fracture and abdominal pain. His mental status is alert, but initially he had a brief loss of consciousness and his vitals signs are R/R 30 and shallow, P/R 110 and B/P 116/56. His skin is warm and moist. Which stage of shock is indicated by the pulse and blood pressure?

    a. compensated
    b. decompensated
    c. distributive
    d. obstructive

29. Based on the scenario in question 28, the most likely cause of the shock is:

    a. head injury.
    b. internal bleeding.
    c. substantial vasodilation.
    d. loss of venous capacitance.

30. Baroreceptors located in the carotid sinuses and _____ are stimulated by decreased blood flow.

    a. intestines
    b. aortic arch
    c. cerebellum
    d. medulla

31. When baroreceptors sense decreased blood flow and activate the vasomotor center, as a result there is:

    a. vasodilation of the peripheral vessels.
    b. vasodilation of the great vessels.
    c. vasoconstriction of the peripheral vessels.
    d. vasoconstriction of the central organs.

32. When the sympathetic nervous system is stimulated as a response to shock, epinephrine and norepinephrine are secreted from the:

    a. thalamus.
    b. hypothalamus.
    c. adrenal gland medulla.
    d. pituitary gland.

33. Which of the following is an early sign of hypovolemic shock?

    a. narrowing pulse pressure
    b. increased peripheral vascular resistance
    c. increased stroke volume
    d. loss of vasomotor tone

34. When the body senses hypovolemia, several regulatory systems are put into play to try to compensate. These include sympathetic responses, vasoconstriction and:

    a. endocrine responses.
    b. CO_2 elimination.
    c. metabolic purging.
    d. osmotic channeling.

35. The maximum amount of intravenous volume expanders prudent for field administration is about _____ liters so as to avoid reducing hematocrit from being effective.

    a. 1–2
    b. 2–3
    c. 4–5
    d. 5–6

36. The indication for the use of PASG/MAST in _____ is still relatively unchanged.

    a. chest trauma
    b. abdominal hemorrhage
    c. stabilization of pelvic fractures
    d. pregnancy

37. Despite the controversies in the use of PASG/MAST the _____ still recommends that the suit be available for immediate use in hospital emergency departments.

    a. National Registry
    b. ACEP
    c. JEMS
    d. NHTSA

38. Decreased perfusion can be caused by an event resulting in blood loss, kinking of the great vessels (i.e., tension pneumo) or:

    a. by release of antidiuretic hormone.
    b. an allergic reaction.
    c. a failure in the buffer system.
    d. loss of vasomotor tone.

39. _____ defends the fluid volume and reduces urine output by promoting sodium reabsorption and water retention in the kidney.

    a. ACTH
    b. Angiotensin I
    c. Aldosterone
    d. Glucagon

40. Renin is released by _____ and catalyzes the conversion of angiotensinogen to angiotensin I.

    a. arterioles in the kidney.
    b. transfer of fatty acids into mitochondria.
    c. cells in the adrenal cortex.
    d. circulating epinephrine.

Test #35 Answer Form

	A	B	C	D		A	B	C	D
1.	❏	❏	❏	❏	21.	❏	❏	❏	❏
2.	❏	❏	❏	❏	22.	❏	❏	❏	❏
3.	❏	❏	❏	❏	23.	❏	❏	❏	❏
4.	❏	❏	❏	❏	24.	❏	❏	❏	❏
5.	❏	❏	❏	❏	25.	❏	❏	❏	❏
6.	❏	❏	❏	❏	26.	❏	❏	❏	❏
7.	❏	❏	❏	❏	27.	❏	❏	❏	❏
8.	❏	❏	❏	❏	28.	❏	❏	❏	❏
9.	❏	❏	❏	❏	29.	❏	❏	❏	❏
10.	❏	❏	❏	❏	30.	❏	❏	❏	❏
11.	❏	❏	❏	❏	31.	❏	❏	❏	❏
12.	❏	❏	❏	❏	32.	❏	❏	❏	❏
13.	❏	❏	❏	❏	33.	❏	❏	❏	❏
14.	❏	❏	❏	❏	34.	❏	❏	❏	❏
15.	❏	❏	❏	❏	35.	❏	❏	❏	❏
16.	❏	❏	❏	❏	36.	❏	❏	❏	❏
17.	❏	❏	❏	❏	37.	❏	❏	❏	❏
18.	❏	❏	❏	❏	38.	❏	❏	❏	❏
19.	❏	❏	❏	❏	39.	❏	❏	❏	❏
20.	❏	❏	❏	❏	40.	❏	❏	❏	❏

36
Soft Tissue Trauma

1. Soft tissue trauma includes all the following, *except*:

    a. bumps and bruises.
    b. hematomas.
    c. lacerations.
    d. spasms and tics.

2. Two common examples of soft tissue trauma that may be fatal are hematomas and:

    a. secondary infections.
    b. abrasions.
    c. genital warts.
    d. insect bites.

3. Any physical activity that increases the exposure of the skin to the environment and _____ will increase the risk of a soft tissue injury.

    a. sea/salt water
    b. physical forces
    c. blood-borne pathogens
    d. airborne pathogens

4. Which of the following is not a layer of the skin?

    a. Cutaneous
    b. Subcutaneous
    c. Superficial lesion
    d. Deep fascia

5. Which section of skin contains the stratum germinativum or basal layer?

    a. Dermis
    b. Epidermus
    c. Subcutaneous lesion
    d. Deep fascia

6. Fibroblasts, macrophages and MAST cells are located in the:

    a. Dermis
    b. Epidermus
    c. Superficial fascia
    d. Deep fascia

7. The _____ is a thick dense layer of fibrous tissue that provides support and protection for the underlying structures.

    a. dermis
    b. epidermus
    c. superficial fascia
    d. deep fascia

8. The skin follows the contours of the underlying structures creating a natural stretch in the skin called:

    a. tension lines.
    b. stretch marks.
    c. relief stretch.
    d. strain outlines.

9. All the following are phases of normal wound healing, *except*:

    a. hemostasis.
    b. inflammation.
    c. neovascularization.
    d. macrophage synthesis.

10. The phase of normal healing that involves fibroblast-forming scar tissue that holds the wound edges together tightly is called:

    a. epithelialization.
    b. collagen synthesis.
    c. stretch marks.
    d. tension lines.

11. _____ is the phase of wound healing through re-establishment of skin layers in the first 12 hours.

    a. Epithelialization
    b. Collagen synthesis
    c. Inflammation
    d. Fibroblast formation

12. Normal wound healing can be altered by which of the following factors?

    a. Skin temperature
    b. Ambient termperature
    c. Body region
    d. Dry skin

13. All the following medications can affect normal wound healing, *except*:

    a. corticosteroids.
    b. penicillin.
    c. laxatives.
    d. anti-coagulants.

14. Which of the following medical conditions does not typically affect normal wound healing?

    a. Severe alcoholism
    b. Diabetes
    c. Acne
    d. Cardiovascular disease

15. What types of wounds are considered high risk for healing problems and infections?

    a. Human bites
    b. Injected wounds
    c. Crush wounds
    d. All of the above

16. Excessive accumulation of scar tissue that extends beyond the original wound borders is called a:

    a. keloid scar.
    b. stretch mark.
    c. suture over-healing.
    d. hypertrophic scar.

17. Plastic surgery is often requested for wound closures for the purpose of:

    a. minimizing the number of stitches used.
    b. cosmetically acceptable healing.
    c. closing gaps that are too large for sutures.
    d. closing gaps that are too small for sutures.

18. Which of the following soft tissue injuries often requires sutures?

    a. Degloving
    b. Abrasions
    c. Ulcers
    d. Abscesses

19. All the following are general categories of closed tissue injuries, *except*:

    a. contusions.
    b. hematomas.
    c. extravasating.
    d. crushing injures.

20. In a/an _____ the epidermis remains intact when cells are damaged and the blood vessels in the dermis are torn, causing swelling and pain. The pain can be delayed for up to 24 to 48 hours after the injury.

    a. contusion
    b. laceration
    c. abrasion
    d. ulcer

21. A/An _____ is a break in the skin of varying depth usually caused by very sharp objects such as a knife.

    a. abrasion
    b. laceration
    c. incision
    d. avulsion

22. A flap of torn loose tissue that may not be viable for reimplantation is called an:

    a. abrasion.
    b. amputation.
    c. impalement.
    d. avulsion.

23. A jagged wound caused by forceful impact with a sharp object, which may cause the ends to bleed freely, is called a/an:

    a. laceration.
    b. amputation.
    c. evisceration.
    d. puncture.

24. Which of the following is not a type of amputation?

    a. Degloving injury
    b. Ring injury
    c. Complete
    d. Partial

25. During which phases of a blast injury would open soft tissue trauma most likely occur?

    a. Primary and secondary
    b. Primary and tertiary
    c. Secondary and tertiary
    d. None of the above

26. A/An _____ injury is an injury from a compressive force sufficient to interfere with the normal metabolic function of the involved tissue.

    a. puncture
    b. crush
    c. impaled
    d. blast

27. Field management for the patient with crush syndrome is focused on aggressive fluid therapy and the administration of:

    a. oxygen to restore hypoxic tissue.
    b. epinephrine to dilate the vessels.
    c. glucagon to metabolize stores of needed glucose.
    d. sodium bicarbonate to neutralize the buildup of acids.

28. All the following are examples of causes of crush injuries, *except*:

    a. a bedridden patient without proper care.
    b. an unconscious patient lying on an extremity.
    c. prolonged application of MAST/PASG.
    d. improperly applied cast.

29. In crush syndrome injury, after the initial damage to soft tissue, the cells in the crushed area become starved for oxygen and _____ occurs.

    a. compartment syndrome
    b. anaerobic metabolism
    c. unconsciousness
    d. respiratory acidosis

30. All the following are included in the pathophysiology of a crush syndrome, *except*:

    a. oxygen free-radicals are released into the blood stream.
    b. various compounds accumulate from systemic inflammation.
    c. lipid peroxidation results.
    d. acute shock and cardiac arrest.

31. In the pathophysiology of compartment syndrome, the tissue pressure rises above the _____ pressure resulting in ischemia to muscle.

    a. venous
    b. arterial
    c. osmotic
    d. capillary hydrostatic

32. Local signs and symptoms of compartment syndrome may include any of the following, *except*:

    a. distal pulses with warm skin.
    b. pain and swelling.
    c. the presentation of a spinal cord injury.
    d. the formation of crystals in the affected tissues.

33. The "Ps" of compartment syndrome, include all the following, *except*:

    a. palpation.
    b. pain.
    c. paresis.
    d. pulselessness.

34. Blast injuries can occur from any explosion, but they are often more serious when they occur:

    a. in a shopping mall.
    b. at a fire scene.
    c. inside a confined space.
    d. in a railroad yard.

35. Initial treatment priorities for soft tissue injuries caused by blasts include:

    a. observing for signs of compartment syndrome.
    b. flushing the patient of combustible materials.
    c. considering that both internal and external injuries are possible.
    d. copious amounts of fluid administration.

36. Which of the following is not a method of hemorrhage control?

    a. Direct pressure
    b. Pressure dressing
    c. Pressure points
    d. Indirect pressure

37. _____ is the quickest and most efficient means of bleeding control.

    a. Direct pressure
    b. Elevation
    c. Tourniquet application
    d. Pressure points

38. The purpose of controlling a hemorrhage by direct pressure is to limit additional significant blood loss and to:

    a. limit exposure to communicable disease.
    b. promote localized clotting.
    c. stop the arterial blood flow.
    d. avoid the use of indirect pressure.

39. Elevation is indicated in all situations where direct pressure is not enough to stop the bleeding, *except* when:

    a. the patient is unconscious.
    b. there is a possible musculoskeletal injury to the involved extremity.
    c. the airway is unprotected or there is a loss of gag reflex.
    d. there is no distal pulse.

40. Which of the following is not correct about the use of pressure dressings?

    a. They provide a continuous mechanical pressure on the wound site.
    b. A circumferential bandage should not be used on the neck.
    c. The bandage should not occlude or impede venous blood flow.
    d. The bandage should not occlude or impede arterial blood flow.

41. Which of the following patients is not recommended to use a pressure dressing?

    a. A patient with a head wound with a suspected head injury.
    b. A pediatric patient with avulsed fingertips.
    c. A patient with an open tib–fib fracture.
    d. A pregnant trauma patient with an eviscerated thigh.

42. A pressure point is a location where a/an:

    a. artery runs over a bone and close to the skin.
    b. artery runs under a vein and close to the skin.
    c. vein runs over a bone and close to the heart.
    d. paramedic can reach with a venous tourniquet.

43. The use of a pressure point to control hemorrhage is indicated in situations where bleeding is not controlled by:

    a. direct pressure.
    b. elevation.
    c. pressure bandage.
    d. all of the above.

44. Do not apply a tourniquet directly around a knee or elbow as _____ in that area, and it will not adequately control the bleeding.

    a. serious nerve damage will result
    b. it may cut the skin or tissue
    c. there is too much bone
    d. there is no artery

45. Once a tourniquet is applied, the decision may be that you will:

    a. take if off once bleeding has been controlled.
    b. lose the limb to save the life.
    c. replace it with an air splint when one is available.
    d. loosen it when the patient experiences paresthesia.

46. The difference between a sterile and non-sterile dressing is that a sterile dressing has gone through:

    a. the process to eliminate bacteria from the dressing material.
    b. hermetically sealed packaging.
    c. special quality control regiments.
    d. a process to apply a residue to the gauze.

47. An occlusive dressing does not allow _____ through the dressing.

    a. passage of air
    b. passage of blood
    c. surfactant
    d. embolism to develop

48. The type of dressing that has been designed to not damage the surface of the wound when it is removed is a(an) _____ dressing.

    a. occlusive
    b. sterile
    c. non-sterile
    d. non-adherent

49. The type of dressing that is designed to stick onto a wound surface by incorporating wound exudates into the dressing mesh is called a/an _____ dressing.

    a. occlusive
    b. adhesive
    c. improperly applied
    d. sterile wrap

50. An improperly applied dressing may result in any of the following, *except*:

    a. decreasing the risk of wound infection.
    b. impeding hemorrhage control.
    c. increasing tissue damage.
    d. unnecessary patient discomfort.

51. Transportation considerations for the patient with an open wound include all the following, *except*:

    a. the patient may need a tetanus shot.
    b. proper cleansing may be needed.
    c. proper insurance authorization may not get approved.
    d. proper dressing of the wound may be needed.

52. Patients with which of the following wounds should be transported for further evaluation in the ED?

    a. Wounds with heavy contamination.
    b. Wounds with nerve, or vascular compromise.
    c. Wounds with cosmetic complications.
    d. All of the above.

53. How often is the immunization for tetanus recommended?

    a. Every year.
    b. Every 5 years.
    c. Every 10 years.
    d. Every 12 years.

54. The paramedic can minimize the risk of infection for a patient with an open wound by:

    a. covering the wound with a dry, sterile dressing.
    b. covering the wound with a wet, sterile dressing.
    c. cleansing and debriding the wound as needed.
    d. placing ice over the sterile dressing.

55. Considerations for the treatment of an amputated part include the amputated part should:

    a. be wrapped in dry sterile dressing.
    b. be wrapped in a sterile moist gauze pad.
    c. be placed in a bag with ice.
    d. always be transported with the patient.

56. Hyperbaric oxygen treatment is sometimes recommended to prevent _____ and improve healing in crush injuries.

    a. respiratory acidosis
    b. pulmonary embolus
    c. gangrene
    d. deep vein thrombosis

57. After the ABCs, the most important treatment in the patient with a crush injury is:

    a. the observation of the presence of ECG changes or dysrhythmias.
    b. to administer 20% solution of mannitol.
    c. transport to a hyperbaric treatment facility.
    d. to administer IV fluid therapy using the Parkland formula.

58. The _____, also called the superficial fascia, contains loose connective tissue and fat that provides both insulation and protection from trauma.

    a. cutaneous layer
    b. subcutaneous layer
    c. basal layer
    d. reticular dermis

59. During the _____ phase of normal wound healing special cells "invade" the blood clot and release mediators that help fight local infections, as well as initiate the healing process.

    a. hemostasis
    b. inflammation
    c. epithelialization
    d. neovascularization

60. _____ is/are an excessive accumulation of scar tissue confined within the original wound borders and is common in areas of high tissue stress such as flexion creases across joints.

    a. Hypertrophic scar
    b. Keloid scar
    c. Stretch marks
    d. Inflammation

Test #36 Answer Form

	A	B	C	D			A	B	C	D
1.	❏	❏	❏	❏		27.	❏	❏	❏	❏
2.	❏	❏	❏	❏		28.	❏	❏	❏	❏
3.	❏	❏	❏	❏		29.	❏	❏	❏	❏
4.	❏	❏	❏	❏		30.	❏	❏	❏	❏
5.	❏	❏	❏	❏		31.	❏	❏	❏	❏
6.	❏	❏	❏	❏		32.	❏	❏	❏	❏
7.	❏	❏	❏	❏		33.	❏	❏	❏	❏
8.	❏	❏	❏	❏		34.	❏	❏	❏	❏
9.	❏	❏	❏	❏		35.	❏	❏	❏	❏
10.	❏	❏	❏	❏		36.	❏	❏	❏	❏
11.	❏	❏	❏	❏		37.	❏	❏	❏	❏
12.	❏	❏	❏	❏		38.	❏	❏	❏	❏
13.	❏	❏	❏	❏		39.	❏	❏	❏	❏
14.	❏	❏	❏	❏		40.	❏	❏	❏	❏
15.	❏	❏	❏	❏		41.	❏	❏	❏	❏
16.	❏	❏	❏	❏		42.	❏	❏	❏	❏
17.	❏	❏	❏	❏		43.	❏	❏	❏	❏
18.	❏	❏	❏	❏		44.	❏	❏	❏	❏
19.	❏	❏	❏	❏		45.	❏	❏	❏	❏
20.	❏	❏	❏	❏		46.	❏	❏	❏	❏
21.	❏	❏	❏	❏		47.	❏	❏	❏	❏
22.	❏	❏	❏	❏		48.	❏	❏	❏	❏
23.	❏	❏	❏	❏		49.	❏	❏	❏	❏
24.	❏	❏	❏	❏		50.	❏	❏	❏	❏
25.	❏	❏	❏	❏		51.	❏	❏	❏	❏
26.	❏	❏	❏	❏		52.	❏	❏	❏	❏

	A	B	C	D		A	B	C	D
53.	❏	❏	❏	❏	57.	❏	❏	❏	❏
54.	❏	❏	❏	❏	58.	❏	❏	❏	❏
55.	❏	❏	❏	❏	59.	❏	❏	❏	❏
56.	❏	❏	❏	❏	60.	❏	❏	❏	❏

37

Burns

1. Approximately 80% of the fire- and burn-related deaths that occur in the United States are a result of a/an _____ fire.

   a. house
   b. automobile
   c. camp
   d. brush

2. Burns are the leading cause of trauma in the _____ age group.

   a. newborn
   b. toddler and preschool
   c. teenage
   d. elderly

3. The elderly are in a high risk group for burns primarily because of:

   a. forgetting to change batteries in smoke detectors.
   b. elder abuse.
   c. smoking in bed.
   d. impairment of mobility or sensation.

4. Prevention strategies to decrease the number of scalding injuries in children include all the following, *except*:

   a. never drinking hot liquids while holding a child.
   b. cooking on backburners whenever possible.
   c. turning down the thermostat on the hot water heater to 120 degrees.
   d. testing the water temperature of a bath before allowing the child to enter.

5. Which of the following is not a pathophysiologic or system complication of a burn injury?

   a. decreased catecholamine release
   b. fluid and electrolyte loss
   c. renal, liver and heart failure
   d. hypothermia

6. All the following are common types of burn injuries, *except*:

   a. thermal.
   b. inhalation.
   c. electrical.
   d. biologic.

7. Which of the following is not a classification of a burn injury?

   a. Superficial
   b. Deep fascia
   c. Partial-thickness
   d. Full-thickness

8. A _____ degree burn involves the outermost layer of skin, the epidermis, as well as the dermal layer.

   a. First
   b. Second
   c. Third
   d. Fourth

9. The three classifications of burn severity do not include:

   a. minor.
   b. moderate.
   c. eschar.
   d. severe.

10. The "rule of nines" is a method of determining:

   a. body surface area burned.
   b. severity of burn.
   c. classification of burn.
   d. type and degree of burn.

11. All the following are examples of severe burns that usually require transport to a burn specialty center, *except*:

   a. burns on the hands or feet.
   b. inhalation burn.
   c. electrical burn.
   d. partial thickness of less than 30%.

12. Which of the following does not have a significant impact on the management and prognosis of the burn-injured patient?

    a. The patient's age.
    b. The patient's gender.
    c. Preexisiting medical problems.
    d. Associated trauma injury.

13. Examples of conditions that are associated with burn injuries include all the following, *except*:

    a. respiratory compromise.
    b. child abuse.
    c. nausea and vomiting.
    d. airway compromise from inhaling super-heated gasses.

14. Signs and symptoms of a burn injury include:

    a. pain in the location of the burn.
    b. chest pain.
    c. edema and/or hemorrhage.
    d. all of the above.

15. The phases of "burn" shock include all the following, *except* the _____ phase.

    a. fluid shift
    b. compensation
    c. resolution
    d. hypermetabolic

16. During the body's initial response to a burn there is a _____ in response to the pain from the burn.

    a. fluid shift
    b. release of catecholamines
    c. burst of energy
    d. decrease in cardiac output

17. During the _____ phase of a burn injury there is a release of vasoactive substances from the burned tissues causing wound edema, fluid loss and hypovolemia.

    a. emergent
    b. compensation
    c. fluid shift
    d. resolution

18. The _____ phase is the final phase of the burn process in which the scar tissue is laid down and healing occurs.

    a. fluid shift
    b. compensation
    c. resolution
    d. hypermetabolic

19. In 60–70% of all thermal burn patients who die, there is an associated inhalation injury when these patients either have cyanide intoxication or:

    a. carbon monoxide poisoning.
    b. asbestosis.
    c. nitrogen narcosis.
    d. thermal inhalation.

20. _____ is the thick and non-elastic scab or immediate scar that forms on the skin following a burn.

    a. Epithelialization
    b. Collagen synthesis
    c. Coagulation synthesis
    d. Eschar

21. When a circumferential scar forms around an extremity, _____ can be the resulting complication.

    a. circulatory compromise
    b. severe fluid loss
    c. rebound acidosis
    d. cosmetic uncertainty

22. When obtaining assessment findings of the patient with a thermal burn, which of the following is least significant?

    a. The MOI.
    b. Fluid replacement amounts.
    c. Preexisting medical conditions.
    d. The classification and severity of the burn.

23. *After* managing the ABCs on the patient with a thermal burn, which of the following is appropriate treatment?

    a. Maintain body heat.
    b. Apply topical analgesia.
    c. Remove the patient to a safe area.
    d. Stop the burning process.

24. The Parkland formula is used my many burn centers to _____ for the burn patient.

    a. measure scar formation
    b. determine fluid replacement
    c. determine the prognosis
    d. measure circulatory compromise

25. Factors that are associated with an increased risk of inhalation injury include all the following, *except*:

    a. standing in a room with a fire.
    b. screaming for help.
    c. crawling on the floor in a room with a fire.
    d. being within an enclosed area involving a fire.

26. Which of the following signs or conditions may indicate that a patient has an inhalation injury?

    a. Singed nasal hairs
    b. Stridor
    c. Inspiratory wheezing
    d. All of the above

27. Regardless of the cause, _____ therapy for carbon monoxide inhalations is beneficial as it helps decrease the time it takes for the hemoglobin to become saturated with oxygen instead of CO.

    a. endotracheal intubation
    b. hyperbaric nitrogen
    c. hyperbaric oxygen
    d. positive pressure ventilation

28. Which of the following do not commonly cause chemical burns?

    a. Acids and bases
    b. Dry chemicals
    c. Saw dust
    d. Phenols

29. When a patient has been burned with a dry powder, special considerations include:

    a. washing it off, then determining what it is.
    b. brushing it off and calling the poison control center for decon procedures.
    c. avoid exposing yourself to the chemical.
    d. waiting for the fire department to do the decon.

30. Which of the following is not appropriate management of a chemical injury to the eye?

    a. Irrigation of most substances is recommended.
    b. Follow local protocols.
    c. Let the patient rub his/her eyes to facilitate drainage.
    d. If possible remove contact lenses.

31. The burning sensation of tear gas lasts for about _____ hour(s), while pepper gas lasts about _____ hour(s).

    a. one: two
    b. four: two
    c. five: four
    d. six: four

32. To minimize the effects of tear gas or pepper spray the paramedic can:

    a. get the patient to blow his/her nose and spit out any residue.
    b. instruct the patient to rub his/her eyes.
    c. use circular strokes to sponge off any residue.
    d. avoid using water to flush the skin.

33. When a patient with contact lenses has an eye injury or burn from a chemical agent the paramedic should:

    a. use the Morgan lens® on the unaffected eye and allow it to drain into the affected eye.
    b. remove the lenses with a gloved hand or assist the patient in doing so.
    c. place the Morgan lens® over the contact and irrigate with normal saline.
    d. never use a Morgan lens® on an eye injury caused by a chemical burn.

34. All the following are true about the severity of electrical burns, *except*:

    a. the body is a good conductor of electricity.
    b. the path of the electricity through the body leads to serious complications.
    c. it can cause internal injuries as well as the entrance and exit burns.
    d. it can cross the heart or brain and cause cancer.

35. In the United States about _____ people die from electrical shock each year.

    a. 100
    b. 1,000
    c. 10,000
    d. 100,000

36. The cause of death from electricity can be attributed to all the following, *except*:

    a. the electrical effect on the heart.
    b. scar tissue formation.
    c. massive muscle destruction from the current passing through the body.
    d. thermal burns from contact with the electrical source.

37. Direct current (DC), which has zero frequency but may be intermittent or pulsating, is:

    a. more dangerous then alternating current (AC).
    b. less dangerous than AC.
    c. causes circumferential burns more often than AC.
    d. causes circumferential burns less often than AC.

38. Alternating current at _____ Hz, which is household current, produces muscle tetany and tends to "freeze" the patient to the current source.

    a. 20
    b. 40
    c. 60
    d. 120

39. _____ is a lifesaving or limb-saving procedure used to allow expansion of the chest or restore circulation to an extremity in which the scar has formed a tight circumferential band.

    a. Circumcision
    b. Escharotomy
    c. Messocision
    d. Lyophilization

40. Which of the following skin conditions has the least resistance to electrical voltage?

    a. Dry, intact skin.
    b. Wet, intact skin.
    c. A thickly calloused palm or sole.
    d. Moist mucous membrane (mouth).

41. When assessing the victim of an electrical burn the paramedic should look for an entry and exit point of the current, because:

    a. anything in the path is "fair game" for injury.
    b. both sites are always easy to find.
    c. the exit wound will indicate how much internal damage is present.
    d. the entry wound will indicate how much internal damage is present.

42. Which of the following signs or symptoms is not commonly found in a person who has sustained an electrical burn?

    a. Trauma from falling.
    b. Hearing impairment or vision loss.
    c. Malocclusion
    d. Muscle contractions or pain.

43. What type of injury does lightening cause?

    a. cardiac asystole or ventricular fibrillation
    b. loss of consciousness or AMS
    c. neuropsychologic problems
    d. all of the above

44. Which of the following electrical burns is least likely to produce both an entry and exit wound?

    a. lightening strike
    b. arc injury
    c. direct contact with an electrical source
    d. indirect contact with an electrical source

45. All the following statements about the management of the patient with an electrical injury are correct, *except*:

    a. Do not touch the patient until you are sure that the power is turned off.
    b. Treatment of an electric injury is the same as for a thermal injury.
    c. The potential for internal injury is less than a thermal injury.
    d. Monitor the patient's ECG to identify hyperkalemia and cell death.

46. The most common entry point for an electrical burn is the:

    a. head.
    b. heart.
    c. hands.
    d. feet.

47. Which of the following is not a common physiologic dysfunction associated with electrical burns?

    a. Involuntary muscular contractions
    b. Singed nasal hairs
    c. Seizures
    d. Respiratory arrest

48. The _____ is/are the most common exit point for an electrical burn.

    a. head
    b. eyes
    c. rectum
    d. feet

49. Ionizing radiation produces immediate chemical effects, known as _____, on human tissue.

    a. ionization
    b. particle density
    c. radionization
    d. micronization

50. Nonionizing radiation includes all the following, *except*:

    a. X-rays.
    b. light.
    c. microwaves.
    d. radar.

51. All the following are types of ionizing radiation that can cause a burn injury, *except*:

    a. neutrons.
    b. gamma rays.
    c. geiger rays.
    d. beta particles.

52. _____ are small particles that are high in energy and can be dangerous if inhaled or ingested.

    a. Alpha particles
    b. Beta particles
    c. Geiger ray
    d. Microwaves

53. The most penetrating particles are _____, for which exposure causes direct tissue damage.

    a. alpha particles
    b. beta particles
    c. gamma rays
    d. neutrons

54. _____ are slow moving and contain low energy so objects such as newspaper or clothing can stop them.

    a. Alpha particles
    b. Beta particles
    c. Geiger rays
    d. Gamma rays

55. A gauge of the likely injury to an irradiated part of an organism is called the:

    a. whole body exposure.
    b. comparable radiation sickness.
    c. radiation absorbed dose (RAD).
    d. roentgen equivalent in man (REM).

56. Radiation sickness results when humans or animals are exposed to excessive doses of _____ radiation.

    a. radio wave
    b. microwave
    c. ionizing
    d. nonionizing

57. The degree of radiation illness is clearly a function of the:

    a. dose.
    b. type of agent one is exposed to.
    c. rate of exposure.
    d. all of the above.

58. _____ is/are very sensitive to radiation and the higher the absorbed dose, the more depressed the count will be.

    a. Red blood cells
    b. White blood cells
    c. Platelets
    d. Hemoglobin

59. A patient that is receiving radiation therapy as a treatment for cancer may experience any of the following symptoms as a direct result of the treatment, *except*:

    a. nausea and vomiting.
    b. hair loss.
    c. pulmonary edema.
    d. sloughing of the skin.

60. What is the difference between a clean and a dirty radiation accident?

    a. In a clean accident the patient has external exposure but not internal.
    b. In a clean accident the patient has internal exposure but not external.
    c. In a dirty accident the patient continues to be a hazard of exposure to responders.
    d. In a dirty accident the patient is exposed to an ionizing source but is not radioactive.

Test #37 Answer Form

	A	B	C	D
1.	❑	❑	❑	❑
2.	❑	❑	❑	❑
3.	❑	❑	❑	❑
4.	❑	❑	❑	❑
5.	❑	❑	❑	❑
6.	❑	❑	❑	❑
7.	❑	❑	❑	❑
8.	❑	❑	❑	❑
9.	❑	❑	❑	❑
10.	❑	❑	❑	❑
11.	❑	❑	❑	❑
12.	❑	❑	❑	❑
13.	❑	❑	❑	❑
14.	❑	❑	❑	❑
15.	❑	❑	❑	❑
16.	❑	❑	❑	❑
17.	❑	❑	❑	❑
18.	❑	❑	❑	❑
19.	❑	❑	❑	❑
20.	❑	❑	❑	❑
21.	❑	❑	❑	❑
22.	❑	❑	❑	❑
23.	❑	❑	❑	❑
24.	❑	❑	❑	❑
25.	❑	❑	❑	❑
26.	❑	❑	❑	❑

	A	B	C	D
27.	❑	❑	❑	❑
28.	❑	❑	❑	❑
29.	❑	❑	❑	❑
30.	❑	❑	❑	❑
31.	❑	❑	❑	❑
32.	❑	❑	❑	❑
33.	❑	❑	❑	❑
34.	❑	❑	❑	❑
35.	❑	❑	❑	❑
36.	❑	❑	❑	❑
37.	❑	❑	❑	❑
38.	❑	❑	❑	❑
39.	❑	❑	❑	❑
40.	❑	❑	❑	❑
41.	❑	❑	❑	❑
42.	❑	❑	❑	❑
43.	❑	❑	❑	❑
44.	❑	❑	❑	❑
45.	❑	❑	❑	❑
46.	❑	❑	❑	❑
47.	❑	❑	❑	❑
48.	❑	❑	❑	❑
49.	❑	❑	❑	❑
50.	❑	❑	❑	❑
51.	❑	❑	❑	❑
52.	❑	❑	❑	❑

	A	B	C	D		A	B	C	D
53.	❏	❏	❏	❏	57.	❏	❏	❏	❏
54.	❏	❏	❏	❏	58.	❏	❏	❏	❏
55.	❏	❏	❏	❏	59.	❏	❏	❏	❏
56.	❏	❏	❏	❏	60.	❏	❏	❏	❏

Head and Facial Trauma

1. Common MOI for blunt trauma to the face and head include all the following, *except*:

   a. MVC.
   b. falls.
   c. GSW.
   d. augmented force.

2. Which of the following is not a common MOI for penetrating injuries to the face and head?

   a. Stabbings
   b. Clubs or bats
   c. Human bites
   d. Animal bites

3. Common associated injuries that accompany face or head injuries include:

   a. airway compromise.
   b. hearing loss.
   c. equilibrium disturbances.
   d. loss of bladder control.

4. Which of the following is not a common MOI for blunt throat injuries?

   a. Hanging
   b. MVC
   c. Strangulation
   d. Stabbing

5. A _____ is hemorrhage in the anterior chamber of the eye.

   a. conjunctival hemorrhage
   b. detached retina
   c. blow-out fracture
   d. hyphema

6. When traumatic pressure is transmitted through the eyeball to the relatively thin bone in the medial and inferior portions of the orbit causing it to break, this is called a:

   a. posterior chamber divide.
   b. detached retina.
   c. blow-out fracture.
   d. hyphema.

7. Isolated injuries to the mouth, such as from a _____, are very common, accounting for as much as 50% of facial trauma.

   a. punch
   b. MVC
   c. penetrating trauma
   d. fishhook

8. The LeFort classifications categorize facial fractures into three types. The higher the number, the more significant the damage, and the more potential there is for a:

   a. complicated airway.
   b. brain injury.
   c. spinal cord injury.
   d. vision disturbance.

9. Lefort fractures are based on:

   a. clinical impression.
   b. history of MOI.
   c. X-ray or CT scan findings.
   d. none of the above.

10. The critical structures in the neck include all the following, *except*:

    a. larynx and trachea.
    b. carotid arteries.
    c. vertebral arteries.
    d. bronchiole arteries.

11. The _____ ear canal is considered a mucous membrane that secretes wax for protection.

    a. pinna
    b. outer
    c. external
    d. inner

12. The middle ear is separated from the external canal by the:

    a. pinna.
    b. eardrum.
    c. cartilage.
    d. inner ear.

13. Light receptors to color vision, which are located in the posterior chamber of the eye, are called:

    a. optic nerve.
    b. retina.
    c. rods.
    d. cones.

14. The _____ is the transparent covering of the iris and pupil, which admits light into the eye.

    a. conjuctiva
    b. lens
    c. sclera
    d. cornea

15. _____ provide protection for the eye and help to lubricate the surface of the eye.

    a. Lens
    b. Eyelids
    c. Lacrimal apparatus
    d. Conjuctiva

16. The _____ are responsible for peripheral vision and low light, night sight conditions.

    a. pupils
    b. rods
    c. cones
    d. retina

17. Which of the following is not a major muscle of the mouth?

    a. Hypoglossal
    b. Tongue
    c. Orbicular oris
    d. Masseter muscles

18. The bones of the mouth include the palate, jawbone and:

    a. hyoid.
    b. teeth.
    c. zygomatic.
    d. mastoid process.

19. When the paramedic examines the patient's face and the jaws and teeth do not meet as they should, this is called:

    a. diplopia.
    b. malocclusion.
    c. a depressed zygoma.
    d. tetany.

20. When a patient has sustained an eye injury, often the recommendation is to cover both eyes to limit or prevent:

    a. the onset of dysconjugate gaze in the unaffected eye.
    b. the onset of dysconjugate gaze in the affected eye.
    c. movement from conjugate gaze of the uninjured eye.
    d. movement from conjugate gaze of the injured eye.

21. In the United States approximately four _____ people sustain a head injury each year.

    a. out of a thousand
    b. thousand
    c. million
    d. hundred million

22. The highest risk of head injury occurs in _____ between _____ years of age.

    a. males: 2 to 12
    b. males: 15 to 24
    c. females: 15 to 24
    d. females: 65 to 85

23. The most common cause of head trauma and subdural hematoma is/are:

    a. MVC.
    b. falls in the elderly.
    c. sports.
    d. falls in the presence of alcohol abuse.

24. The scalp has an important freely moveable sheet of connective tissue called _____ that helps to deflect blows.

    a. parietal fold
    b. mastoid sheath
    c. emissary
    d. galea

25. The actual bones that comprise the skull are double layered with a spongy middle layer allowing them to:

    a. facilitate drainage in the event of a hemorrhage.
    b. aerate the meninges.
    c. be strong yet light in weight.
    d. recycle cerebrospinal fluid.

26. Trauma to the _____ may cause interference to the voluntary skeletal movement and may result in extremity paralysis, paresthesia or weakness.

    a. medulla
    b. cerebrum
    c. brainstem
    d. occiput

27. When a person is struck in the _____ lobe it may cause seeing "stars," blurred vision or other visual disturbances.

    a. temporal
    b. parietal
    c. occipital
    d. frontal

28. The cranial nerves (CN) that can be affected in head injury are the oculomotor nerve CN _____ and the vagus nerve CN _____.

    a. II: X
    b. III: V
    c. III: X
    d. IV: XII

29. The _____ is responsible for the level of arousal and must be an intact cortical function for the level of awareness to be present.

    a. foraman magnum
    b. vagus nerve
    c. hypothalamus
    d. reticular activating system

30. The arachnoid membrane, which appears to look like a web of blood vessels, is actually composed of:

    a. venous blood vessels that reabsorb CSF.
    b. venous blood vessels that drain the cerebral sinuses.
    c. arteries that stimulate cerebral function.
    d. arteries that manufacture CSF.

31. The brain has a very high metabolic rate and consumes _____% of the body's oxygen supply.

    a. 5
    b. 10
    c. 20
    d. 50

32. A mechanism called _____ is responsible for regulating the body's blood pressure to maintain the cerebral perfusion pressure (CPP).

    a. intercerebral pressure
    b. intracerebral pressure
    c. autoregulation
    d. mean arterial force

33. The general categories of head injuries include all the following, *except*:

    a. coup.
    b. contra coup.
    c. diffuse axonal injury.
    d. peripheral injury.

34. Which of the following is not a type of brain injury?

    a. Peripheral injury
    b. Focal injury
    c. Subarachnoid hemorrhage
    d. Diffuse axonal injury

35. Cerebral contusion, intracranial hemorrhage and epidural hematoma are all examples of _____ brain injuries.

    a. peripheral
    b. focal
    c. subarachnoid
    d. diffuse axonal

36. _____ is the effect of acceleration or deceleration on the brain.

    a. Coup
    b. Contra coup
    c. Focal
    d. Diffuse axonal injury

37. A _____ is a mild diffuse axonal injury, which results in a transient episode of neuronal dysfunction with rapid return to normal neurologic activity.

    a. subarachnoid injury
    b. concussion
    c. epidural hematoma
    d. contusion

38. Which of the following is not a type of skull fracture that can be determined by an X-ray?

    a. linear
    b. depressed
    c. battle's sign
    d. basilar

39. All the following are types of intracranial hemorrhage, *except*:

    a. epidural.
    b. intracerebral.
    c. basilar.
    d. subdural.

40. _____ hematomas are bleeds that are more common in elderly and alcoholic patients who fall down and hit their heads often.

    a. Acute subdural
    b. Chronic subdural
    c. Acute epidural
    d. Chronic epidural

41. All the following are assessment findings that are consistent with rising ICP caused by downward pressure on the brain, *except* pressure on the:

    a. respiratory center causing irregular respirations.
    b. hypothalamus causing vomiting.
    c. brain stem causing tachycardia.
    d. oculomotor nerve causing unequal or unreactive pupils.

42. The "Cushing" response in brain herniation with hypotension and bradycardia is a late response and usually precedes death by only _____ minutes.

    a. 4 to 6
    b. 10
    c. 15
    d. 20

43. When there is pressure on the cerebral cortex and upper brainstem from an enlarging hematoma, which of the following assessment findings may be present?

    a. Pupils are still reactive.
    b. The BP rises and pulse rate slows.
    c. Cheyne-Stokes respirations.
    d. All of the above.

44. When an enlarging hematoma asserts pressure on the middle brain stem, which of the following assessment findings may be present?

    a. Pupils are still reactive.
    b. Wide pulse pressure.
    c. Decorticate posturing.
    d. Slowed respirations.

45. Which of the following statements is not correct regarding the impact of pressure from ICP on the lower brainstem or medulla?

    a. Vegetative functions are temporarily impaired because of the pressure.
    b. The patient's injury is not considered survivable.
    c. The respirations are ataxic or absent.
    d. The ECG will have QRS, S-T and T wave changes.

46. With GCS being an objective measure of eye opening, verbal response and motor response in a numerical score, a moderate head injury would be:

    a. 13 to 15.
    b. 8 to 12.
    c. 5 to 8.
    d. < 8.

47. The severe _____ was formerly called a brainstem injury, and it involved severe mechanical disruption of many axons in both cerebral hemispheres, extending to the brainstem.

    a. peripheral injury
    b. focal injury
    c. subarachnoid hemorrhage
    d. diffuse axonal injury

48. When assessing a patient's head for possible depressed and open skull fractures, the paramedic should be careful to use the _____ to palpate and not "poke" into the fracture site.

    a. pads of the fingers
    b. flat side of a tongue depressor
    c. stethoscope with a sterile gauze
    d. palm of the hand

49. The signs and symptoms of an intracranial hematoma include any of the following, *except*:

    a. headache which is getting increasingly severe.
    b. nausea and vomiting.
    c. tachycardia and tachypnea.
    d. changes in mental status.

50. Signs of brain irritation include:

    a. change in personality.
    b. irritability.
    c. repeating words or phrases.
    d. all of the above.

51. The appropriate management of a head injury by the paramedic includes all the following, *except*:

    a. assure an adequate airway, ventilation and oxygenation.
    b. aggressive hyperventilation.
    c. assure adequate circulation.
    d. conduct serial neurologic assessments.

52. If hypotension develops in the patient with a head injury, it is most likely caused by bleeding from:

    a. another organ or injuries besides the brain.
    b. the middle meningeal artery.
    c. a subarachnoid hemorrhage.
    d. the circle of Willis.

53. Studies have shown that _____ improves outcome in combative head trauma patients.

   a. the use of steroids
   b. osmotic diuretics given in the field
   c. aggressive hyperventilation
   d. paralysis prior to intubation

54. In the patient with a head injury, the use of glucose is recommended:

   a. after intubation of a combative patient.
   b. only when hypoglycemia is confirmed.
   c. only when given simultaneously with steroids.
   d. prior to sedation for intubation.

55. When treating a patient with increased ICP the paramedic should first:

   a. paralyze then intubate the patient.
   b. assure adequate tidal volume.
   c. hyperventilate the patient.
   d. administer an osmotic diuretic.

56. In the management of a head injury patient the paramedic should assure that the cerebral perfusion pressure is maintained by making sure to keep the _____ BP over _____ mmHg.

   a. systolic: 70
   b. systolic: 100
   c. diastolic: 50
   d. diastolic: 70

57. While assuring a patent airway in the patient with head trauma, the paramedic should avoid _____ as it may increase the ICP.

   a. inserting an OPA
   b. using a water soluble jelly
   c. nasal intubation
   d. oral tracheal intubation

58. When assessing a patient suspected of having an intracranial hematoma developing which of the following is the most important finding?

   a. The history of the MOI.
   b. The past medical history.
   c. The patient's current medications.
   d. When the patient ate last.

59. Which of the following types of head injury may present with confusion, disorientation and amnesia of the event?

   a. a mild diffuse axonal injury
   b. a moderate diffuse axonal injury
   c. a severe diffuse axonal injury
   d. none of the above

60. Which of the following types of skull fractures are easily missed in the absence of symptoms from an underlying hematoma developing?

   a. Linear
   b. Depressed
   c. Battle's sign
   d. Basilar

Test #38 Answer Form

	A	B	C	D			A	B	C	D
1.	❏	❏	❏	❏		27.	❏	❏	❏	❏
2.	❏	❏	❏	❏		28.	❏	❏	❏	❏
3.	❏	❏	❏	❏		29.	❏	❏	❏	❏
4.	❏	❏	❏	❏		30.	❏	❏	❏	❏
5.	❏	❏	❏	❏		31.	❏	❏	❏	❏
6.	❏	❏	❏	❏		32.	❏	❏	❏	❏
7.	❏	❏	❏	❏		33.	❏	❏	❏	❏
8.	❏	❏	❏	❏		34.	❏	❏	❏	❏
9.	❏	❏	❏	❏		35.	❏	❏	❏	❏
10.	❏	❏	❏	❏		36.	❏	❏	❏	❏
11.	❏	❏	❏	❏		37.	❏	❏	❏	❏
12.	❏	❏	❏	❏		38.	❏	❏	❏	❏
13.	❏	❏	❏	❏		39.	❏	❏	❏	❏
14.	❏	❏	❏	❏		40.	❏	❏	❏	❏
15.	❏	❏	❏	❏		41.	❏	❏	❏	❏
16.	❏	❏	❏	❏		42.	❏	❏	❏	❏
17.	❏	❏	❏	❏		43.	❏	❏	❏	❏
18.	❏	❏	❏	❏		44.	❏	❏	❏	❏
19.	❏	❏	❏	❏		45.	❏	❏	❏	❏
20.	❏	❏	❏	❏		46.	❏	❏	❏	❏
21.	❏	❏	❏	❏		47.	❏	❏	❏	❏
22.	❏	❏	❏	❏		48.	❏	❏	❏	❏
23.	❏	❏	❏	❏		49.	❏	❏	❏	❏
24.	❏	❏	❏	❏		50.	❏	❏	❏	❏
25.	❏	❏	❏	❏		51.	❏	❏	❏	❏
26.	❏	❏	❏	❏		52.	❏	❏	❏	❏

	A	B	C	D		A	B	C	D
53.	❏	❏	❏	❏	57.	❏	❏	❏	❏
54.	❏	❏	❏	❏	58.	❏	❏	❏	❏
55.	❏	❏	❏	❏	59.	❏	❏	❏	❏
56.	❏	❏	❏	❏	60.	❏	❏	❏	❏

39

Spinal Trauma

1. Which age group has the highest incidence of spinal cord injury?

   a. men 31–50
   b. men 16–30
   c. women 31–50
   d. women 16–30

2. It is estimated that _____ % of spinal cord injury is caused by improper handling of the patient.

   a. 5
   b. 10
   c. 25
   d. 35

3. The spine consists of interconnected bone and:

   a. ligaments.
   b. muscles.
   c. tendons.
   d. all of the above.

4. The ligament that prevents hyperflexion in the spine is the:

   a. anterior longitudinal.
   b. posterior longitudinal.
   c. cruciform.
   d. atlantoaxial.

5. A ligament that supports the atlas vertebrae is the:

   a. anterior longitudinal.
   b. posterior longitudinal.
   c. cruciform.
   d. atlantoaxial.

6. The second cervical vertebrae is also called the:

   a. cribiform.
   b. atlas.
   c. axis.
   d. pivotal.

7. The ligament that serves to hold the odontoid process close to the anterior arch is the:

   a. anterior longitudinal.
   b. posterior longitudinal.
   c. cruciform.
   d. atlantoaxial.

8. The five groups of vertebrae include each of the following, *except*:

   a. cervical.
   b. thoracic.
   c. odontoid.
   d. lumbar.

9. The area of the spine that is the most protected from injury is the:

   a. cervical.
   b. thoracic.
   c. lumbar.
   d. abdominal.

10. The _____ spine provides a balance point for the torso.

    a. coccyx
    b. thoracic
    c. cervical
    d. sacrum

11. The coccyx, which is a fusion of _____ bones, is commonly called the _____.

    a. 3; sacrum
    b. 4; tailbone
    c. 5; tailbone
    d. 6; buttock

12. The vertebrae consist of the body, vertebral arch, and the:

    a. foramen magnum.
    b. transverse process.
    c. spina bifida.
    d. spinous foramen.

13. The posterior aspect of the vertebrae that projects back from the junction of two lamina is called the:

   a. vertebral arch.
   b. spinous process.
   c. intercerebral disk.
   d. transverse process.

14. The relatively soft, gel-like internal portion of the disk is called the:

   a. annulus fibrosis.
   b. lamina.
   c. odontoid.
   d. nucleus pulposus.

15. Where does the spinal cord end?

   a. C-6
   b. T-5
   c. L-2
   d. L-6

16. Where does CSF come from?

   a. The intervertebral disks.
   b. It is manufactured in the ventricles of the brain.
   c. It is manufactured in the pancreas.
   d. It is stored in the bile duct.

17. The material that is located in the anatomical spinal tracts is called:

   a. white matter.
   b. melanin.
   c. myelin sheath.
   d. gray matter.

18. Information from body parts and sensory information are carried to the brain by the:

   a. sensory system.
   b. ascending nerve tracts.
   c. descending nerve tracts.
   d. parasympathetic NS.

19. Corticospinal and reticulospinal are two types of:

   a. sensory system nerves.
   b. ascending nerve tracts.
   c. descending nerve tracts.
   d. parasympathetic NS.

20. What is a funiculus?

   a. A group of nerve fibers with a similar function.
   b. A ligament found in the spinal column.
   c. The key to the corticospinal tract.
   d. The center of the reticulospinal tract.

21. The lateral spinothalamic tracts:

   a. conduct sensory impulses of touch and pressure to the brain.
   b. send muscular impulses from the brain to muscle.
   c. conduct impulses of pain and temperature to the brain.
   d. coordinate impulses necessary for muscular movements.

22. A particular area where the spinal nerve provides either motor stimulation, sensations, or both is called a:

   a. ganglion.
   b. dermatome.
   c. axon.
   d. nerve band.

23. Motor nerve deficits at the level of the umbilicus can be caused by nerve root damage to:

   a. C-4
   b. L-4
   c. T-10
   d. T-12

24. The motor nerve root for knee flexion is located at:

   a. C-6
   b. S-1
   c. T-8
   d. L-4

25. Sensation in the little finger is located in which nerve root?

   a. C-2
   b. C-8
   c. T-5
   d. L-1

26. Sensation in the inguinal crease is located in which nerve root?

   a. C-8
   b. T-4
   c. L-2
   d. S-1

27. All the following suggest a spinal cord injury, *except*:

    a. pain, tenderness, and painful movement.
    b. deformity, cuts, or bruises over the spine.
    c. weakness on one side of the body.
    d. paralysis and weakness of the legs.

28. Each of the following is a positive MOI for spinal injury, *except*:

    a. sports injuries such as golf and bowling.
    b. shooting or stabbing injuries near the spine.
    c. falls greater than three times the patient's height.
    d. high-speed motor vehicle collisions.

29. Prior to an X-ray being taken in the ED, if a patient is cleared of a spinal injury by a physician, there should be:

    a. no distracting injuries.
    b. a reliable patient with no signs and symptoms of injury.
    c. no altered mental status or intoxication.
    d. all of the above.

30. When is partial spinal immobilization used in the field?
    a. when the distance a patient fell is < 30 feet
    b. when the MOI is not severe
    c. if the patient prefers not to lie down
    d. it should not be used at all

31. You are treating a toddler who fell out of a shopping cart and lacerated his head. He was initially unconscious, but now is crying and covered with blood. How best should he be managed?

    a. Cervical collar application and hemorrhage control.
    b. Full spinal immobilization with the parent providing support.
    c. Hemorrhage control and transport in a child car seat.
    d. Backboard and manual head stabilization by the parent.

32. When considering not to immobilize a patient, the patient must be considered reliable. Which of the following would make a patient reliable?

    a. A belligerent patient.
    b. An alert patient with a communication problem.
    c. A patient who is alert and has always been alert.
    d. An alert patient having an acute stress reaction.

33. If a patient with an "uncertain MOI" does complain of some minor pain upon moving his head you should:

    a. determine the range of motion.
    b. continue your assessment and document the complaint.
    c. fully immobilize the spine.
    d. be sure to throw a collar on before arriving at the ED.

34. Why should you palpate the spinous process if you suspect a neck injury?

    a. because this will rule out neck injury
    b. tender areas do not hurt unless palpated
    c. patients appreciate the extra care
    d. the vertebrae may be dislocated even though there is still movement

35. Assessment of the upper extremities include all the following, *except*:

    a. assess for finger abduction and adduction.
    b. assess for finger and hand extension.
    c. ask the patient to make a fist in the air.
    d. assess sensory function in the upper extremities.

36. You are treating a construction worker who did not have a helmet on while he was walking under a platform and was struck on the head by a large falling brick. Which of the following types of injury do you suspect this patient might have?

    a. Vertical compression of the spine.
    b. Hyperflexion of the head and neck.
    c. Hyperextension of the head and neck.
    d. Distraction of the neck.

37. You and your partner are immobilizing a patient who attempted to hang himself. Which of the following injuries do you associate with a hanging?

    a. Rotational neck injury.
    b. Flexion of the neck.
    c. Vertical compression of the neck.
    d. Distraction of the neck.

38. You arrive at the scene of a vehicle that was T-boned in an intersection. The EMT–Bs are short-boarding the driver who is complaining of neck and back pain. Which of the following injuries do you suspect?

    a. Rotational neck injury.
    b. Flexion of the neck.
    c. Vertical compression of the neck.
    d. Distraction of the neck.

39. The type of spinal cord injury that is characterized by a temporary disruption of cord-mediated functions is a cord:

a. concussion.
b. contusion.
c. compression.
d. transection.

40. The type of spinal cord injury that is characterized by hypotension and vasodilation, loss of bladder and bowel control, and priaprism in male patients is:

a. spinal hemorrhage.
b. spinal shock.
c. neurogenic shock.
d. cord laceration.

41. You are called to assist a patient who has fallen, but has no complaint of injury. The patient has a preexisting spinal cord injury, which has left him with a loss of motor function, motion and light touch, but only on the left side of his body. Which of the following conditions does this patient have?

a. anterior cord syndrome
b. central cord syndrome
c. incomplete spinal cord transection
d. brown–Sequard syndrome

42. All the following are common non-traumatic spinal conditions, *except*:

a. low back pain syndrome.
b. degenerative disk disease.
c. spondylolysis.
d. epidural abscess.

43. It is estimated that between _____ percent of the population experience some degree of low back pain during their lifetime.

a. 20–30
b. 40–50
c. 60–90
d. 80–100

44. All the following are risk factors for low back injury, *except*:

a. EMS personnel.
b. truck drivers.
c. people with osteoporosis.
d. golfers.

45. In which of the following spinal disorders is heredity considered to be a significant factor?

a. degenerative disk
b. spondylolysis
c. low back pain syndrome
d. spinal cord tumors

46. What is the primary management of a patient with severe low back pain?

a. palliative care
b. full spinal immobilization
c. partial spinal immobilization
d. rapid transport to an ED

47. What is the most common cause of spinal cord tumors?

a. trauma
b. heredity
c. metastasis
d. PCBS

48. The diameter of the spinal cord is approximately _____ mm and the diameter of the spinal column is approximately _____ mm.

a. 5;10
b. 10;15
c. 15;20
d. 20;25

49. Which of the following statements is not correct about rigid cervical collars?

a. They are also referred to as extrication collars.
b. They limit movement of the neck.
c. They totally eliminate neck movement.
d. They are the standard for cervical immobilization.

50. Which of the following is the primary reason for removing a helmet from a patient with a potential SCI?

a. the paramedic is trained to do it
b. airway management
c. patient needs to be immobilized
d. ED staff does not have sufficient training to do it

51. Which of the following is not an indication for rapid extrication?

a. compensating shock
b. decompensating shock
c. penetrating chest wound
d. penetrating abdominal wound

52. For which of the following patients should the paramedic perform a rapid takedown?

    a. An ambulatory patient who tripped and fell and broke her nose.
    b. An ambulatory driver involved in a MVC with airbag deployed w/o injury that was belted and had no LOC.
    c. An ambulatory passenger of a high speed MVC complaining of a headache.
    d. A toddler in the arms of a parent walking around at a collision scene.

53. When should a child be removed from a car seat to immobilize the spine?

    a. when the child is crying
    b. when the parents are distressed
    c. when it is necessary for the patient to be supine
    d. when you cannot palpate the child's back

54. Patients are immobilized in the neutral, in-line anatomic position for all the following reasons, *except* this:

    a. position allows for the most space for the cord.
    b. position is the most comfortable for the patient.
    c. is the most stable position for the spinal column.
    d. position will help to reduce cord hypoxia.

55. Which of the following is not a principle of spinal immobilization?

    a. The goal is to prevent further injury.
    b. 15% of secondary spinal injuries are preventable with immobilization.
    c. Spinal immobilization should begin after the initial assessment.
    d. Spinal immobilization should begin with the initial assessment.

56. Patients with herniated intervertebral disks are commonly affected in which two areas of the spine?

    a. cervical and thoracic
    b. thoracic and lumbar
    c. lumbar and sacral
    d. lumbar and cervical

57. What is the preferred method for assessing a patient for spinal tenderness?

    a. palpate over each of the spinal processes
    b. palpate over each of the vertebral bodies
    c. ask the patient to move all four extremities
    d. ask the patient if he/she has any back pain

58. The evaluation of motor function of the lower extremities includes assessment of plantar flexion and:

    a. great toe flexion.
    b. foot dorsiflexion.
    c. Babinski reflex.
    d. plantar reflex.

59. The causes of traumatic spinal cord injury include direct trauma, excessive movement, and:

    a. directions of force.
    b. inflammation of arch.
    c. Achilles' heel.
    d. blight reflexes.

60. You are assessing a 20-year-old male that was removed from a pool on a backboard by lifeguards on the scene. Your assessment findings include hypotension, bradycardia, and skin that is pink and warm. What do you suspect with these findings?

    a. spinal shock
    b. neurogenic shock
    c. spinal cord compression
    d. disk prolapse

Test #39 Answer Form

	A	B	C	D		A	B	C	D
1.	❏	❏	❏	❏	27.	❏	❏	❏	❏
2.	❏	❏	❏	❏	28.	❏	❏	❏	❏
3.	❏	❏	❏	❏	29.	❏	❏	❏	❏
4.	❏	❏	❏	❏	30.	❏	❏	❏	❏
5.	❏	❏	❏	❏	31.	❏	❏	❏	❏
6.	❏	❏	❏	❏	32.	❏	❏	❏	❏
7.	❏	❏	❏	❏	33.	❏	❏	❏	❏
8.	❏	❏	❏	❏	34.	❏	❏	❏	❏
9.	❏	❏	❏	❏	35.	❏	❏	❏	❏
10.	❏	❏	❏	❏	36.	❏	❏	❏	❏
11.	❏	❏	❏	❏	37.	❏	❏	❏	❏
12.	❏	❏	❏	❏	38.	❏	❏	❏	❏
13.	❏	❏	❏	❏	39.	❏	❏	❏	❏
14.	❏	❏	❏	❏	40.	❏	❏	❏	❏
15.	❏	❏	❏	❏	41.	❏	❏	❏	❏
16.	❏	❏	❏	❏	42.	❏	❏	❏	❏
17.	❏	❏	❏	❏	43.	❏	❏	❏	❏
18.	❏	❏	❏	❏	44.	❏	❏	❏	❏
19.	❏	❏	❏	❏	45.	❏	❏	❏	❏
20.	❏	❏	❏	❏	46.	❏	❏	❏	❏
21.	❏	❏	❏	❏	47.	❏	❏	❏	❏
22.	❏	❏	❏	❏	48.	❏	❏	❏	❏
23.	❏	❏	❏	❏	49.	❏	❏	❏	❏
24.	❏	❏	❏	❏	50.	❏	❏	❏	❏
25.	❏	❏	❏	❏	51.	❏	❏	❏	❏
26.	❏	❏	❏	❏	52.	❏	❏	❏	❏

	A	B	C	D		A	B	C	D
53.	❏	❏	❏	❏	57.	❏	❏	❏	❏
54.	❏	❏	❏	❏	58.	❏	❏	❏	❏
55.	❏	❏	❏	❏	59.	❏	❏	❏	❏
56.	❏	❏	❏	❏	60.	❏	❏	❏	❏

40

Thoracic Trauma

1. Chest injuries are the _____ leading cause of trauma deaths each year in the United States.

   a. primary
   b. second
   c. third
   d. fifth

2. The MOI of a thoracic injury involves blunt trauma, caused by all the following, *except*:

   a. penetrating.
   b. compression.
   c. deceleration.
   d. acceleration.

3. The major problem with the injury to the mediastinum is:

   a. tearing of a great vessel.
   b. contusion of the heart.
   c. esophageal spasm.
   d. aortic seizure.

4. An esophageal injury such as a _____ may occur to the esophagus when the throat or upper chest is perforated.

   a. spasm
   b. tear
   c. flare-up
   d. fracture

5. When an explosion occurs within a confined space, the pressure injures the lung tissue causing:

   a. necrosis.
   b. petechial impressions.
   c. massive lung contusions to develop.
   d. tears.

6. The anterior chest is made up of the rib cage, consisting of all the following, *except* the:

   a. sternum.
   b. clavicles.
   c. twelve pairs of ribs.
   d. twelve thoracic vertebrae.

7. Which of the following is not a muscle of the thorax?

   a. External intercostals
   b. Medial intercostals
   c. Internal intercostals
   d. Trapezius

8. _____ is a major muscle that moves the head and is also an accessory muscle of breathing as it helps to lift the chest cage.

   a. Sternocleidomastoid
   b. Rhomboids
   c. Pectoralis major
   d. Latissimus dorsi

9. The muscle that originates in the occipital bone and inserts into the clavicle, with its function being to raise and lower the shoulders, is called the:

   a. rhomboid.
   b. trapezius.
   c. external costals.
   d. sternocleidomastoid.

10. The trachea extends from the anterior throat into the chest cavity and then bifurcates at the carina into the:

    a. parenchyma.
    b. anterior rhomboid major.
    c. distal rhomboid minor.
    d. mainstem bronchi.

11. _____ is the lung tissue itself rather than all the supporting connective tissues.

    a. Parenchyma
    b. Bronchi
    c. Alveoli
    d. Pleura

12. All the following are major arteries of the chest, *except* the:

    a. aorta.
    b. internal mammary artery.
    c. carotid artery.
    d. inferior vena cava.

13. Which of the following is not a major vein of the chest?

   a. Aorta
   b. Internal jugular
   c. External jugular
   d. Subclavian

14. The _____ is located in the mediastinum, or center of the chest.

   a. heart
   b. trachea
   c. esophagus
   d. all of the above

15. The mechanical process of ventilation involves all the following, *except*:

   a. during inspiration, the diaphragm and intercostal muscles contract.
   b. diaphragmatic contraction creates a vacuum in the chest cavity.
   c. positive intrathoracic pressure pushes air out of the lungs.
   d. negative intrathoracic pressure "sucks" air into the lungs, expanding them.

16. Any injury that affects the diaphragm, intercostal muscles, or _____ can affect the mechanics of ventilation severely.

   a. vagus nerve
   b. accessory muscles of breathing
   c. aortic arch
   d. lumbar spine

17. The ability to exchange gas during respiration is a function of all the following elements, *except*:

   a. serous pleural fluid.
   b. alveolar capillary interface.
   c. pulmonary circulation.
   d. acid-base balance.

18. Chemoreceptors, located in the aortic arch and _____, measure carbon dioxide levels in the blood.

   a. capillary beds
   b. carotid sinus
   c. parenchyma
   d. alveoli

19. All the following are examples of impairments in gas exchange from thoracic trauma, *except*:

   a. atelectasis from inadequately inflating all the alveoli.
   b. contusion to the lung tissue from compression of the chest.
   c. disruption of the respiratory tract from a cut to the trachea.
   d. disassociation of the alveoli from the parenchyma.

20. Assessment findings of the patient who has experienced thoracic trauma may include a pulse that is:

   a. tachycardic from shock.
   b. bradycardic from a conduction problem.
   c. in deficit from damage to a great vessel.
   d. all of the above.

21. Typical chest wall injuries include all the following, *except*:

   a. conduction disturbances.
   b. rib fractures.
   c. flail segment.
   d. sternal fracture.

22. Complications from rib fractures increase with any of the following, *except*:

   a. age.
   b. sexual preference.
   c. number of fractures.
   d. location of the fractures.

23. Ribs _____ are most often fractured because they are thin and poorly protected.

   a. 1 to 3
   b. 4 to 9
   c. 10 to 12
   d. none of the above

24. Fractures of the 1st and 2nd ribs indicate _____ and may also involve a rupture of the aorta, tracheo-bronchial tree injury, or a vascular injury.

   a. mild trauma
   b. moderate trauma
   c. severe trauma
   d. all of the above

25. A flail segment is a very serious chest injury and has mortality rates of _____% because of the associated injuries and impact on ventilations.

   a. 5 to 10
   b. 10 to 20
   c. 20 to 40
   d. 40 to 50

26. Which of the following statements about the pathology of a flail segment is incorrect?

    a. If the flail segment is small, the paradoxical movement is minimal because of muscle spasm.
    b. Pain is a contributing factor to the severity of this injury.
    c. Pain can reduce thoracic expansion and decrease ventilation.
    d. The arterial blood flow is impaired resulting in a ventilation–perfusion mismatch.

27. Which of the following is a common associated complication of a flail segment?

    a. Pulmonary contusion
    b. Subcutaneous emphysema
    c. Pericardial effusion
    d. Pulmonary edema

28. The most common cause of a sternal fracture is a _____ injury caused by an MVC.

    a. severe hyperflexion
    b. blunt blow to the chest
    c. acceleration
    d. deceleration compression

29. The main reason why a sternal fracture has such a high mortality rate is:

    a. because of the high incidence of vomiting.
    b. that nearly all these patients lose consciousness.
    c. because of the associated injuries.
    d. these patients are often given too much fluid prehospitally.

30. When assessing the patient with a simple pneumothorax, the patient may have decreased chest wall movement and slight pleuritic chest pain, which may be referred to the:

    a. shoulder or arm on the unaffected side.
    b. shoulder or arm on the affected side.
    c. abdomen and upper thighs.
    d. neck.

31. In an open pneumothorax, a ventilation perfusion mismatch can occur from:

    a. shunting.
    b. hypoventilation and hypoxia.
    c. a large functional dead space developing.
    d. all of the above.

32. The management of the patient with an open pneumothorax includes all the following, *except*:

    a. aggressive fluid replacement.
    b. occluding the open wound.
    c. airway and ventilation control.
    d. evaluation of the need for endotracheal intubation.

33. The pathophysiology of a tension pneumothorax includes all the following, *except*:

    a. the lung collapses on the affected side with mediastinal shift to the contralateral side.
    b. a serious reduction in cardiac output by the deformation of the vena cava, reducing preload.
    c. the lung collapse leads to right-to-left intrapulmonary shunting and hypoxia.
    d. the lung collapse leads to left-to-right intrapulmonary shunting and hypercarbia.

34. Which of the following assessment findings will most likely not be present in a patient with a tension pneumothorax?

    a. Unilateral decreased or absent breath sounds.
    b. Hyporesonance and mediastinal shift to the ipsilateral side.
    c. Tachypnea, cyanosis, and extreme anxiety.
    d. Narrow pulse pressure and JVD.

35. It is not uncommon for an intercostal artery to bleed as much as _____ cc per minute into the chest.

    a. 10
    b. 20
    c. 40
    d. 50

36. Bleeding from a pulmonary contusion generally causes 1,000 to 1,500 cc of blood loss, although the chest cavity can hold some _____ cc of blood.

    a. 2,000 to 3,000
    b. 3,000 to 4,000
    c. 4,000 to 5,000
    d. 5,000 to 6,000

37. Intrapulmonary hemorrhage occurs in either the bronchus or the:

    a. alveoli.
    b. aorta.
    c. parenchyma.
    d. pleural space.

38. When evaluating the patient with a hemothorax, expect to find the signs and symptoms of shock as well as:

    a. decreased breath sounds.
    b. respiratory distress.
    c. a chest that is dull on percussion.
    d. all of the above.

39. The management of a hemopneumothorax includes:

    a. aggressive fluid replacement.
    b. the same management as a pulmonary contusion.
    c. the same management as a hemothorax.
    d. all of the above.

40. Pulmonary contusions are very common with blunt thoracic trauma, but are often missed on evaluation because of:

    a. an overexpansion effect.
    b. an inertial effect.
    c. the high incidence of other associated injuries.
    d. the Spalding effect.

41. Any of the following assessment findings may be present in the patient who has a lung contusion, *except*:

    a. decreased SpO$_2$.
    b. coughing and hemoptysis.
    c. collapsed alveoli.
    d. tachypnea and dyspnea.

42. Patients with pulmonary contusions also tend to have other severe thoracic and _____ injuries, so always assume multiple potential injuries are present.

    a. head
    b. neck
    c. spinal cord
    d. abdominal

43. The purpose of the pericardium is to anchor the heart and restrict excess movement, as well as:

    a. prevent the kinking of the great vessels.
    b. facilitate right to left pulmonary shunting.
    c. link the lymphatic system.
    d. conduct electrical impulses.

44. The major problem in pericardial tamponade is the impairment of _____, which significantly decreases the amount of blood the heart is able to pump out.

    a. pulmonic systolic filling
    b. ventricular diastolic filling
    c. pulmonic diastolic emptying
    d. ventricular diastolic emptying

45. Upon examination of a patient who has a cardiac tamponade, the paramedic may locate many of the following findings, *except*:

    a. narrow pulse pressure.
    b. Cushing's triad.
    c. pulsus paradoxus.
    d. Kussmual's sign.

46. The pathophysiology of a myocardial contusion may include any of the following, *except*:

    a. when the epicardium or endocardium are lacerated, a hemopericardium can develop.
    b. the areas of contusion are usually clearly demarcated.
    c. the areas of contusion are rarely defined.
    d. the areas of contusion may cause conduction defects on the ECG.

47. Many patients with myocardial contusion are relatively asymptomatic initially in the absence of associated injuries. Helpful signs include ECG changes, if present, and persistent:

    a. sinus tachycardia without obvious hypovolemia.
    b. right bundle branch block.
    c. atrial flutter.
    d. atrial fibrillation.

48. The management of the patient with a myocardial contusion after airway and ventilation control includes _____ according to local protocols.

    a. administration of fluids
    b. considering antidysrhythmics
    c. considering vasopressor agents
    d. all of the above

49. The management of a patient with a myocardial rupture includes supportive care of the ABCs and observing for the onset of _____ following trauma.

    a. severe headache
    b. abdominal distention
    c. CHF or pulmonary edema
    d. neurologic deficits

50. The primary causes of aortic dissection/rupture are primarily MVCs and:

    a. GSWs.
    b. falls.
    c. rib fractures.
    d. associated diaphragmatic rupture.

51. Aortic dissection/rupture is a very critical injury where _____% of the patients die instantaneously.

    a. 10 to 20
    b. 40 to 60
    c. 60 to 80
    d. 85 to 95

52. When examining a patient who is suspected of having an aortic dissection/rupture, any of the following findings may be present, *except*:

    a. a different BP on each arm.
    b. retrosternal or interscapular pain.
    c. pleuritic pain in the neck.
    d. ischemic pain of the extremities.

53. All the following are appropriate management for the patient suspected of having a diaphragmatic rupture, *except*:

    a. be alert for vomiting.
    b. place the shock patient in Trendelenburg's position.
    c. assess the need for positive pressure.
    d. support airway and ventilation.

54. Upon examination of the patient with an esophageal injury, the paramedic may find that the patient is having a:

    a. cardiac event.
    b. CVA.
    c. seizure.
    d. tension pneumothorax.

55. All the following are typical assessment findings in a patient with traumatic asphyxia, *except*:

    a. cyanosis to the face and upper neck.
    b. JVD.
    c. the skin below the affected area is cyanotic.
    d. petechia in the upper chest, neck, and face.

56. The management of the patient with traumatic asphyxia includes:

    a. IV fluids for hypotension.
    b. needle decompression prior to the release of compression.
    c. needle decompression after the release of compression.
    d. none of the above.

57. Tracheobronchial injury is rare and occurs in:

    a. blunt chest trauma.
    b. penetrating chest trauma.
    c. both blunt and penetrating chest trauma.
    d. high incidents in COPD patients.

58. Which of the following is not a typical assessment finding in a patient with a tracheo-bronchial injury?

    a. The patient is difficult to intubate.
    b. Signs of tension pneumothorax that do not respond to a needle decompression.
    c. Dyspnea and hemoptysis.
    d. Brady-block dysrhythmias.

59. The most frequent cause of an esophageal injury is from:

    a. Mallory-Weiss tear.
    b. blunt trauma.
    c. penetrating trauma.
    d. all of the above.

60. You are assessing a 33-year-old female who was the driver of a vehicle involved in a moderate speed rear-end MVC. She is complaining of increased difficulty breathing and pain in the lower chest and upper abdomen. She has the presence of a scaffold abdomen, there are bowel sounds in the lower right chest, and the area is dull to percussion. You suspect:

    a. diaphragmatic injury.
    b. tension pneumothorax.
    c. ectopic pregnancy.
    d. none of the above.

Test #40 Answer Form

	A	B	C	D
1.	❏	❏	❏	❏
2.	❏	❏	❏	❏
3.	❏	❏	❏	❏
4.	❏	❏	❏	❏
5.	❏	❏	❏	❏
6.	❏	❏	❏	❏
7.	❏	❏	❏	❏
8.	❏	❏	❏	❏
9.	❏	❏	❏	❏
10.	❏	❏	❏	❏
11.	❏	❏	❏	❏
12.	❏	❏	❏	❏
13.	❏	❏	❏	❏
14.	❏	❏	❏	❏
15.	❏	❏	❏	❏
16.	❏	❏	❏	❏
17.	❏	❏	❏	❏
18.	❏	❏	❏	❏
19.	❏	❏	❏	❏
20.	❏	❏	❏	❏
21.	❏	❏	❏	❏
22.	❏	❏	❏	❏
23.	❏	❏	❏	❏
24.	❏	❏	❏	❏
25.	❏	❏	❏	❏
26.	❏	❏	❏	❏

	A	B	C	D
27.	❏	❏	❏	❏
28.	❏	❏	❏	❏
29.	❏	❏	❏	❏
30.	❏	❏	❏	❏
31.	❏	❏	❏	❏
32.	❏	❏	❏	❏
33.	❏	❏	❏	❏
34.	❏	❏	❏	❏
35.	❏	❏	❏	❏
36.	❏	❏	❏	❏
37.	❏	❏	❏	❏
38.	❏	❏	❏	❏
39.	❏	❏	❏	❏
40.	❏	❏	❏	❏
41.	❏	❏	❏	❏
42.	❏	❏	❏	❏
43.	❏	❏	❏	❏
44.	❏	❏	❏	❏
45.	❏	❏	❏	❏
46.	❏	❏	❏	❏
47.	❏	❏	❏	❏
48.	❏	❏	❏	❏
49.	❏	❏	❏	❏
50.	❏	❏	❏	❏
51.	❏	❏	❏	❏
52.	❏	❏	❏	❏

	A	B	C	D		A	B	C	D
53.	❏	❏	❏	❏	57.	❏	❏	❏	❏
54.	❏	❏	❏	❏	58.	❏	❏	❏	❏
55.	❏	❏	❏	❏	59.	❏	❏	❏	❏
56.	❏	❏	❏	❏	60.	❏	❏	❏	❏

41

Abdominal Trauma

1. Abdominal trauma is the _____ leading cause of preventable trauma death.

   a. second
   b. third
   c. fourth
   d. fifth

2. The abdominal cavity can hide significant blood loss. As much as _____ can be lost before any signs of distention are apparent.

   a. 1 liter
   b. 1.5 liters
   c. 2 liters
   d. 2.5 liters

3. Immediate concerns, after the ABCs in the management of the patient with abdominal trauma, are hemorrhage, major organ damage, and:

   a. the possibility of peritonitis.
   b. the possible use of vasopressors.
   c. IV fluid replacement.
   d. associated chest injuries.

4. Abdominal trauma often goes unrecognized because the _____ is/are often unrecognized.

   a. signs of shock
   b. golden hour
   c. MOI
   d. platinum ten minutes

5. Motor vehicle crashes often involve _____ forces that compress internal organs and cause shearing of organs that are suspended by ligaments.

   a. rapid acceleration
   b. twisting
   c. rapid deceleration
   d. sublexation

6. The _____ is the section of the small intestine that is approximately 8 feet in length, absorbing the majority of the food we eat.

   a. duodenum
   b. jejunum
   c. ileum
   d. colon

7. The _____ is the last section of the small intestine and varies in length from 15 to 25 feet.

   a. duodenum
   b. jejunum
   c. ileum
   d. colon

8. The retroperitoneal space is a/an _____ behind the peritoneal space.

   a. actual space
   b. potential space
   c. solid organ
   d. hollow organ

9. The _____ is the largest organ in the body and often sustains injuries during rapid deceleration forces.

   a. liver
   b. kidney
   c. heart
   d. lung

10. Abnormal physical findings of the abdomen include all the following, *except*:

   a. a pulsating mass.
   b. a non-pulsating mass.
   c. muscle spasm.
   d. distention.

11. You have just finished a light palpation of all four quadrants of a patient with an MOI suggestive of possible internal injury. You discovered that the patient had pain on palpation in the ULQ without rebound tenderness. What type of pain does the examination reflect?

    a. somatic
    b. visceral
    c. guarded
    d. obstructive

12. What organ(s) may be injured in the patient described in question 11?

    a. appendix and small intestine
    b. liver and stomach
    c. stomach and spleen
    d. liver and gallbladder

13. Kehr's sign is an assessment finding of pain in the abdomen that radiates to the left shoulder. This finding indicates:

    a. acute bowel obstruction.
    b. intra-peritoneal bleeding and/or irritation.
    c. aortic aneurysm.
    d. ileus.

14. When a patient has ecchymosis in the umbilical area caused by peritoneal bleeding, this is known as:

    a. Cullen's sign.
    b. Grey–Turner's sign.
    c. periumbilical guarding.
    d. peritoneal's sign.

15. You and your crew have been dispatched to a football game at a local high school for a traumatic injury. Upon arrival you find a diaphoretic 29-year-old male who is doubled over in severe pain. He tells you that suddenly, without warning while he was sitting on the bench, he starting having excruciating pain in his left testicle. He also says he feels like he is going to vomit. What do you suspect is the cause of his pain?

    a. kidney stone
    b. renal colic
    c. testicular torsion
    d. intra-abdominal bleeding

16. How would you assess the patient described in question 15?

    a. Lay him supine on a backboard while removing his pants on the field.
    b. Gently move him on a stretcher into the ambulance before examining him.
    c. Administer morphine before moving him.
    d. Administer oxygen and walk him to the ambulance.

17. How would you treat the patient described in question 15?

    a. Treat for shock and begin a rapid transport.
    b. Administer oxygen and transport on a backboard.
    c. Manage his pain and transport gently.
    d. Apply ice, and place him in Trendelenburg's position.

18. The definitive treatment for his condition in most cases is:

    a. prompt surgery.
    b. pain management and bed rest.
    c. manual repositioning in the ED.
    d. rest, abundant hydration, and pain management.

19. After arriving on the scene of a possible assault, you find a 26-year-old male who denies being assaulted but confesses that he has a large foreign body stuck in his anus. He is bleeding from the rectum, has acute abdominal pain, and is tachycardic. The immediate complications associated with this type of emergency include:

    a. perforations and hemorrhage.
    b. traumatic peristalsis.
    c. alimentary spasms.
    d. acute peritonitis.

20. What do you suspect is the cause of the abdominal pain and tachycardia in the patient described in question 19?

    a. The patient is unable to pass gas.
    b. Contamination from fecal matter.
    c. Peritonitis from blood loss.
    d. Ischemia from bowel strangulation.

21. What is your management plan for the patient described in question 19?

    a. Keep the patient in a position of comfort.
    b. Attempt to remove the foreign object and control bleeding.
    c. Keep the patient supine with knees flexed.
    d. Apply ice and elevate the legs.

22. Associated signs and symptoms that should be anticipated by the paramedic for the patient described in question 19 include:

    a. dysrhythmias.
    b. narrowed pulse pressure.
    c. widening pulse pressure.
    d. nausea and vomiting.

23. You are on the scene of an MVC and find that the driver was apparently ejected from the vehicle after it crashed into a guardrail. The patient looks about 50 years old, is unconscious, but has no outward signs of trauma. Her breathing is shallow, clear and equal, pulse is 130 and weak, B/P is 76/24. Your initial field impression is a/an:

    a. potential head injury.
    b. aortic aneurysm.
    c. intra-abdominal bleed.
    d. spinal cord injury.

24. Initial treatment for the patient in question 23 includes all the following, *except*:

    a. airway management.
    b. hyperventilation.
    c. IV fluid replacement.
    d. rapid transport to a trauma center.

25. Traumatic injuries associated with consensual sex include all the following, *except*:

    a. restraint injuries.
    b. tears from pierced body jewelry.
    c. fractured penis.
    d. emotional withdrawal.

26. During your assessment of a third trimester female who was the driver of a vehicle involved in a moderate-speed collision, you recall that the patient can lose up to _____ of her blood volume before signs of shock are evident.

    a. 15%
    b. 25%
    c. 35%
    d. 45%

27. Direct trauma to the abdomen of the pregnant patient may result in all the following conditions, *except*:

    a. uterine inversion.
    b. premature labor.
    c. abruptio placenta.
    d. uterine rupture.

28. During the assessment of a patient that has pain from irritation of the diaphragm, to what area would you expect the patient's pain to radiate?

    a. back
    b. shoulder
    c. lower abdomen
    d. It will not radiate anywhere.

29. Besides the kidneys and spleen, which of the following organs are partially located within the retroperitoneal cavity?

    a. liver
    b. gallbladder
    c. pancreas
    d. duodenum

30. _____ is the term for decreased motility of the intestine.

    a. Alimentary
    b. Viscus
    c. Excursion
    d. Ileus

Test #41 Answer Form

	A	B	C	D		A	B	C	D
1.	❏	❏	❏	❏	16.	❏	❏	❏	❏
2.	❏	❏	❏	❏	17.	❏	❏	❏	❏
3.	❏	❏	❏	❏	18.	❏	❏	❏	❏
4.	❏	❏	❏	❏	19.	❏	❏	❏	❏
5.	❏	❏	❏	❏	20.	❏	❏	❏	❏
6.	❏	❏	❏	❏	21.	❏	❏	❏	❏
7.	❏	❏	❏	❏	22.	❏	❏	❏	❏
8.	❏	❏	❏	❏	23.	❏	❏	❏	❏
9.	❏	❏	❏	❏	24.	❏	❏	❏	❏
10.	❏	❏	❏	❏	25.	❏	❏	❏	❏
11.	❏	❏	❏	❏	26.	❏	❏	❏	❏
12.	❏	❏	❏	❏	27.	❏	❏	❏	❏
13.	❏	❏	❏	❏	28.	❏	❏	❏	❏
14.	❏	❏	❏	❏	29.	❏	❏	❏	❏
15.	❏	❏	❏	❏	30.	❏	❏	❏	❏

42

Musculoskeletal Trauma

1. The anatomic components of the musculoskeletal system include all the following, *except*:

   a. axial skeleton.
   b. muscles.
   c. tendons.
   d. hamstrings.

2. The axial skeleton consists of the skull, vertebral column, and:

   a. bony thorax.
   b. pelvis.
   c. rhomboids.
   d. soleus.

3. The pectoral girdle is composed of the:

   a. scapula and manubrium.
   b. latissimus dorsi.
   c. pubis.
   d. clavicle and scapula.

4. When muscles contract, they pull the _____, which then causes the bones to move at the joints.

   a. tendons
   b. ligaments
   c. marrow
   d. Haversian canals

5. Long bones are broken down into groups, which include all the following, *except*:

   a. diaphysis.
   b. periosteum.
   c. epiphysis.
   d. elasteum.

6. The scapula is broken down into the following areas, *except* for the:

   a. upper division.
   b. median division.
   c. lower division.
   d. glenoid fassa.

7. The sternoclavicular joint and the acromioclavicular joint are two important joints of the:

   a. metaphysis.
   b. scapula.
   c. clavicle.
   d. pelvic girdle.

8. _____ is the area between the epiphysis and diaphysis.

   a. Metaphysis
   b. Periosteum
   c. Haversian canals
   d. Bone marrow sheds

9. Which of the following is not a part of the humerus?

   a. The neck and shaft.
   b. Medial and lateral condyle.
   c. The olecranon.
   d. The elbow.

10. The _____ is located on the little finger side of the lower arm and is part of the wrist joint.

    a. radius head
    b. radius shaft
    c. ulna head
    d. ulna shaft

11. You have been called to transport a football player who has separated his shoulder. This injury is actually a dislocation of the:

    a. acromioclavicular joint.
    b. sternoclavicular joint.
    c. metaphysis.
    d. olecranon.

12. Which of the following joints is not part of the phalanges?

    a. Metacarpalphalangeal
    b. Proximal intraphalangeal
    c. Medial intraphalangeal
    d. Distal intraphalangeal

13. Of the following components, which is not part of the pelvis?

    a. Ilium
    b. Ischium
    c. Acetabulum
    d. Femur

14. A _____ is a rounded protuberance at the articulation of a bone, similar to a knuckle.

    a. trochanter
    b. condyle
    c. phalange
    d. fossa

15. The tibia, located in the _____ lower leg, is made up of the tibia plateau, the shaft, and the _____

    a. anterior; medial malleolus
    b. anterior; lateral condyle
    c. posterior; medial malleolus
    d. posterior; lateral condyle

16. Along with muscles and tendons, the long bones are involved in:

    a. flexion.
    b. extension.
    c. rotation.
    d. all of the above.

17. The fibula, which is located in the _____leg, is made up of the head, shaft, and the _____ malleolus.

    a. upper; medial
    b. lower; lateral
    c. anterior; medial
    d. posterior; lateral

18. Which of the following is not a type of muscle?

    a. Smooth
    b. Skeletal
    c. Axial
    d. Cardiac

19. _____ muscle is found in the lower airways, blood vessels, and intestines.

    a. Smooth
    b. Skeletal
    c. Axial
    d. Cardiac

20. Connective tissue covering the epiphysis, which acts as a surface for articulation, is called:

    a. tendon.
    b. cartilage.
    c. ligament.
    d. muscle.

21. _____ is/are connective tissue which support the joints and allow for range of motion.

    a. Tendons
    b. Cartilage
    c. Ligaments
    d. Muscles

22. _____ can relax or contract to alter the inner lumen diameter of vessels.

    a. Gomphoses
    b. Smooth muscle
    c. Tendons
    d. Cardiac muscle

23. Bones are responsible for all the following, *except*:

    a. producing red blood cells.
    b. storing salts.
    c. protecting vital organs.
    d. producing white blood cells.

24. The attribute of a muscle being able to generate an impulse is referred to as:

    a. automaticity.
    b. excitability.
    c. conduction.
    d. rhythm.

25. _____ is(are) under conscious control and includes the major muscle mass of the body and allows for mobility.

    a. Smooth muscle
    b. Skeletal muscle
    c. Cartilage
    d. Ligaments

26. Structural classifications of joints include all the following, *except*:

    a. fibrous.
    b. cartilaginous.
    c. tendon.
    d. synovial.

27. A _____ is a line of fusion between two bones that are separate in early development.

    a. symphysis
    b. gomphosis
    c. syndesmosis
    d. condyloid

28. Immovable joints where one bone is fitted into a socket of another which is not intended for movements, such as a tooth, is/are:

    a. symphysis.
    b. gomphoses.
    c. syndesmoses.
    d. condyloid.

29. _____ are articulations in which the bones are united by ligaments.

    a. Fusions
    b. Cartilage
    c. Syndesmoses
    d. Condyloids

30. A _____ joint is a joint filled with fluid, which lubricates the articulated surfaces.

    a. cartilaginous
    b. synchondrosis
    c. symphysis
    d. synovial

31. A _____ is a fracture that tears away the outer covering of the bone, often most of the length of the bone.

    a. spiral
    b. comminuted
    c. greenstick
    d. oblique

32. Flexion, extension, abduction, and circumduction are all movement allowed by what type of joint?

    a. Sychondrosis
    b. Gomphosis
    c. Transvere
    d. Synovial

33. A fracture where the break is at a right angle to the axis of the long bone is called a _____ fracture.

    a. epiphyseal
    b. transverse
    c. oblique
    d. comminuted

34. An uncomplicated tibia/fibula fracture can bleed about _____ cc over the first two hours.

    a. 500
    b. 1,000
    c. 1,500
    d. 2,000

35. A partial dislocation of a joint is called a:

    a. subluxation.
    b. luxation.
    c. sprain.
    d. stress fracture.

36. A complete disruption of the integrity of a joint is called a:

    a. sprain.
    b. dislocation.
    c. fracture.
    d. subluxation.

37. All the following are typical causes of pathologic fractures, *except*:

    a. osteoporosis.
    b. metastasis from cancer.
    c. cancer of the bone.
    d. repeated abnormal stress.

38. The knee dislocation can completely disrupt the blood supply to the lower leg when the _____ is displaced to the _____, compressing the posterior tibial artery.

    a. tibia; anterior
    b. tibia; posterior
    c. fibula; anterior
    d. fibula; posterior

39. The elbow when dislocated is very serious and can threaten the:

    a. brachial plexus, causing paralysis.
    b. radial plexus, causing paralysis.
    c. brachial artery and blood supply to the arm.
    d. radial artery and blood supply to the arm.

40. A fracture is considered complicated if it involved any one or more of the following conditions, *except*:

    a. a crushing injury.
    b. painful, swollen deformity.
    c. decreased distal pulse.
    d. diminished distal sensory or motor function.

41. All the following are examples of conditions that can cause inflammation and degeneration of the joints, *except*:

    a. decreased distal pulse.
    b. bursitis.
    c. tendonitis.
    d. gouty arthritis.

42. All the following traction splints are unipolar, *except* the _____, which is bipolar.

   a. Sager®
   b. KTD®
   c. Hare®
   d. None of the above

43. Realignment of dislocations should be considered if distal circulation is impaired or:

   a. if the patient is in pain.
   b. when the deformity is gross.
   c. when the patient signs a release first.
   d. transportation is long or delayed.

44. The difference between a knee dislocation and a patella dislocation is that:

   a. a knee dislocation involves the tibia popping out of the knee joint.
   b. a patella dislocation is much more dangerous than a knee dislocation.
   c. the knee dislocation requires surgery and the patella dislocation does not.
   d. the patella dislocation should never be manipulated in the field.

45. The combination of a long board and PASG/MAST should be used for a _____ fracture, because of the normal blood loss accompanying this type of fracture.

   a. pelvic
   b. mid-shaft femur
   c. proximal femur
   d. tibia/fibula

46. A sling and swathe type of splint is commonly used with all the following injuries, *except*:

   a. shoulder dislocation.
   b. forearm fracture.
   c. humerus fracture.
   d. elbow dislocation.

47. Cold is used initially to reduce the swelling and pain of a fracture. Heat can be useful to improve circulation, but only after the:

   a. initial swelling has gone down.
   b. first hour.
   c. first 12 hours.
   d. first 24 hours.

48. A Colles' fracture is a common fracture of the:

   a. shoulder.
   b. hand.
   c. wrist.
   d. forearm.

49. The key objective in the management of a closed long bone fracture is to carefully splint the long bone in a straight position without:

   a. causing the patient any pain.
   b. the use of analgesics.
   c. allowing the bone to protrude through the skin.
   d. forgetting to assess for DCAP-BTLS.

50. Which of the following is not a typical finding at the site of a musculoskeletal injury?

   a. Pain or tenderness
   b. Crepitation
   c. Diaphoresis
   d. Capillary refilling

Test #42 Answer Form

	A	B	C	D			A	B	C	D
1.	❑	❑	❑	❑		26.	❑	❑	❑	❑
2.	❑	❑	❑	❑		27.	❑	❑	❑	❑
3.	❑	❑	❑	❑		28.	❑	❑	❑	❑
4.	❑	❑	❑	❑		29.	❑	❑	❑	❑
5.	❑	❑	❑	❑		30.	❑	❑	❑	❑
6.	❑	❑	❑	❑		31.	❑	❑	❑	❑
7.	❑	❑	❑	❑		32.	❑	❑	❑	❑
8.	❑	❑	❑	❑		33.	❑	❑	❑	❑
9.	❑	❑	❑	❑		34.	❑	❑	❑	❑
10.	❑	❑	❑	❑		35.	❑	❑	❑	❑
11.	❑	❑	❑	❑		36.	❑	❑	❑	❑
12.	❑	❑	❑	❑		37.	❑	❑	❑	❑
13.	❑	❑	❑	❑		38.	❑	❑	❑	❑
14.	❑	❑	❑	❑		39.	❑	❑	❑	❑
15.	❑	❑	❑	❑		40.	❑	❑	❑	❑
16.	❑	❑	❑	❑		41.	❑	❑	❑	❑
17.	❑	❑	❑	❑		42.	❑	❑	❑	❑
18.	❑	❑	❑	❑		43.	❑	❑	❑	❑
19.	❑	❑	❑	❑		44.	❑	❑	❑	❑
20.	❑	❑	❑	❑		45.	❑	❑	❑	❑
21.	❑	❑	❑	❑		46.	❑	❑	❑	❑
22.	❑	❑	❑	❑		47.	❑	❑	❑	❑
23.	❑	❑	❑	❑		48.	❑	❑	❑	❑
24.	❑	❑	❑	❑		49.	❑	❑	❑	❑
25.	❑	❑	❑	❑		50.	❑	❑	❑	❑

43

Neonatology

1. Vessels of fetal circulation include all the following, *except*:

   a. umbilical arteries.
   b. umbilical vein.
   c. ductus venosus.
   d. foramen arteriosus.

2. After birth fetal circulation changes and the _____ turns into a fibrous cord that serves as a ligament.

   a. umbilical arteries
   b. umbilical vein
   c. ductus venosus
   d. foramen arteriosus

3. After the baby takes its first breath, the _____ closes and shunts blood to the lungs.

   a. foramen ovale
   b. ductus venosus
   c. ductus arteriosus
   d. foramen arteriosus

4. Newborns are very sensitive to hypoxia and if they experience hypoxia or severe acidosis, a serious condition called _____ may occur.

   a. persistent fetal circulation
   b. hypoxic apnea
   c. neonatal pulmonary syndrome
   d. hypoxic drive syndrome

5. The condition described in the previous question can be corrected or avoided by:

   a. performing CPR as needed.
   b. intubating the newborn after birth.
   c. stimulating the newborn to breathe.
   d. administering epinephrine.

6. When apnea occurs in infants that were born full term where no cause for the apnea can be determined, this condition is called:

   a. primary apnea.
   b. secondary apnea.
   c. ALTE.
   d. apnea of infancy.

7. There are three causes of infant apnea: central, obstructive, and:

   a. anomaly.
   b. mixed.
   c. complete.
   d. incomplete.

8. The most common cause of Down syndrome occurs when a baby is born with _____ rather than two copies of chromosome 21.

   a. one
   b. three
   c. four
   d. five

9. A paramedic can recognize a newborn with Down syndrome by all the following characteristics, *except*:

   a. small tongue in relationship to the size of the mouth.
   b. small ears with an abnormal shape.
   c. flat facial profile with a small nose.
   d. small fold on the inner corners of the eyes.

10. Other distinguishing characteristics of Down syndrome include all the following, *except*:

    a. joint hypermobility.
    b. an excessive space between the large and second toe.
    c. a single deep crease across the palm of the hand.
    d. a downward slant of the eyes.

11. The paramedic can recognize a newborn that is born with the birth defect spina bifida because the infant will have a/an:

    a. overall weak body muscle tone.
    b. exposed spinal structures.
    c. excessively large fontanels.
    d. exceedingly small fontanels.

12. Significant antepartum factors that can affect child-birth include all the following, *except*:

    a. the mother's use of drugs.
    b. the mother's age is <16 years old.
    c. diabetes.
    d. the father's age is >65 years old.

13. Significant antepartum factors that classify the new-born as "High Risk" include all the following, *except*:

    a. post-term gestation.
    b. premature labor.
    c. prolonged labor.
    d. excessive false labor.

14. Factors that are associated with premature births include all the following, *except*:

    a. prolapsed cord.
    b. the mother's use of tabacco.
    c. multiple fetuses.
    d. third trimester hemorrhage.

15. Factors that are associated with low birth weights include all the following, *except*:

    a. gestational diabetes.
    b. prolonged labor.
    c. the mother's use of alcohol.
    d. multiple fetuses.

16. Babies born with a low birth weight range from _____ grams.

    a. 500–2,500
    b. 1,000–3,500
    c. 1,500–4,500
    d. 2,000–5,000

17. Which of the following is not a risk factor associated with crack/cocaine use by a pregnant woman?

    a. Miscarriage
    b. Premature labor
    c. Placenta previa
    d. Abruptio placenta

18. The use of crack/cocaine by a pregnant woman puts the fetus at risk for all the following, *except*:

    a. sickle cell disease.
    b. birth defects.
    c. feeding problems.
    d. sleep disorders.

19. Immediately after birth the paramedic should assess the newborn for:

    a. level of consciousness, respiratory rate, and heart rate.
    b. respiratory effort, heart rate, and skin color.
    c. respiratory rate, heart rate, and approximate weight.
    d. level of consciousness, respiratory effort, and meconium staining.

20. In the clinical setting newborns are screened for genetic and _____ disorders.

    a. teratogenic
    b. cardiovascular
    c. infectious
    d. metabolic

21. When a baby is born without enough thyroid hormone (congenital hypothyroidism), this condition can lead to:

    a. myxedema.
    b. poor growth and mental retardation.
    c. abnormal protrusion of the eyes.
    d. goiter.

22. The newborn that is born with fetal alcohol syndrome (FAS) can be distinguished by which of the following characteristics?

    a. Low birth weight, small head, and small eye openings.
    b. Low birth weight, large head, and thick upper lip.
    c. Upward slant of eyes and small head.
    d. Protruding upper jaw and thinned lips.

23. Which of the following statements about FAS is not correct?

    a. FAS does not occur with consumption of very small amounts of alcohol during pregnancy.
    b. FAS is distinguished by developmental disabilities.
    c. FAS can result in infant and fetal death.
    d. Cardiovascular defects are associated with FAS.

24. Your patient is a 23-year-old female, who is in custody of the police. She is in active labor. The police state she is high on heroin. Which of the following complications can you expect with this delivery?

    a. Prolonged labor and fetal distress.
    b. Prolapsed cord.
    c. Decreased mental status of the newborn.
    d. Breach presentation and delivery.

25. How would you manage the delivery for the patient described in question 24?

   a. Monitor, transport, and consider administration of Pitocin®.
   b. Attempt to prevent delivery and begin a rapid transport.
   c. Administer oxygen, assist ventilations, and administer Narcan®.
   d. Assist with the delivery of the breach baby.

26. Common traumatic injuries to the newborn associated with childbirth include all the following, *except*:

   a. hyperthermia.
   b. CVA.
   c. spinal cord injury.
   d. forceps trauma to the head.

27. Which of the following injuries is associated with shoulder dystocia?

   a. Spinal cord injury
   b. Fractured clavicle
   c. Brachial plexus injury
   d. Hypothermia

28. Your partner has just assisted with the delivery of a 38-week gestation newborn. You have assessed the infant after one minute and have determined that the infant's heart rate is 60 bpm even after you have warmed, dried, stimulated, and provided blow-by oxygen. What would you do next?

   a. Suction for meconium.
   b. Assist with ventilations by BVM.
   c. Intubate the newborn.
   d. Start CPR.

29. In continuing with the care of the newborn in question 28, after 30 seconds you assess the heart rate, which has not increased from 60 bpm. What would you do next?

   a. Administer high flow oxygen.
   b. Assist with ventilations by BVM.
   c. Intubate the newborn.
   d. Start CPR.

30. The initial steps of post-arrest stabilization for the neonate include:

   a. keeping the baby warm and continuing oxygen delivery.
   b. starting an IV drip of lidocaine.
   c. administering an epinephrine bolus every 5 minutes.
   d. placing a nasogastric tube.

31. Major risk factors associated with premature birth include all the following, *except*:

   a. hypoxia.
   b. hypothermia.
   c. hypoglycemia.
   d. hyperglycemia.

32. Premature infants often have immature lungs and lack enough _____, a chemical that prevents the alveoli from collapsing when a baby exhales.

   a. fibrolactin
   b. surfactant
   c. ficin
   d. fibrinectin

33. Neonates can lose body heat rapidly for all the following reasons, *except* that they have:

   a. excessive heat loss through breathing.
   b. a larger body surface area.
   c. smaller amounts of subcutaneous fat.
   d. temperature regulation mechanisms that are immature.

34. The most common causes of neonatal seizures are hypoxia, fever, infection, and:

   a. hypoglycemia.
   b. alcohol.
   c. drugs.
   d. genetic disorders.

35. Any fever in neonates is serious and requires evaluation because of their:

   a. immature lungs.
   b. immature thermoregulatory system.
   c. high risk of seizures from fever.
   d. high risk of aspiration.

36. The neonate can develop infection from the mother _____ birth.

   a. before and during
   b. during
   c. during and after
   d. before, during, and after

37. Jaundice occurs when a baby's immature liver cannot dispose of excess:

   a. insulin.
   b. glycogen.
   c. bilirubin.
   d. urine.

38. Approximately 60% of full-term infants and 80% of premature infants develop jaundice in the first _____ of life.

    a. 2–3 minutes
    b. 2–3 hours
    c. 2–3 days
    d. 2–3 weeks

39. The most common causes of vomiting in the neonate include: infections, increased ICP, and:

    a. drug withdrawal.
    b. genetic disorders.
    c. metabolic disorders.
    d. pyloric stenosis.

40. Complications from vomiting in the neonate include: aspiration, dehydration, and:

    a. seizures.
    b. lactose intolerance.
    c. increased ICP.
    d. electrolyte imbalance.

41. Diarrhea in neonates is difficult to assess because:

    a. of residual meconium.
    b. all stools are loose.
    c. diapers can change stool consistency.
    d. the large amount of bile excretion.

42. Neonates are prone to abdominal distention because of gastric and fluid distention caused by immature digestive systems. Other causes of distention include all the following, *except*:

    a. intestinal obstruction.
    b. hernias.
    c. congenital abnormalities.
    d. neurologic abnormalities.

43. ALS transport has been requested for a 20-day-old baby, from a pediatrician's office to the hospital. The baby is crying persistently and the transport is for severe distention of the abdomen caused by a possible bowel obstruction. Your primary concern during the transport is:

    a. to prevent infectious exposure.
    b. to watch the baby's airway.
    c. to stop the baby's crying.
    d. to infuse at least 20 cc saline per kg.

44. During an emergency involving a neonate, medication administration via the _____ route can lead to low plasma levels and should be the last choice.

    a. ETT
    b. IV
    c. IO
    d. rectal

45. Complication of positive pressure ventilations in neonates includes all the following, *except*:

    a. distended abdomen.
    b. diaphragmatic herniation.
    c. barotraumas.
    d. pneumothorax.

46. The most common type of hernia associated with neonates is a/an _____ hernia.

    a. diaphragmatic
    b. inguinal
    c. umbilical
    d. hiatal

47. Using the inverted pyramid of newborn resuscitation, ALS interventions are begun only after airway, ventilation, and _____ are performed.

    a. suction
    b. oxygenation
    c. CPR
    d. initial transport

48. Besides airway problems, _____ problems are the most common potentially life-threatening disorder that affects neonates.

    a. hypoglycemia
    b. hypothermia
    c. fluid imbalance
    d. congenital heart

49. Of the following list of drugs or agents, which is not a teratogen?

    a. Alcohol
    b. Lithium
    c. Concentrated lemon juice
    d. Vitamin A and its derivatives

50. During the delivery of twins, the paramedic can tell if the babies are fraternal or identical because fraternal twins:

    a. develop from the same zygote.
    b. always have their own placenta.
    c. (one) will present as a breach.
    d. have their own umbilical cords.

Test #43 Answer Form

	A	B	C	D			A	B	C	D
1.	❏	❏	❏	❏		26.	❏	❏	❏	❏
2.	❏	❏	❏	❏		27.	❏	❏	❏	❏
3.	❏	❏	❏	❏		28.	❏	❏	❏	❏
4.	❏	❏	❏	❏		29.	❏	❏	❏	❏
5.	❏	❏	❏	❏		30.	❏	❏	❏	❏
6.	❏	❏	❏	❏		31.	❏	❏	❏	❏
7.	❏	❏	❏	❏		32.	❏	❏	❏	❏
8.	❏	❏	❏	❏		33.	❏	❏	❏	❏
9.	❏	❏	❏	❏		34.	❏	❏	❏	❏
10.	❏	❏	❏	❏		35.	❏	❏	❏	❏
11.	❏	❏	❏	❏		36.	❏	❏	❏	❏
12.	❏	❏	❏	❏		37.	❏	❏	❏	❏
13.	❏	❏	❏	❏		38.	❏	❏	❏	❏
14.	❏	❏	❏	❏		39.	❏	❏	❏	❏
15.	❏	❏	❏	❏		40.	❏	❏	❏	❏
16.	❏	❏	❏	❏		41.	❏	❏	❏	❏
17.	❏	❏	❏	❏		42.	❏	❏	❏	❏
18.	❏	❏	❏	❏		43.	❏	❏	❏	❏
19.	❏	❏	❏	❏		44.	❏	❏	❏	❏
20.	❏	❏	❏	❏		45.	❏	❏	❏	❏
21.	❏	❏	❏	❏		46.	❏	❏	❏	❏
22.	❏	❏	❏	❏		47.	❏	❏	❏	❏
23.	❏	❏	❏	❏		48.	❏	❏	❏	❏
24.	❏	❏	❏	❏		49.	❏	❏	❏	❏
25.	❏	❏	❏	❏		50.	❏	❏	❏	❏

44

Pediatrics

1. Because of the child's stage of emotional development in the _____ age group, this group is the most difficult to evaluate.

   a. neonate
   b. infant
   c. toddler
   d. adolescent

2. In the _____ age group, feelings of guilt and fear of pain often dominate the thinking of these children.

   a. infant
   b. toddler
   c. preschool
   d. school-age

3. Children in the _____ age group are extremely concerned about modesty and are terrified of disfigurement and death.

   a. toddler
   b. preschool
   c. school-age
   d. adolescent

4. Which of the following statements about an infant's airway is incorrect?

   a. The infant's tongue is very large in relation to the size of the mouth.
   b. The small trachea of an infant is more anterior than in an adult's airway.
   c. The smallest diameter of the airway in an infant is at the cricoid ring.
   d. The largest diameter of the airway in an infant is at the cricoid ring.

5. Infants are obligate nose breathers until _____ months of age, and they might not open their mouths to breathe even when their nose becomes obstructed from a cold, creating periods of apnea.

   a. 3
   b. 6
   c. 9
   d. 12

6. In the infant, the fontanels are used as a diagnostic aid in assessing for shock, dehydration, and:

   a. head injury.
   b. hypoglycemia.
   c. hyperthermia.
   d. hypothermia.

7. All the following are characteristics of an infant's chest, *except*:

   a. respiratory muscles are not well developed.
   b. in respiratory distress the infant can compensate for long periods.
   c. abdominal or "belly breathing" is normal.
   d. sternal retractions are a sign of distress.

8. Which of the following is correct about the infant's thermoregulatory system?

   a. They do not have the ability to shiver to create body heat.
   b. Skin color is a poor indicator of hyperthermia.
   c. Skin color is a poor indicator of hypothermia.
   d. Full term infants are born with a mature temperature regulation.

9. _____ is the number one cause of death in children over one year of age.

   a. SIDS
   b. Abuse
   c. Infection
   d. Trauma

10. Which of the following is the immediate concern for the paramedic when treating a child that has a poisoning or drug overdose?

   a. Respiratory depression
   b. Anaphylaxis
   c. Vomiting and aspiration
   d. Shock

11. All the following statements about pediatric trauma are correct, *except*:

a. Pediatric trauma often presents with certain predictable types of injuries in each age group.
b. The child's head, face, and neck are areas injured more frequently than an adult's.
c. Pneumothorax and hemothorax are injuries that do not occur in children.
d. Pediatric trauma care training for EMS providers is not as extensive as adult trauma training.

12. The incidence of pediatric suicide has increased significantly in recent years for all the following risk factors, *except*:

a. easier access to lethal weapons.
b. higher incidents of abuse and neglect.
c. greater access to drugs and alcohol.
d. greater access to motor vehicles.

13. Risk factors for pediatric suicide, that are generally out of the child's control, include all the following, *except*:

a. the use of alcohol and drugs.
b. inadequate support system.
c. exposure to domestic violence.
d. breakup of a romantic relationship.

14. Risk factors for adolescent depression include all the following, *except*:

a. chronic illness.
b. stress.
c. female 2:1 over males.
d. males 3:1 over females.

15. Physical complaints associated with depression in children include:

a. headache and muscle ache.
b. nausea and vomiting.
c. dizziness.
d. delay in puberty.

16. A child abuse or neglect injury can be physical, sexual, or _____ in nature.

a. emotional
b. financial
c. self-destructive
d. congenital

17. When a paramedic notes the presence of multiple bruises of various ages on a child during a physical examination, he/she should document the findings by noting:

a. the estimated age of each bruise.
b. the location and color of each bruise.
c. who he/she suspects caused the bruising.
d. the detailed story behind every bruise.

18. Which of the following is an example of child neglect?

a. Burns on the genitalia.
b. Signs of malnourishment.
c. Signs of shaken baby syndrome.
d. A central nervous system injury.

19. All the following are signs of shaken baby syndrome, *except*:

a. irritability or AMS.
b. increased appetite.
c. limp extremities.
d. inability to lift his/her own head.

20. Risk factors identified for children at risk for shaken baby syndrome include any of the following, *except*:

a. children with young parents.
b. children under one year old.
c. families that are below poverty level.
d. children that are sexually abused simultaneously.

21. Signs and symptoms of stroke are the same in a child as in an adult. However, the risk factors for stroke in children include all the following, *except*:

a. heart disease.
b. sickle cell anemia.
c. congenital heart disease.
d. trauma.

22. All the following childhood diseases are preventable, *except*:

a. tetanus.
b. rubeola.
c. poliomyelitis.
d. meningitis.

23. Your patient is a 7-year-old with Coxsackie virus (hand, foot, and mouth syndrome). You are aware that this condition is highly contagious so you don gloves and avoid contact with:

a. rash and feces.
b. discharge from the eyes.
c. cuts or open wounds.
d. respiratory secretions.

24. Dispatched to a local high school, you have been asked to transport a teenager with infectious mononucleosis. The nurse tells you that this condition is mildly contagious and to wear gloves and avoid contact with:

    a. urine or feces.
    b. discharge from blisters.
    c. saliva or blood.
    d. rash or hives.

25. Which of the following conditions requires isolation technique for PPE?

    a. Whooping cough (pertussis)
    b. Viral meningitis
    c. Meningococcemia meningitis
    d. Impetigo

26. All the following statements about febrile seizures in children are correct, *except*:

    a. Most febrile seizures are focalized and last several minutes.
    b. They are associated with a rapid rise in body temperature.
    c. There are no lasting neurologic deficits.
    d. The postictal period is usually brief, but the child is very tired.

27. _____ is the number one reason for children missing school and the number one reason for pediatric ED visits caused by chronic illness.

    a. Allergies
    b. Diabetes
    c. Croup
    d. Asthma

28. Your patient is a 5-year-old male with symptoms of an upper respiratory infection, nausea, vomiting, and confusion. The parents tell you that the child has been sick with the flu, but the confusion is new. The child's medications include nebulized Albuterol® as needed for the last week and over the counter Bayer® Children's aspirin as needed for fevers. You suspect the child is:

    a. developing pneumonia.
    b. presenting with Reye's syndrome.
    c. having an AMS caused by dehydration.
    d. may have had a seizure.

29. Your management of the patient discussed in question 28 will include support and care of the ABCs and:

    a. administration of Albuterol® and Solumedrol®.
    b. IV fluids and seizure precautions.
    c. considering the use of acetaminophen.
    d. administration of prophylactic rectal diazepam.

30. Common triggers of asthma in children include all the following, *except*:

    a. allergies.
    b. seizures.
    c. exposure to smoke.
    d. stress.

31. When asthma is triggered, changes in the airways occur. Which of the following is the correct sequence of airway changes?

    a. Bronchoconstriction, inflammation, and excess mucus production.
    b. Wheezing, excess mucus production, and bronchoconstriction.
    c. Inflammation, excess mucus production, and bronchoconstriction.
    d. Mucus production, wheezing, bronchoconstriction.

32. The most common causes of respiratory distress in the infant age group include all the following, *except*:

    a. epiglottitis.
    b. croup.
    c. bronchiolitis.
    d. asthma.

33. _____ is a condition characterized by infections of the bronchioles that results in swelling of the lower airways and tachypnea, retractions, and cyanosis.

    a. Epiglottitis
    b. Croup
    c. Bronchiolitis
    d. Pneumonia

34. Your patient is a 5-year-old that is having difficulty breathing. The patient has difficulty exhaling, the SpO_2 is 94% with oxygen, and there are decreased breath sounds bilaterally with no wheezing. Which of the following conditions do you suspect?

    a. Allergic reaction
    b. Bronchiolitis
    c. Foreign body airway obstruction
    d. Asthma attack

35. Your management plan for the patient discussed in question 34 includes continued oxygenation and:

   a. supportive care and reassessment.
   b. gentle transport with a parent close by.
   c. nebulized Albuterol®.
   d. epinephrine and Benadryl®.

36. _____ is a condition precipitated by a viral or bacterial infection and is characterized by fever, tachypnea, rales, consolidation in one or more lobes, and cough.

   a. Asthma
   b. Croup
   c. Bronchiolitis
   d. Pneumonia

37. Croup causes the tissue _____ the glottal opening to swell compared to epiglottitis, which causes the tissue _____ the glottal opening to swell, resulting in a higher risk of complete airway obstruction.

   a. under; above
   b. above; under
   c. lateral to; under
   d. lateral to; above

38. Why does the prevalence of asthma decrease as children get older?

   a. As the immune system matures, some children outgrow the condition.
   b. Some children outgrow the condition with the use of steroids.
   c. Natural antibodies develop with the use of steroids.
   d. As airways enlarge, some children outgrow the condition.

39. The most prominent indicator of respiratory failure in children is:

   a. increased use of accessory muscles.
   b. low SpO$_2$ levels.
   c. decreased level of consciousness.
   d. decreased capillary filling.

40. Besides fever, common causes of seizures in children include all the following, *except*:

   a. epilepsy.
   b. dehydration.
   c. poison ingestion.
   d. idiopathic conditions.

41. Besides cool or cold temperatures, hypothermia in children can be caused by:

   a. prolonged infection.
   b. diarrhea.
   c. vomiting.
   d. seizures.

42. Brain disorders affecting the thermoregulatory center in children may present as a finding of _____ upon physical examination.

   a. hyperactivity
   b. hypothermia
   c. hyperthermia
   d. hypoxia

43. Children that are diagnosed with a new onset of diabetes mellitus will usually present to the paramedic as being:

   a. hyperactive.
   b. hypothermic.
   c. hyperglycemic.
   d. hypoglycemic.

44. Congenital heart defects are deformities of the structures of the heart that occur:

   a. after the first month of life.
   b. after six months of life.
   c. only when the mother has used drugs during pregnancy.
   d. while the fetus is developing in utero.

45. The significant problem associated with heart defects is that they:

   a. disrupt normal blood flow.
   b. cause murmurs.
   c. cause dysrhythmias.
   d. cause arrhythmias.

46. A defect of the heart that is characterized by valves that are absent, too small, or do not close completely is called:

   a. stenosis.
   b. coarctation.
   c. truncus.
   d. valvosis.

47. The most common cardiac dysrhythmias seen in children are tachycardias, bradycardias, and:

   a. ventricular fibrillation.
   b. bundle branch blocks.
   c. heart blocks.
   d. asystole.

48. Always consider _____ to be the underlying cause of cardiac dysrhythmias in children until proven otherwise.

    a. hypoglycemia
    b. hypothermia
    c. hypoxia
    d. heredity

49. A highly contagious bacterial or viral disease in children that is characterized by discharge from the eyes is:

    a. impetigo.
    b. conjunctivitis.
    c. Lyme disease.
    d. German measles.

50. The pediatric patient that presents with sunken eyes, recent weight loss, and tachycardia should be evaluated to rule out:

    a. polio.
    b. pertussis.
    c. naphylaxis.
    d. dehydration.

51. You are transporting an infant to the ED for evaluation of an URI. The child has been sick with fever, decreased PO intake, and vomiting. During the transport, the child experiences a febrile seizure. Which of the following is the most appropriate treatment for the child?

    a. Apply ice packs to the torso and head.
    b. Administer IV fluids.
    c. Administer Valium®.
    d. Gentle cooling measures.

52. You are dispatched at 3 a.m. for a 4-year-old sick child. Upon arrival at the residence, the parents tell you that the child has been sick with a cold, but tonight it suddenly got worse when the child spiked a temperature. The child is having difficulty breathing, and has a sore throat and difficulty swallowing. You suspect the child has:

    a. croup.
    b. bronchiolitis.
    c. epiglottitis.
    d. a partial obstruction.

53. Which of the following is not appropriate management for the patient discussed in question 52?

    a. Keep a parent with the child at all times.
    b. Visualize the airway for an obstruction.
    c. Permit the child to sit up.
    d. Minimize handling and examining to prevent agitation.

54. While attempting to apply an oxygen mask to the patient discussed in question 52, the child resists. How should you proceed next?

    a. consider the use of blow-by oxygen
    b. insist that the parent hold the mask in place
    c. turn up the liter flow so it feels like a fan
    d. consider RSI

55. Transportation considerations for the patient discussed in question 52 should include:

    a. immediate, but calm transport.
    b. rapid transport with lights only.
    c. lie the child down on the stretcher with the parent nearby.
    d. strap the parent into the stretcher with the child in his/her lap.

56. Police have called you to care for a teenager who has overdosed on methadone. The 14-year-old is unconscious with shallow respirations and no signs of outward trauma. After managing the ABCs, your primary concern is:

    a. to begin a rapid transport.
    b. the patient's mental status.
    c. to be prepared for seizures.
    d. to administer IV fluids.

57. Appropriate ALS management for the patient described in question 56 includes administering:

    a. 5 mg Valium®.
    b. 2–4 ml/kg D-50 W.
    c. 0.1 mg/kg naloxone.
    d. atropine 0.5–1.0 mg.

58. You arrive at the scene of a motor vehicle collision to find a six-year-old male lying supine on the pavement. A witness tells you the child ran out in front of a moving car and was struck. What type of injuries do you suspect?

    a. Head, chest, and upper extremities.
    b. Head, chest, and lower extremities.
    c. Chest, abdomen, and upper extremities.
    d. Chest, abdomen, and lower extremities.

59. The injury pattern for the patient described in question 58 is common and is also described as:

    a. Cushing's triad.
    b. Waddel's triad.
    c. Hendrick's triage.
    d. Greenstick pattern.

Test #44 Answer Form

	A	B	C	D			A	B	C	D
1.	❏	❏	❏	❏		27.	❏	❏	❏	❏
2.	❏	❏	❏	❏		28.	❏	❏	❏	❏
3.	❏	❏	❏	❏		29.	❏	❏	❏	❏
4.	❏	❏	❏	❏		30.	❏	❏	❏	❏
5.	❏	❏	❏	❏		31.	❏	❏	❏	❏
6.	❏	❏	❏	❏		32.	❏	❏	❏	❏
7.	❏	❏	❏	❏		33.	❏	❏	❏	❏
8.	❏	❏	❏	❏		34.	❏	❏	❏	❏
9.	❏	❏	❏	❏		35.	❏	❏	❏	❏
10.	❏	❏	❏	❏		36.	❏	❏	❏	❏
11.	❏	❏	❏	❏		37.	❏	❏	❏	❏
12.	❏	❏	❏	❏		38.	❏	❏	❏	❏
13.	❏	❏	❏	❏		39.	❏	❏	❏	❏
14.	❏	❏	❏	❏		40.	❏	❏	❏	❏
15.	❏	❏	❏	❏		41.	❏	❏	❏	❏
16.	❏	❏	❏	❏		42.	❏	❏	❏	❏
17.	❏	❏	❏	❏		43.	❏	❏	❏	❏
18.	❏	❏	❏	❏		44.	❏	❏	❏	❏
19.	❏	❏	❏	❏		45.	❏	❏	❏	❏
20.	❏	❏	❏	❏		46.	❏	❏	❏	❏
21.	❏	❏	❏	❏		47.	❏	❏	❏	❏
22.	❏	❏	❏	❏		48.	❏	❏	❏	❏
23.	❏	❏	❏	❏		49.	❏	❏	❏	❏
24.	❏	❏	❏	❏		50.	❏	❏	❏	❏
25.	❏	❏	❏	❏		51.	❏	❏	❏	❏
26.	❏	❏	❏	❏		52.	❏	❏	❏	❏

	A	B	C	D			A	B	C	D
53.	❏	❏	❏	❏		57.	❏	❏	❏	❏
54.	❏	❏	❏	❏		58.	❏	❏	❏	❏
55.	❏	❏	❏	❏		59.	❏	❏	❏	❏
56.	❏	❏	❏	❏						

Geriatrics

1. _____ is the study of the problems of all aspects of aging.

    a. Oldentology
    b. Agentology
    c. Genealogy
    d. Gerontology

2. As the body ages, the skin begins to sag and wrinkles develop because of the:

    a. increased vascularity in the skin.
    b. loss of elastic fiber.
    c. loss of T cell function.
    d. loss of sebaceous glands.

3. With aging, the musculoskeletal system is affected by:

    a. the forming of opacities.
    b. decreased muscle and bone mass.
    c. hypertrophy of muscles.
    d. increasing bone marrow production.

4. Changes in the respiratory system caused by the effects of aging include all the following, *except*:

    a. decreased gag reflex responses increase the risk of aspiration.
    b. lung capacity diminished with the loss of elasticity.
    c. the chest wall becomes stiff and rigid increasing the risk for fractures.
    d. decreased cilia increase the risk of infectious pulmonary diseases.

5. With aging comes a decreased _____ response, which affects the ability to increase the heart rate in response to stress and exercise.

    a. estrogen
    b. catecholamine
    c. androgen
    d. progesterone

6. Which of the following is not a psychologic change associated with aging?

    a. loss of support system
    b. increased isolation
    c. increased depression
    d. decreased depression

7. The changes in the endocrine system caused by aging include decreased reproductive functions and:

    a. decrease in thyroid function.
    b. atrophy of hormone receptors.
    c. surgical removal of the pancreas.
    d. excessive sympathetic stimulation.

8. During perimenopause (the years before menopause) about 90% of women experience irregular menses and begin to experience the symptoms of menopause. This is caused by:

    a. excessive hormone production.
    b. the drop in sexual hormone levels.
    c. increased release of catecholamines.
    d. decreased release of catecholamines.

9. In addition to the classic symptoms of hot flashes and irregular menstrual periods, nearly 80% of menopausal women experience other symptoms that are collectively called:

    a. post-maternal pattern.
    b. menacing disorder.
    c. menopausal syndrome.
    d. PMS.

10. In the year 2030, it is projected that one in _____ people will be age 65 or older in the United States.

    a. three
    b. five
    c. ten
    d. twenty-five

11. Which of the following groups are living longer?

    a. married people
    b. cohabitating people
    c. people who have attained higher education
    d. all of the above

12. As the baby boomers grow older it is estimated that treating psychiatric illnesses will become a crises in the United States with the numbers of mentally ill seniors expected to _____ by the year 2030.

    a. double
    b. triple
    c. quadruple
    d. none of the above

13. The actual number of people dying from _____ has risen 37% since 1950 and remains the number one cause of death in the United States.

    a. heart disease
    b. cancer
    c. COPD
    d. diabetes

14. The most prevalent chronic diseases for older Americans include all the following, *except*:

    a. arthritis.
    b. hypertension.
    c. stroke.
    d. hyperthyroidism

15. What is the difference in the pathology of cardiovascular emergencies in older adults compared to that of younger adults?

    a. The catecholamine response in cardiac emergencies increases with age.
    b. Younger adults tend to die from AMI rather than heart failure.
    c. Coronary artery disease predisposes the elderly to superior outcomes.
    d. There is really no difference when an older or younger adult experiences an AMI.

16. Subtle assessment findings associated with cardiac emergencies in the older patient may include any of the following, *except*:

    a. mild dyspnea.
    b. confusion.
    c. back pain.
    d. weakness or fatigue.

17. Currently the single greatest health problem in the United States, it is estimated that nearly 55% of all Americans will have _____ by age 60.

    a. a stroke
    b. diabetes
    c. hypertension
    d. cancer

18. Typical emergencies with Parkinson's patients include which of the following causes?

    a. Falls
    b. Dementia
    c. Medication toxicity
    d. All of the above

19. All of the following statements about Alzheimer's disease are accurate, *except*:

    a. This disease is more prevalent in men than women.
    b. It is the fourth leading case of death in American adults.
    c. It strikes over 21,000 people in the United States each year.
    d. The incidence is higher in women.

20. Emergencies with Alzheimer's patients fall into three categories. Which of the following is not one of those categories?

    a. Behavioral
    b. Psychiatric
    c. Metabolic
    d. Neurologic

21. All the following are examples of physiologic factors that can cause depression in older Americans, *except*:

    a. medications.
    b. organic brain disease.
    c. fear of dying.
    d. dehydration.

22. _____ is a chronic and progressive neurologic condition that robs memory and intellect.

    a. Parkinson's
    b. Alzheimer's
    c. Hypothyroidism
    d. Hyperthyroidism

23. Physical complaints in the elderly patient are often vague and may include:

    a. muscle ache.
    b. joint pain.
    c. sleeplessness.
    d. any of the above.

24. Thyroid disease, such as hypothyroidism, in elders can predispose them to risks such as:

    a. hypothermia.
    b. cholecystitis.
    c. diverticulitis.
    d. malnutrition.

25. Special considerations for diabetes in the elderly include all the following, *except*:

   a. cognitive impairments may hinder an older person from preparing meals.
   b. the elderly have decreased susceptibility to certain infections.
   c. neuropathy is more prevalent in the elderly.
   d. slower metabolism affects carbohydrate absorption.

26. The most common causes of minor GI bleeds in the elderly are:

   a. peptic ulcer and angiodysplasia.
   b. diverticular diseases.
   c. hemorrhoids and colorectal cancer.
   d. none of the above.

27. Common GI problems in the elderly such as _____ are most often caused by cancer, adhesions, or hernias.

   a. bowel obstruction
   b. hemorrhoids
   c. gastritis
   d. all of the above

28. Symptoms associated with alcohol abuse in the elderly typically include all the following, *except*:

   a. tremors.
   b. hyperglycemia.
   c. chronic diarrhea.
   d. memory loss.

29. Factors that increase the risk for developing osteoarthritis include all the following, *except*:

   a. heredity.
   b. obesity.
   c. kyphosis.
   d. diabetes.

30. _____ is a chronic inflammatory disease of the bones that results in thickening, softening, and eventual bowing of the bone.

   a. Osteoporosis
   b. Paget's disease
   c. Osteoarthritis
   d. Gout

31. All the following are common signs or symptoms of adverse drug interactions in the elderly, *except*:

   a. potentiation.
   b. confusion.
   c. depression.
   d. falls.

32. Elderly patients with slowed metabolism can get increased amounts of medications in the body from normal doses that can reach lethal levels. This is commonly referred to as:

   a. concurrent disease overdose.
   b. altered hepatic function.
   c. depressed renal function.
   d. drug toxicity.

33. Which of the following is not a type of nursing home regulated by state and federal standards?

   a. Intermediate care facilities.
   b. Residential care facilities.
   c. Skilled nursing facilities.
   d. Senior retirement facilities.

34. Independent living with limited nursing care, social, recreation, and rehabilitation activities is an example of a/an _____ nursing home.

   a. intermediate care facility
   b. residential care facility
   c. skilled nursing facility
   d. senior retirement facility

35. Which of the following statements about "falls" that occur among elderly people is least accurate?

   a. Injuries resulting from falls are the sixth leading cause of death in those over 65.
   b. In the elderly falling is widely recognized as a major life and health-threatening problem.
   c. Fractures from falls cost an estimated one billion dollars annually in the United States.
   d. Common injuries from falls include hip and upper limb fractures.

36. Affective disorders increase the risk of injury in the elderly by interfering with:

   a. thermoregulation.
   b. the tasks of daily living.
   c. the immune response.
   d. cardiac output.

37. Contributing factors to the rate of completed suicide in the elderly being higher than in the general population include all the following, *except*:

   a. disfigurement.
   b. the increased change to home health care.
   c. reduction or loss of mobility.
   d. lower self-esteem.

38. _____ is/are ischemic and sometimes necrotic damage to the skin, subcutaneous tissue, and often muscle caused by prolonged periods of immobilization.

   a. Folliculitis
   b. Ulcers
   c. Pressure sores
   d. Abscesses

39. The elderly are at increased risk for morbidity and mortality from burns, because of:

   a. changes in the skin.
   b. decreased immune response.
   c. preexisting illness.
   d. all of the above.

40. Any older person can become a victim of abuse with the most common abusers being:

   a. landlords.
   b. neighbors.
   c. friends.
   d. family members.

41. Which of the following is not typically considered a form of abuse in the elderly?

   a. Financial abuse
   b. Emotional neglect
   c. Resistance abuse
   d. Institutional abuse

42. All the following are typical reasons why elderly patients can be difficult to assess, *except*:

   a. the presence of concurrent illnesses can present with confusing signs and symptoms.
   b. the caretaker limits access to the patient.
   c. normal physiologic changes, such as loss of sensation, can obscure physical findings.
   d. serious problems for the patient are often underestimated.

43. During the physical examination the older patient must be handled gently so as not to:

   a. cause any additional injury.
   b. confuse the patient with your specialized equipment.
   c. overwhelm the caretaker with your techniques.
   d. force the patient to receive unwanted care.

44. Unless there is an obvious environmental explanation, assume that hypothermia in the elderly is caused by _____ until proven otherwise.

   a. severe infection
   b. hypothyroidism
   c. osmotic diuresis
   d. hypoglycemia

45. The most common complications that result from osteoporosis include hip fractures and:

   a. sepsis.
   b. vertebral fractures.
   c. deep vein thrombosis.
   d. pulmonary embolism.

46. All the following increase the risk of infectious pulmonary disease in the elderly, *except*:

   a. diminished cough reflex.
   b. diminished gag reflex.
   c. decrease in cilia.
   d. loss of accommodation.

47. When formulating a field impression for the patient with diseases of the nervous system, the paramedic should always consider _____ early, as a potential cause of AMS.

   a. hypothyroidism
   b. hypothermia
   c. hypoglycemia
   d. dementia

48. Non-acute causes of confusion in the elderly include:

   a. dementia.
   b. delirium.
   c. depression.
   d. all of the above.

49. _____ is the leading cause of new onset blindness and end-stage renal disease in the elderly.

   a. Stroke
   b. Diabetes
   c. Hypertension
   d. Adverse medication reaction

50. _____ is/are a service for home care patients who require palliative and supportive care for terminal illnesses.

   a. Mental health daycare
   b. Case management
   c. Hospice programs
   d. Day hospitals

Test #45 Answer Form

	A	B	C	D			A	B	C	D
1.	❏	❏	❏	❏		26.	❏	❏	❏	❏
2.	❏	❏	❏	❏		27.	❏	❏	❏	❏
3.	❏	❏	❏	❏		28.	❏	❏	❏	❏
4.	❏	❏	❏	❏		29.	❏	❏	❏	❏
5.	❏	❏	❏	❏		30.	❏	❏	❏	❏
6.	❏	❏	❏	❏		31.	❏	❏	❏	❏
7.	❏	❏	❏	❏		32.	❏	❏	❏	❏
8.	❏	❏	❏	❏		33.	❏	❏	❏	❏
9.	❏	❏	❏	❏		34.	❏	❏	❏	❏
10.	❏	❏	❏	❏		35.	❏	❏	❏	❏
11.	❏	❏	❏	❏		36.	❏	❏	❏	❏
12.	❏	❏	❏	❏		37.	❏	❏	❏	❏
13.	❏	❏	❏	❏		38.	❏	❏	❏	❏
14.	❏	❏	❏	❏		39.	❏	❏	❏	❏
15.	❏	❏	❏	❏		40.	❏	❏	❏	❏
16.	❏	❏	❏	❏		41.	❏	❏	❏	❏
17.	❏	❏	❏	❏		42.	❏	❏	❏	❏
18.	❏	❏	❏	❏		43.	❏	❏	❏	❏
19.	❏	❏	❏	❏		44.	❏	❏	❏	❏
20.	❏	❏	❏	❏		45.	❏	❏	❏	❏
21.	❏	❏	❏	❏		46.	❏	❏	❏	❏
22.	❏	❏	❏	❏		47.	❏	❏	❏	❏
23.	❏	❏	❏	❏		48.	❏	❏	❏	❏
24.	❏	❏	❏	❏		49.	❏	❏	❏	❏
25.	❏	❏	❏	❏		50.	❏	❏	❏	❏

46

The Challenged Patient

1. You are assessing a patient who has a hearing impairment. The patient tells you that he lost his hearing when he had meningitis as a child. What type of deafness do you suspect he has?

   a. Conductive
   b. Pagetoid
   c. Sensorineural
   d. Paradoxic

2. Accommodations that a paramedic may find helpful during the care of a patient with a hearing disability may include all the following, *except*:

   a. shouting at the patient.
   b. speaking slowly while looking at the patient.
   c. using written communication.
   d. the use of an amplifying device.

3. Which of the following actions are inappropriate when communicating with a deaf patient who reads lips?

   a. Making eye contact prior to speaking.
   b. Speaking slowly with exaggerated lip movement.
   c. Speaking slowly without exaggerated lip movement.
   d. Speaking normally without exaggerated lip movement.

4. Acute causes of visual impairment include:

   a. optic neuritis or neurosis.
   b. cataracts and glaucoma.
   c. strokes and CNS infections.
   d. diabetic retinopathy or MS.

5. Which of the following conditions may result in a transient blindness for the patient?

   a. Acute head injury
   b. Near drowning
   c. TIA
   d. Acute hypothermia

6. All the following are types of speech impairments, *except* _____ disorders.

   a. language
   b. articulation
   c. voice production
   d. tongue

7. The group of speech disorders that affect understanding of language, forming language, or expressing language are collectively referred to as:

   a. aphasia.
   b. dysarthria.
   c. fluency disorders.
   d. amentia.

8. When a patient is able to understand language and form speech patterns but is unable to express them properly because of physical impairment of the speech pathways, this condition is called:

   a. aphasia.
   b. dysarthria.
   c. fluency disorders.
   d. amentia.

9. Fluency disorders, such as stuttering, may be associated with all the following, *except*:

   a. organic basis.
   b. deficiency of a neurotransmitter.
   c. psychiatric disorder.
   d. traumatic laryngeal injury.

10. Which of the following is the most significant finding of a speech impairment for a patient in the emergency setting?

    a. Hearing loss with an acute onset.
    b. Hearing loss with a slow onset.
    c. A possible associated psychiatric disorder.
    d. Chronic slurred speech.

11. Etiologies of obesity in humans have been associated with all the following, *except*:

   a. a low metabolic rate.
   b. a high basal metabolic rate.
   c. excess insulin production.
   d. the use of steroids.

12. The patient you are assessing states that he is hearing voices and his caretaker confirms that the patient has no concept of reality. Which of the following conditions does the patient have?

   a. Hyalosis
   b. Telepathy
   c. Psychoses
   d. Neuroses

13. When dealing with a patient who is experiencing hallucinations the best management is to gently calm and reassure the patient that everything is all right using a technique called _____ down.

   a. stand
   b. talk
   c. take
   d. show

14. When caring for patients with a history of mental illness the paramedic should avoid which of the following: asking:

   a. about their history of mental illness.
   b. permission to assess them.
   c. about physical problems not associated with mental illness.
   d. permission to enter their personal space.

15. When managing patients with Down syndrome the paramedic should keep in mind all the following, *except*:

   a. these patients have a below average IQ.
   b. that many have a congenital heart defect.
   c. they have a unique airway anatomy.
   d. they have abnormal intestines.

16. Psychoses are often associated with an underlying biochemical brain disease such as:

   a. brainwashing.
   b. TIA.
   c. stroke.
   d. deficiency of neurotransmitters.

17. The more practical and current term for emotional or mental impairment is:

   a. maladaptive behavior.
   b. misunderstood manners.
   c. cerebrally challenged.
   d. comprehension deficit.

18. When treating a patient with a history of chronic arthritis the paramedic should give consideration to all the following, *except*:

   a. decreased ROM may limit the PE.
   b. decreased MS may limit the focused history.
   c. the patient may have a limited ability for motility.
   d. taking a complete medication history prior to giving meds.

19. While performing a physical examination on a cancer patient it would not be uncommon to find:

   a. transdermal pain medications.
   b. a medical alert tag with cancer information.
   c. spastic paralysis of extremities.
   d. multiple lesions on the torso.

20. When caring for a patient with cerebral palsy the paramedic should anticipate all the following, *except*:

   a. assume the patient understands everything you say and do.
   b. may need suctioning, because of increased oral secretions.
   c. may need to pad contractures.
   d. to consider the need for respiratory support.

21. Common problems encountered with a patient with multiple sclerosis who may require medical intervention include all the following, *except*:

   a. UTI.
   b. stroke.
   c. sepsis.
   d. muscle spasm.

22. You are assessing a patient who is hypertensive and complaining of weakness. The patient has a history of myasthenia gravis, so you contact medical control because:

   a. many common medications may worsen an exacerbation.
   b. the patient will probably refuse any treatment.
   c. these symptoms do not require treatment with her history.
   d. you may have to give the patient additional doses of her own medication.

23. A patient with spina bifida may require special attention to _____, which are often present with these patients.

    a. catheters
    b. open sores
    c. contractures
    d. muscle spasms

24. For the paramedic the phrase "terminally ill" usually means that the patient has a condition that will result in his or her death within the next:

    a. 6 to 12 months.
    b. 12 to 18 months.
    c. 1 to 2 years.
    d. 5 years.

25. When caring for the patient with a terminal illness such as cancer, a major issue for the paramedic is:

    a. DNAR status.
    b. pain control.
    c. "end of life" priorities.
    d. living will status.

26. The patient you are caring for is competent but very sick. He states that he is going to refuse transport because he cannot afford to pay. To get him to go to the hospital you should:

    a. tell him that the care will be free this time.
    b. tell him that this time his bill will be reduced.
    c. try to convince him that his health should be the first priority.
    d. tell him that he will die if he does not come with you.

27. If the patient described in question 27 still refuses to go to the hospital despite all your efforts, what should you do next?

    a. Call the police and ask for restraints.
    b. Acknowledge that the competent patient has a right to refuse care.
    c. Force him to go anyway.
    d. Call medical control for consent to restrain the patient.

28. Common causes of conductive hearing loss include:

    a. injury or earwax.
    b. birth defects and aging.
    c. medications and tumors.
    d. mumps or measles.

29. Approximately 80% of hearing loss is related to the loss of _____ sounds.

    a. low pitched
    b. high pitched
    c. distant
    d. isolated

30. All the following diseases are associated with progressive chronic vision loss, *except*:

    a. multiple sclerosis.
    b. diabetes.
    c. congenital cataracts.
    d. cerebral palsy.

31. A nursing home resident requires transport for evaluation of a possible UTI. You observe that the patient's extremities are grossly contracted and that she will not fit on your stretcher like most patients. Which of the following would be appropriate for this patient?

    a. Only force the extremities to move enough to fit the patient on the stretcher.
    b. Refuse to transport the patient.
    c. Pad the contractures and use extra care during the move.
    d. Consider administering a muscle relaxant prior to moving the patient.

32. Transport of the patient with cystic fibrosis may require which of the following accommodations by the paramedic?

    a. respiratory support
    b. management of catheters
    c. padding of contractures
    d. medical consent by a caregiver

33. Cultural differences in patients vary. The paramedic should be aware of each patient's private/personal space needs. Assessment is best initiated by:

    a. examining the patient with no one else present.
    b. pointing to an area of the body before touching it.
    c. asking the patient's spouse for permission to examine.
    d. only perform the physical exam while in the ambulance.

34. When caring for patients with cultural backgrounds that differ from your own, the most important concept for the paramedic is:

   a. language barriers will never compound cultural differences.
   b. cultural differences will limit the paramedic's judgment.
   c. patient's with cultural differences have different needs and wants.
   d. cultural-based preferences may conflict with a paramedics learned medical practice.

35. Which of the following statements about cultural diversity is incorrect?

   a. All people share common problems or situations.
   b. People identify with their ethnic cultural background.
   c. The paramedic should respect the integrity of cultural beliefs.
   d. Different individuals within the same family may have different sets of beliefs.

36. When caring for an obese patient additional manpower may be required as well as:

   a. specialized assessment skills.
   b. extra PPE for unique physical ailments.
   c. specialized management skills.
   d. appropriately sized diagnostic devices.

37. When caring for a patient who speaks a different language, which of the following should the paramedic do first?

   a. Use a phrase or picture book.
   b. Speak in English first to determine if he/she can understand even a little of the language.
   c. Let the patient put on your stethoscope and speak into the bell.
   d. Give the patient a paper and pen and encourage them to draw a picture.

38. When caring for a patient with a visual impairment, to lessen the patient's fear or anxiety, the paramedic should:

   a. describe everything he/she is going to do before actually doing it.
   b. not ask the patient about his/her visual impairment.
   c. leave his/her leader dogs at the residence, as the ambulance is unsafe.
   d. avoid explaining what care may be in store for him/her.

39. A patient with stroke-like symptoms is unable to say what he means. What type of speech disorder is the patient most likely experiencing?

   a. expressive aphasia
   b. receptive aphasia
   c. dysarthria
   d. fluency disorder

40. All the following are common causes of voice production disorders, *except*:

   a. laryngitis.
   b. stuttering.
   c. tumors.
   d. polyps.

41. The most common cause of either para- or quadriplegia is:

   a. muscular dystrophy.
   b. multiple sclerosis.
   c. trauma.
   d. birth defect.

42. Special accommodations for the care of a patient with a preexisting quadriplegia include:

   a. involving the alert and oriented patient in any decisions regarding movement and transport.
   b. obtaining consent for treatment from the patient's caregiver.
   c. full spinal immobilization.
   d. complete neurologic assessment and documentation.

43. Which of the following patients is most likely to develop hyperactivity or become dangerous while in the care of EMS?

   a. Psychotic person
   b. Neurotic person
   c. Homeless person
   d. Financially impaired person

44. Obesity is defined as being _____ above ideal body weight.

   a. 5–10%
   b. 10–20%
   c. 20–30%
   d. 30–40%

45. It is estimated that one in _____ Americans meets the definition for obesity.

   a. two
   b. three
   c. four
   d. five

46. Causes of mental retardation include all the following, *except*:

    a. birth defects.
    b. poverty.
    c. childhood disease.
    d. gender.

47. A child with spina bifida may have associated abnormalities, which include all the following, *except*:

    a. mental retardation.
    b. epilepsy.
    c. cerebral palsy.
    d. poliomyelitis.

48. Classic signs and symptoms of myasthenia gravis include:

    a. chest pain and shortness of breath.
    b. drooping eyelids and difficulty swallowing.
    c. headache and hypertension.
    d. memory loss and cognitive dysfunction.

49. In most cases prehospital care of the patient with myasthenia gravis will include:

    a. oxygen and nitroglycerin.
    b. supportive care and transport.
    c. oxygen and lopressor.
    d. reorientation to time and place.

Test #46 Answer Form

	A	B	C	D			A	B	C	D
1.	❏	❏	❏	❏		26.	❏	❏	❏	❏
2.	❏	❏	❏	❏		27.	❏	❏	❏	❏
3.	❏	❏	❏	❏		28.	❏	❏	❏	❏
4.	❏	❏	❏	❏		29.	❏	❏	❏	❏
5.	❏	❏	❏	❏		30.	❏	❏	❏	❏
6.	❏	❏	❏	❏		31.	❏	❏	❏	❏
7.	❏	❏	❏	❏		32.	❏	❏	❏	❏
8.	❏	❏	❏	❏		33.	❏	❏	❏	❏
9.	❏	❏	❏	❏		34.	❏	❏	❏	❏
10.	❏	❏	❏	❏		35.	❏	❏	❏	❏
11.	❏	❏	❏	❏		36.	❏	❏	❏	❏
12.	❏	❏	❏	❏		37.	❏	❏	❏	❏
13.	❏	❏	❏	❏		38.	❏	❏	❏	❏
14.	❏	❏	❏	❏		39.	❏	❏	❏	❏
15.	❏	❏	❏	❏		40.	❏	❏	❏	❏
16.	❏	❏	❏	❏		41.	❏	❏	❏	❏
17.	❏	❏	❏	❏		42.	❏	❏	❏	❏
18.	❏	❏	❏	❏		43.	❏	❏	❏	❏
19.	❏	❏	❏	❏		44.	❏	❏	❏	❏
20.	❏	❏	❏	❏		45.	❏	❏	❏	❏
21.	❏	❏	❏	❏		46.	❏	❏	❏	❏
22.	❏	❏	❏	❏		47.	❏	❏	❏	❏
23.	❏	❏	❏	❏		48.	❏	❏	❏	❏
24.	❏	❏	❏	❏		49.	❏	❏	❏	❏
25.	❏	❏	❏	❏						

47

Acute Interventions in the Home Care Patient

1. The roles of the home care professional and the paramedic are similar in that they both:

   a. offer supportive health care of the patient living at home.
   b. can provide emergency advance cardiac life support.
   c. offer palliative care.
   d. offer routine monitoring at home.

2. The roles of the home care professional and the paramedic are different in that only the paramedic can:

   a. offer supportive health care of the patient living at home.
   b. can provide emergency advanced cardiac life support.
   c. offer palliative care.
   d. offer routine monitoring at home.

3. Examples of patients that require home health care include all the following, *except*:

   a. chronic pain management.
   b. patients enrolled in hospice.
   c. cystic fibrosis patients.
   d. patients with diabetes mellitus.

4. Examples of diseases or conditions typical to the home care patient include:

   a. complications from infections.
   b. post MI insufficiency.
   c. sleep apnea.
   d. all of the above.

5. Community services that can provide care at home can be any of the following, *except*:

   a. profit.
   b. non-profit.
   c. church affiliated.
   d. politically rivaled.

6. Which of the following home health services is not a skilled service?

   a. Shopping service
   b. Infant care
   c. Case management
   d. Nursing

7. Home health services that are considered as support services include all the following, *except*:

   a. housekeeping.
   b. dental care.
   c. companions.
   d. personal care for grooming and dressing.

8. Palliative and support services for the terminally ill patient under medical supervision are provided by:

   a. hospice programs.
   b. church groups.
   c. HMOs.
   d. community centers.

9. Circulatory pathologies that are typical to the home care patient include:

   a. wound care.
   b. sleep apnea.
   c. obstructed shunts.
   d. sepsis.

10. Why are home health care services becoming the preference for patients and their families?

   a. These services help to reduce expensive inpatient stays.
   b. The HMOs are quicker to pay for these services than hospitalizations.
   c. There is no room left in the nursing homes.
   d. None of the above.

11. Hospice care emphasizes comfort measures and counseling to provide physical, spiritual, social, and _____ needs.

   a. financial
   b. long distance
   c. long-term
   d. economic

12. _____ care provides supportive care, comfort care, and referral for patient conditions such as chemotherapy, pain management, or daily activities.

   a. Acute
   b. Home
   c. Hospice
   d. HMO

13. _____ care provides services such as help with DNARs, advanced directives, and bereavement care.

   a. Acute
   b. Home
   c. Hospice
   d. HMO

14. Which of the following is an example of a type of patient that has the potential to become a detriment to the quality of care for in-home care?

   a. high maintenance patients
   b. neglected patients
   c. abused patients
   d. all of the above

15. Which of the following are examples of complications of in-home care that would result in the patient having to be hospitalized?

   a. Bed-wetting
   b. Anxiety
   c. Sleeplessness
   d. None of the above

16. _____ care is the work towards the relief of pain and suffering and provision of care for chronically ill patients and their family and friends.

   a. Palliative
   b. Modified
   c. Advanced
   d. Progressive

17. Which of the following situations with airway devices in the home would EMS most likely be called to assist?

   a. Discontinued use
   b. Obstructed tubing
   c. Properly placed tubing
   d. Routine suctioning

18. Which of the following devices is an example of an enhanced alveolar ventilation device found in the home?

   a. Nasal canula
   b. Simple face mask
   c. Pulmonary function meter
   d. Oxygen purifier

19. Which of the following is not a modification of traditional positive pressure ventilation?

   a. BiPAP
   b. CPAP
   c. PPEK
   d. PEEP

20. Which of the following is considered noninvasive ventilation?

   a. ETT
   b. EOA
   c. BiPAP
   d. PEEP

21. A home monitoring device which detects changes in thoracic or abdominal movement and heart rate is called a/an:

   a. apnea monitor.
   b. nebulizer.
   c. ventilator.
   d. pulmonary function meter.

22. All the following assessment findings would help identify failure of a home ventilatory device, *except*:

   a. decreased hypoxia.
   b. dyspnea.
   c. decreased tidal volume.
   d. decreased peak flow.

23. Vascular access devices (VADs) are common in home care settings and are used for all the following, *except*:

   a. medication administration.
   b. long-term vascular access.
   c. volume replacement.
   d. nutritional support.

24. While caring for a patient with a VAD, which of the following complications would not be a reason to transport the patient to the hospital?

    a. Dislodgement
    b. A too rapid infusion rate
    c. Embolism
    d. Extravastion

25. Which of the following is not a common VAD found in the home care setting?

    a. Port-A-Cath®.
    b. Hickman®
    c. Groshon®
    d. Extracath®

26. Your patient is having an acute onset of respiratory distress. She is tachypnic, cyanotic, and diaphoretic, and states the symptoms came on suddenly. Your assessment reveals that the patient has a VAD in place because she is a cancer patient who is receiving chemotherapy. Which of the following complications do you suspect?

    a. Embolism
    b. AMI
    c. Infection
    d. Sepsis

27. After providing high flow oxygen, your management plan for the patient described in question 27 should include:

    a. ventilatory support as needed and rapid transport.
    b. IV fluid challenge, ASA, and MS.
    c. NTG, ASA, and MS.
    d. NTG, lasix, and rapid transport.

28. All the following are devices for the GU tract that are commonly found in home care settings, *except*:

    a. Canadian catheter®.
    b. suprapubic catheters.
    c. Condom catheter®.
    d. Foley catheter®.

29. Which of the following GI tract devices is not commonly found in the home care setting?

    a. Colostomy bags
    b. J-tubes
    c. G-tubes
    d. P-tubes

30. The primary reasons patients are sent home with urinary catheters include:

    a. trauma and paralysis.
    b. UTI and urinary retention.
    c. immobilization and sedation.
    d. pregnancy and postoperative care.

31. GI/GU crisis in the home care setting can result from any of the following, *except*:

    a. improper patient positioning.
    b. gastric feeding.
    c. urosepsis.
    d. flatulence.

32. When a patient in the home care setting has a failure of a GU device, the paramedic may find any of the following assessment findings, *except*:

    a. changes in compulsion.
    b. dysuria.
    c. changes in urine color.
    d. changes in urine output.

33. The rights of the terminally ill patient include all the following, *except* the right to:

    a. know the truth.
    b. know justice.
    c. consent to treatment.
    d. choose the place to die and time of death.

34. There are _____ stages a dying person goes through, much like the stages in the grieving process after death.

    a. four
    b. five
    c. six
    d. seven

35. During the first stage of dying, a person experiences "shock and disbelief" and finally acceptance. This first stage can take moments or months before moving on to the second stage which is:

    a. bargaining.
    b. anger.
    c. depression.
    d. detachment.

36. For the dying person, acquiescence is achieved in the final stage of:

   a. bargaining.
   b. anger.
   c. depression.
   d. detachment.

37. Examples of wound closure techniques that the paramedic may be called to assess in the home care patient include all the following, *except*:

   a. squamous.
   b. sutures.
   c. wires.
   d. staples.

38. Which of the following is not a gastric emptying or feeding device?

   a. NG tube
   b. Colostomy
   c. Urostomy
   d. Peg tube

39. The general term for an operation in which an artificial opening in the body is formed is:

   a. incisure.
   b. ostomy.
   c. ectomy.
   d. intomy.

40. When assessing a patient in the home care setting who receives dialysis regularly, which of the following devices would you expect to find?

   a. VAD
   b. Feeding tube
   c. Pulmonary function meter
   d. Suprapubic catheter

41. A home health aide has called you to transport a home resident with chronic MS who has a urostomy and a feeding tube. The patient is tachypnic, febrile, and tachycardic. The aide tells you the urine output is decreased and the feeding schedule has been normal. Which of the following complications do you suspect first?

   a. local infection of the urostomy
   b. local infection of the feeding tube
   c. systemic infection
   d. respiratory infection

42. Your patient is a 66-year-old male complaining of abdominal pain with a slow and progressive onset over two days. His vital signs, including temperature, are normal. He denies any chest pain or shortness of breath. PO intake has been normal. What other information from the patient would be pertinent now?

   a. Any changes in bowels.
   b. Any changes in medications.
   c. Any nausea or vomiting.
   d. All of the above.

43. A physical examination of the patient described in question 43 reveals a distended abdomen with diffuse pain on palpation. The patient has had no nausea or vomiting, but has not had a bowel movement in two days. What do you suspect is the cause of his abdominal pain?

   a. GI bleed
   b. Hemorrhoids
   c. Obstruction
   d. Diverticulitis

44. Your management plan for the patient described in question 44 includes:

   a. oxygen, IV fluids, and rapid transport.
   b. oxygen and pain management.
   c. position of comfort and supportive care.
   d. suppository and transport.

45. You have been called to evaluate a bedridden home care patient. The visiting nurse discovered the patient had hematuria this morning when she was checking the patient's Foley catheter®. Which of the following might be the cause of the hematuria?

   a. Cystitis
   b. Infection
   c. Urethritis
   d. Any of the above

46. Your management plan for the patient described in question 46 includes:

   a. oxygen, IV fluids, and rapid transport.
   b. supportive care and routine transport.
   c. change the catheter and return to service.
   d. treating for shock.

47. The paramedic should respectfully interact with family members of the home care patient when present, because:

   a. they often know more about the patient's special needs than anyone else.
   b. they have the patient's advanced directives.
   c. most often they will not let the patient speak for him/herself.
   d. you are required to do so.

48. Which of the following is not an example of an airway condition typical to the home care setting?

   a. Sleep apnea
   b. Cystic fibrosis
   c. Asthma
   d. Lung transplant candidates

49. You have been called to a residence for a respiratory distress call. Upon arrival the family tells you that the patient does not want to be transported because the patient has an end stage terminal illness. They allow you in to assess, but state, "Hospice is on the way and that they made a mistake by calling EMS." What would be appropriate management for this patient?

   a. Wait for Hospice to arrive and then leave.
   b. Insist to the family that the patient should be transported.
   c. Call for police assistance.
   d. Offer assistance to the patient and then insist on transport.

Test #47 Answer Form

	A	B	C	D			A	B	C	D
1.	❏	❏	❏	❏		26.	❏	❏	❏	❏
2.	❏	❏	❏	❏		27.	❏	❏	❏	❏
3.	❏	❏	❏	❏		28.	❏	❏	❏	❏
4.	❏	❏	❏	❏		29.	❏	❏	❏	❏
5.	❏	❏	❏	❏		30.	❏	❏	❏	❏
6.	❏	❏	❏	❏		31.	❏	❏	❏	❏
7.	❏	❏	❏	❏		32.	❏	❏	❏	❏
8.	❏	❏	❏	❏		33.	❏	❏	❏	❏
9.	❏	❏	❏	❏		34.	❏	❏	❏	❏
10.	❏	❏	❏	❏		35.	❏	❏	❏	❏
11.	❏	❏	❏	❏		36.	❏	❏	❏	❏
12.	❏	❏	❏	❏		37.	❏	❏	❏	❏
13.	❏	❏	❏	❏		38.	❏	❏	❏	❏
14.	❏	❏	❏	❏		39.	❏	❏	❏	❏
15.	❏	❏	❏	❏		40.	❏	❏	❏	❏
16.	❏	❏	❏	❏		41.	❏	❏	❏	❏
17.	❏	❏	❏	❏		42.	❏	❏	❏	❏
18.	❏	❏	❏	❏		43.	❏	❏	❏	❏
19.	❏	❏	❏	❏		44.	❏	❏	❏	❏
20.	❏	❏	❏	❏		45.	❏	❏	❏	❏
21.	❏	❏	❏	❏		46.	❏	❏	❏	❏
22.	❏	❏	❏	❏		47.	❏	❏	❏	❏
23.	❏	❏	❏	❏		48.	❏	❏	❏	❏
24.	❏	❏	❏	❏		49.	❏	❏	❏	❏
25.	❏	❏	❏	❏						

Ambulance Operations and Medical Incident Command

1. _____ standards are minimum standards and not considered the "gold standard."

   a. National
   b. State
   c. Local
   d. Regional

2. The U.S. General Services Administration's Automotive Commodity Center issues the federal regulations specifying:

   a. the required response times for high rise buildings.
   b. BLS equipment that is mandatory on all ambulances.
   c. ALS equipment that is required on ambulances.
   d. ambulance design and manufacturing requirements.

3. All the following are accountable reasons for completing an ambulance equipment/supply checklist on each shift, *except* it:

   a. helps to make the work environments safer for the EMS personnel.
   b. serves to assure the ambulance is in proper driving condition.
   c. serves to assure the warning devices are all operating.
   d. serves to make the patient comfortable during transport.

4. Which of the following is not typically found on a vehicle/equipment checklist?

   a. Oxygen therapy and suction equipment.
   b. Supplies for childbirth.
   c. Restock items to be obtained from the hospital.
   d. Equipment for the transfer of the patient.

5. Special considerations for EMS providers who carry medications on their vehicles include:

   a. routinely checking expiration dates.
   b. having the junior EMS provider restock.
   c. getting the Medical Director to authorize medication purchases.
   d. billing the patients to recoup the cost of the medications.

6. OSHA requires that the ambulance be properly disinfected:

   a. once every twenty-four hours.
   b. on a weekly basis, even if there were no transports that week.
   c. after the transport of any patients with a potentially communicable disease.
   d. after the transport of any patient.

7. Each service is required, by OSHA or the state equivalent of OSHA, to have an exposure control plan that specifies:

   a. which mask to place on a TB patient.
   b. cleaning requirements.
   c. when to open vents in the ambulance.
   d. how to transfer potentially communicable patients.

8. The strategy used by an EMS agency to maneuver its ambulances and crews in an effort to reduce response times is referred to as:

   a. line of response.
   b. ambulance deployment.
   c. ambulance stratagem.
   d. zoning.

9. _____ is the ability to muster additional crews, should all the regularly staffed ambulances be on calls or a multiple casualty incident overtaxes the system's resources.

   a. Standards of reliability
   b. System status management
   c. Peak-load backup
   d. Reserve capacity

10. A computerized personnel and ambulance deployment system designed to meet service demands with fewer resources and to ensure appropriate response time and vehicle locations is called:

    a. standards of reliability.
    b. system status management.
    c. peak-load backup.
    d. reserve capacity.

11. Appropriate response time has to be determined by each community based on:

    a. its resources.
    b. ACLS standards.
    c. American Heart Association standards.
    d. National standards.

12. The number one rule of medicine, "Do no harm!" relates to all the following people, *except* the:

    a. ambulance operator.
    b. EMT–B.
    c. paramedic.
    d. patient.

13. In addition to personal injury and vehicle repair or replacement, the costs of ambulance collisions include:

    a. increased insurance premiums.
    b. down time.
    c. lawsuits.
    d. all of the above.

14. One concept that appears in most laws in statutes that deal with emergency vehicle operation is the concept of:

    a. res ipsa locquitor.
    b. negligence.
    c. due regard.
    d. causation.

15. The language described in the concept in question 14, sets up a _____ standard for the operator of an emergency vehicle than for any other driver on the road.

    a. safer
    b. higher
    c. lower
    d. liberal

16. Typical laws allow the operator of an ambulance, while in emergency operation, to be exempt from:

    a. passing over railroad crossings with the gates down.
    b. passing a school bus operator with the blinking red lights on.
    c. the posted parking regulations.
    d. none of the above.

17. Studies have shown that most other motorists do not see or hear your ambulance until it is within _____ feet of their vehicles.

    a. 10 to 25
    b. 25 to 50
    c. 50 to 100
    d. 100 to 200

18. All the following are recommended guidelines for the proper use of a siren, *except*:

    a. do not pull up close to a vehicle and then sound your siren.
    b. use the siren sparingly and only when you must.
    c. use the siren at all times while the lights are on.
    d. never assume all motorists will hear your siren.

19. Whenever the ambulance is on the road, day or night, the headlights should be turned on to:

    a. increase its visibility.
    b. comply with insurance stipulations.
    c. receive lower insurance premiums.
    d. annoy other motorists.

20. When your ambulance is the first to arrive at the scene of a highway incident and no potential hazards are apparent, you should park your emergency vehicle at least _____ the wreckage.

    a. 50 feet in front of
    b. 100 feet in front of
    c. 50 feet behind
    d. 100 feet behind

21. In 1969, R. Adams Cowley, MD convinced the _____ state legislature to fund the first statewide state police "medevac" program.

    a. New York
    b. California
    c. Florida
    d. Maryland

22. An MCI is a _____, which results in casualties severely burdening or exceeding the normal EMS resources of an agency in whose area the event occurs.

    a. mass casualty incident
    b. multiple casualty incident
    c. many citizens injured
    d. mixed community incident

23. When you are the first to arrive at the scene of an MCI, the first size-up radio report to the dispatcher is very important and should include all the following, *except*:

    a. specific location of the incident.
    b. location of the triage sector.
    c. extent of the incident.
    d. approximate number of patients.

24. A _____ incident is one where the patients need rescue or extrication to gain access to them.

    a. dangerous
    b. safe
    c. continued
    d. closed

25. Though originally developed for fire services, the incident command system (ICS) has been adopted to serve all emergency response disciplines and consists of procedures for controlling:

    a. personnel.
    b. equipment and facilities.
    c. communications.
    d. all of the above.

26. ICS is designed to begin developing from the time an incident occurs until:

    a. all victims are safely away from the incident.
    b. the fire or hazard is extinguished or contained.
    c. the requirement for management and operations no longer exists.
    d. all emergency medical responders are safely away.

27. Depending on the size of the incident, any of the following functional components of an IMS may be implemented, *except*:

    a. public relations.
    b. operations.
    c. planning.
    d. logistics.

28. A key component of ICS is _____, which is the desired number of subordinates that one supervisor can manage effectively at an incident.

    a. consolidated action plan
    b. span of control
    c. singular command
    d. unified command

29. The incident commander is the individual with overall responsibility for managing the incident, which includes all the following, *except*:

    a. assessing incident priorities.
    b. determining the strategic goals.
    c. designating hospital bed priorities.
    d. developing the incident action plan.

30. While working in an MCI, the use of bibs and vests serve a value in:

    a. making it easy to identify the command officers.
    b. making the command officers safer with better visibility.
    c. keeping order and avoiding chaos.
    d. identifying the priority of the patients.

31. It is not uncommon for physicians and nurses to stop at the scene of an MCI and offer assistance. Besides utilizing them in the treatment sector, what other area may be appropriate for their expertise?

    a. Safety
    b. Communications
    c. Triage
    d. Rescue

32. A very useful aspect to the use of triage tags at an MCI is that:

    a. patients can fill them out themselves.
    b. they do not take any training to use.
    c. they are inexpensive.
    d. they help to eliminate the need to reassess each patient over and over again.

33. Performing a post-incident critique is commonly done after an MCI because:

a. it serves the same function as a CISD.
b. every incident has something to teach.
c. it may involve media coverage.
d. commanders can critique without the fear of offending anyone.

34. Because there may be units from many different jurisdictions at an MCI, it is easier to use simple sector titles based on:

a. preference of the incident commander.
b. geographic location.
c. available resources.
d. the function they serve.

35. The role of the EMS provider and their agencies in planning for MCIs is:

a. active participation.
b. to be involved in drilling.
c. to be involved in planning and education.
d. all of the above.

36. An incident involving a residential house fire where all the patients are out on the front lawn of the home is an example of a(an) _____ incident.

a. open
b. closed
c. continuing
d. dangerous

37. The _____ section at an MCI is responsible for providing services and materials, such as communications unit, medical unit, or food unit, for the incident.

a. operations
b. planning
c. logistics
d. command

38. When all the involved agencies at an MCI contribute to the command process by determining the overall goals and objects, and use joint planning for tactical activities, they are working under:

a. OHSA CFR 29.
b. NFPA standard 1500.
c. singular command.
d. unified command.

39. During an MCI, a consolidated action plan should be developed at the:

a. dispatch center.
b. unified command post.
c. first arriving emergency vehicle.
d. discretion of the incident commander.

40. The use of a staging sector at an MCI is important because:

a. personnel arriving to assist can report to staging and avoid entering the scene.
b. congestion at the scene can be minimized.
c. it helps to minimize freelancing at the scene.
d. all of the above.

41. At an MCI, triage is done on all patients in an effort to assure that:

a. the most serious patients are treated and transported first.
b. all the critical patients go to the best hospitals.
c. the most important patients get the ALS care.
d. all low priority patients receive a different standard of care.

42. One of the most helpful tips that can smooth out operations at an MCI is:

a. to never let the driver, keys, or stretcher get separated from their ambulance.
b. use multiple radios with multiple channels to avoid confusion at the scene.
c. drive directly into the incident and look around to see where you are needed.
d. talk to the media and keep them advised of the evolving events.

43. Each corner of the ambulance should have flashers that are large and blinking in tandem or unison to help oncoming vehicles:

a. identify the name of the EMS service.
b. identify the location and size of the ambulance.
c. know where the EMS personnel are going to place the cones.
d. anticipate the placement of flares.

44. While working at the scene of a highway incident, beware that the _____ of the ambulance often obstructs the view of the warning lights to other motorists.

a. lighted flares
b. reflector tape
c. open rear doors
d. inexperienced driver

45. Fixed wing aircraft are used as the primary means of emergency transport in:

    a. remote regions such as parts of Alaska.
    b. missions under 50 miles distance from a hospital facility.
    c. search and rescue missions.
    d. none of the above.

46. Special consideration for aeromedical transport includes the need to intubate the patient prior to flight because of:

    a. the pressure changes during assent and decent.
    b. limited treatment area in the aircraft.
    c. the temperature changes during the flight.
    d. the various altitudes that the helicopter flies.

47. A helicopter requires a landing zone of approximately _____ feet on relatively level ground.

    a. 50 × 50
    b. 50 × 100
    c. 100 × 100
    d. 100 × 200

48. All the following are general rules to follow when approaching a helicopter that has landed to transport your patient, *except*:

    a. do not allow anyone to smoke within 200 feet of the aircraft.
    b. stay clear of the tail rotor at all times.
    c. when working at night shine a flashlight at the pilot to signal you are ready.
    d. allow the flight crew to direct the loading on board of the patient.

49. The Commission of Accreditation of Air Medical Services (CAAMS) was developed as a voluntary process for air medical services to:

    a. enforce the FAA standards for air travel.
    b. enforce standards for worker safety.
    c. help communities obtain funding for aeromedical programs.
    d. strengthen the safety of the aviation transport environment.

50. Disadvantages of aeromedic evacuation include all the following, *except*:

    a. access to remote areas.
    b. weather and environmental restrictions to flying.
    c. altitude limitations.
    d. airspeed limitations.

Test #48 Answer Form

	A	B	C	D		A	B	C	D
1.	❏	❏	❏	❏	26.	❏	❏	❏	❏
2.	❏	❏	❏	❏	27.	❏	❏	❏	❏
3.	❏	❏	❏	❏	28.	❏	❏	❏	❏
4.	❏	❏	❏	❏	29.	❏	❏	❏	❏
5.	❏	❏	❏	❏	30.	❏	❏	❏	❏
6.	❏	❏	❏	❏	31.	❏	❏	❏	❏
7.	❏	❏	❏	❏	32.	❏	❏	❏	❏
8.	❏	❏	❏	❏	33.	❏	❏	❏	❏
9.	❏	❏	❏	❏	34.	❏	❏	❏	❏
10.	❏	❏	❏	❏	35.	❏	❏	❏	❏
11.	❏	❏	❏	❏	36.	❏	❏	❏	❏
12.	❏	❏	❏	❏	37.	❏	❏	❏	❏
13.	❏	❏	❏	❏	38.	❏	❏	❏	❏
14.	❏	❏	❏	❏	39.	❏	❏	❏	❏
15.	❏	❏	❏	❏	40.	❏	❏	❏	❏
16.	❏	❏	❏	❏	41.	❏	❏	❏	❏
17.	❏	❏	❏	❏	42.	❏	❏	❏	❏
18.	❏	❏	❏	❏	43.	❏	❏	❏	❏
19.	❏	❏	❏	❏	44.	❏	❏	❏	❏
20.	❏	❏	❏	❏	45.	❏	❏	❏	❏
21.	❏	❏	❏	❏	46.	❏	❏	❏	❏
22.	❏	❏	❏	❏	47.	❏	❏	❏	❏
23.	❏	❏	❏	❏	48.	❏	❏	❏	❏
24.	❏	❏	❏	❏	49.	❏	❏	❏	❏
25.	❏	❏	❏	❏	50.	❏	❏	❏	❏

49

Rescue Awareness and Operations

1. The level of rescue training that all paramedics should be trained in is the _____ level.

   a. technical
   b. command
   c. awareness
   d. operations

2. What should set the priority of each rescue?

   a. The time police are able to hold back traffic.
   b. The abilities of the heavy rescue team.
   c. The patient's medical condition.
   d. The EMS providers need to return to service.

3. Awareness level training involves the ability to:

   a. comprehend the hazards.
   b. command the incident.
   c. mitigate all hazards.
   d. discern the causes of the reactions.

4. A successful rescue requires:

   a. medical training.
   b. mechanical training.
   c. a combination of A & B.
   d. a patient with minor injuries.

5. In general, all paramedics should have the proper training and PPE to:

   a. allow them to access the patient.
   b. provide assessment of the patient.
   c. provide management of the patient at the scene.
   d. all of the above.

6. It is essential that the paramedic know:

   a. when to enter an unstable situation.
   b. when it is or is not safe to gain access.
   c. how to stabilize a toxic atmosphere.
   d. how to enter a below grade rescue.

7. What PPE should be immediately available to all the paramedics?

   a. helmets and eye protection
   b. turnout gear and lights
   c. SCBA
   d. back country survival gear

8. Why are construction hard hats inappropriate for rescue work?

   a. Their duckbill brim is removable.
   b. They do not withstand severe impact.
   c. They are not warm enough.
   d. They have no ANSI rating.

9. What type of helmets are often used in confined space rescue?

   a. Standard type fire helmets
   b. Kayaking helmets
   c. Leather fire helmets
   d. Climbing helmets

10. Eye protection should be approved by:

    a. ANSI.
    b. EPA.
    c. NFPA.
    d. EDNA.

11. Eye protection is best provided by:

    a. regular glasses.
    b. a fire helmet face shield.
    c. contact lenses.
    d. industrial safety glasses.

12. The best gloves for rescue work by paramedics are:

    a. latex.
    b. rubber.
    c. leather work gloves.
    d. heavy gauntlet style firefighting gloves.

13. Limited flash protection in turnout gear is provided by:

   a. Nomex®.
   b. PBI®.
   c. flame retardant cotton.
   d. all of the above.

14. What is the best blanket to use for patient protection from heat and glass dust?

   a. Inexpensive vinyl tarps
   b. Aluminized rescue blankets
   c. Wool blankets
   d. Plastic sheeting

15. What should be used to shield the patient from sharp-edged objects or glass during a rescue?

   a. Plastic sheeting
   b. Sheets
   c. Backboards
   d. Vinyl tarps

16. The eye protection required for a rescue includes all the following, *except*:

   a. industrial safety glasses.
   b. a fire helmet face shield.
   c. goggles that are ANSI approved.
   d. all of the above.

17. Which is the last technique to employ in a water rescue?

   a. Reach
   b. Row
   c. Throw
   d. Go

18. The most common associated problem in water rescue is:

   a. strainers.
   b. hydraulics.
   c. eddies.
   d. hypothermia.

19. Another name for written safety procedures used by rescue teams is:

   a. protocols.
   b. regulations.
   c. SOPs.
   d. Bylaws.

20. The safety procedures discussed in question 19 should include:

   a. required safety equipment.
   b. requiring or prohibiting certain actions.
   c. the role of the safety officer.
   d. all of the above.

21. The person responsible for making the "go/no go" decision for a rescue operation is called the:

   a. incident commander.
   b. lead medic.
   c. team leader.
   d. safety officer.

22. Each of the following are phases of a rescue operation, *except*:

   a. size-up.
   b. elevation of control.
   c. disentanglement.
   d. medical treatment.

23. What is the value of a rescue plan?

   a. It describes how to respond to every incident.
   b. Improvement of personnel safety and operational success.
   c. There are fewer rescuers needed at incidents.
   d. The location to which units respond are specified.

24. Rescues that will take an extended amount of time may require:

   a. staging with protection from weather.
   b. food and hydration for personnel.
   c. rotation of personnel.
   d. all of the above.

25. Fluid for rehydration of personnel should consist of any of the following, *except*:

   a. water.
   b. Gatorade®.
   c. coffee.
   d. Power Aide®.

26. Upon arrival at the rescue incident, the EMS crew should:

   a. conduct a scene size-up.
   b. determine the hospital destination.
   c. disentangle the patient.
   d. set out flares on the roadway.

27. Upon arrival at a rescue search, what is the purpose of doing a risk versus benefit analysis?

   a. To determine the cause of the incident.
   b. To determine if it is a body recovery.
   c. To determine the full damage of the incident.
   d. To be eligible for federal funding.

28. Examples of on-scene hazards that need to be controlled by the paramedic upon arrival at the scene include:

    a. a car fire.
    b. chemical spills.
    c. creating a safe perimeter.
    d. downed electrical wires.

29. What safety precautions should be taken at all rescue scenes?

    a. Ensure all rescuers wear PPE.
    b. Make sure EMS personnel are visible.
    c. Be alert to traffic at the scene.
    d. All of the above.

30. Examples of potential hazards that may exist at the scene of a rescue include each of the following, *except*:

    a. more than two patients in the collision.
    b. poisonous or caustic substances.
    c. confined spaces such as a mine or cave.
    d. urban violence or a hostage scene.

31. Examples of rescue situations that "hide" patients include:

    a. avalanches.
    b. structural mishaps.
    c. cave-ins.
    d. all of the above.

32. When dispatched to incidents described in question 31, the paramedic should consider requesting:

    a. a surgeon to the scene.
    b. medical control be activated.
    c. an on-scene SAR specialist.
    d. a helicopter to the scene.

33. Paramedics should not enter an area to provide patient care unless they are:

    a. trained in all aspects of rescue.
    b. authorized by medical control to do so.
    c. protected from hazards with PPE.
    d. responding in a two medic unit.

34. The rescue term that means to remove the debris or parts of the vehicle from around the patient(s) so the patient may be freed for removal is:

    a. evacuation.
    b. extrication.
    c. disentanglement.
    d. gaining access.

35. The initial ALS interventions may be held off and only BLS provided when patients are found in any of the following situations, except:

    a. stranded in swift moving water.
    b. entrapped in vehicles with a fire.
    c. just removed from a pool.
    d. overcome by life-threatening atmospheres.

36. In the situations listed in question 35, rapid transport of a non-stabilized patient to a safer location, is justified based on the:

    a. high volume of patients.
    b. risk of injury to the rescuers.
    c. expense of the cost of care.
    d. age of the patient involved.

37. The most technical and time consuming part of a rescue is the _____ phase.

    a. hazard control
    b. extrication
    c. disentanglement
    d. removal

38. The patient packaging should take into consideration the:

    a. distance the ambulance will travel to the hospital.
    b. means of egress.
    c. number of crew members available.
    d. none of the above.

39. If it is necessary to lift a patient vertically out of a narrow hole, the best device to consider using is a:

    a. scoop stretcher.
    b. SKED.
    c. KED.
    d. Stokes® basket.

40. The term "special rescue operations" usually includes any of the following, *except*:

    a. hazardous atmosphere rescue.
    b. highway operations/vehicle rescue.
    c. hazardous terrain rescue.
    d. aeromedical transport.

41. Paramedics should consider which of the following to prepare for a water rescue incident?

    a. Learn to swim.
    b. Wear a PFD around water or ice.
    c. Take a basic water rescue course.
    d. All of the above.

42. With the exception of hot tubs, most bodies of water are considered cold water. What is the problem with being immersed in cold water?

   a. The patient inhales water faster.
   b. The patient loses salts and electrolytes rapidly.
   c. The patient's body is less buoyant.
   d. Hypothermia can rapidly set in.

43. Humans cannot maintain body temperature in water that is less than _____ degrees F.

   a. 98
   b. 96
   c. 94
   d. 92

44. Compared to the air, water causes heat _____ at a rate _____ times faster.

   a. loss; 5
   b. loss; 25
   c. gain; 10
   d. gain; 15

45. The contributing factors to the patient's demise when immersed in a body of water that is 35°F for more than 10 minutes include all the following, *except*:

   a. inability to attempt self-rescue.
   b. inability to follow simple directions.
   c. shivering causes muscle cramps.
   d. sudden immersion may trigger laryngospasm.

46. Why should hypothermic patients be removed from water in a horizontal position?

   a. They may have too much blood in the periphery.
   b. They may be dehydrated from cold diuresis.
   c. They do not tolerate the vagal stimuli.
   d. They can not tolerate the increased ICP.

47. When suddenly submerged while waiting for rescue, you should assume the _____ position.

   a. sniffing
   b. HELP
   c. tripod
   d. floating

48. A survivability estimate should be done quickly after arriving at the scene of a water rescue incident. Of the following which is not relevant to the estimate?

   a. Number of trained and equipped rescuers.
   b. Past history of submersion.
   c. Any known trauma to the patient.
   d. Age of the patient.

49. The water rescue model includes:

   a. reach.
   b. throw.
   c. row.
   d. all the above before a "go" rescue.

50. What is the danger of a low head dam?

   a. The water can rise above the dam.
   b. The water tends to throw objects clear.
   c. It is easy to get stuck on large rocks or boulders.
   d. Recirculating water is difficult to get out of.

51. If you accidentally fall into a body of swiftly moving water, what should you do?

   a. Float downstream feet first.
   b. Assume the HELP position.
   c. Attempt to walk out.
   d. Float downstream head and hands first.

52. Water moving through obstructions is sometimes called a "strainer." Examples include each of the following, *except*:

   a. a large boulder in the water.
   b. downed trees.
   c. grating over a pipe entry.
   d. wire rebar.

53. When water turns a bend in the river, the _____ of the curve moves _____ of the curve.

   a. inside: faster than the outside
   b. inside: slower than the outside
   c. outside: slower than the inside
   d. outside: faster than the inside

54. Alcohol is a contributory factor to as many as _____ % of boating fatalities.

   a. 10
   b. 50
   c. 30
   d. 75

55. What is the most effective strategy at preventing deaths from boating accidents?

   a. Requiring boating education.
   b. Enforcing anti-drinking laws.
   c. Carrying a PFD for each boater.
   d. Each boater wearing a PFD.

56. The protective response of the human body to cold water submersion is called the:

    a. mainstream reflex.
    b. mammalian diving reflex.
    c. immersion factor.
    d. HELP response.

57. Upon arrival at a water rescue, the paramedic should ask the bystanders:

    a. the precise location where the patient went under.
    b. how long the patient was in the water.
    c. if the patient seemed intoxicated.
    d. what the patient was wearing.

58. If a 25-year-old male patient is found unconscious in a swimming pool, what should his care entail?

    a. Spinal immobilization prior to removal.
    b. Oxygen therapy prior to removal from the pool.
    c. CPR while in the water if he has no pulse.
    d. None of the above.

59. What affects the patient's survivability "profile?"

    a. Age
    b. Posture
    c. Body fat
    d. All of the above

60. When a patient is found in a pool and is suspected to have a neck injury, to properly apply a backboard in the pool takes at least _____ rescuers in the water.

    a. 1
    b. 2
    c. 3
    d. 4

61. When applying a backboard on a patient who is in the water, the team should do all the following, *except*:

    a. secure with straps or cravats.
    b. maintain neck and head stabilization.
    c. lift the patient onto the board.
    d. extricate the patient head first.

62. According to NIOSH, it is estimated that _____ % of the fatalities associated with confined spaces are people attempting to rescue the patient.

    a. 10
    b. 20
    c. 40
    d. 60

63. The definition of a confined space is a space:

    a. not designated for human habitation.
    b. with limited access/egress.
    c. not designated for human occupancy.
    d. all of the above.

64. Each of the following are considered confined spaces, except:

    a. wells and cisterns.
    b. silos.
    c. hoppers.
    d. jail cells.

65. What is the biggest problem with confined spaces?

    a. They are oxygen deficient.
    b. They are difficult to crawl through.
    c. They are not well lit.
    d. They contain hazardous materials.

66. Problems associated with confined space rescue include:

    a. engulfment hazards.
    b. entrapment in machinery.
    c. limited access caused by structural concerns.
    d. all of the above.

67. What is the hazard associated with dust?

    a. It has a terrible odor.
    b. It can damage emergency equipment.
    c. It can create an explosive hazard.
    d. It is difficult to see.

68. Typical gases found in confined spaces include:

    a. carbon monoxide.
    b. methane.
    c. ammonia.
    d. all of the above.

69. Water seepage, ground vibrations, and disregarding safety regulations are some of the reasons for:

    a. structural collapse.
    b. vehicle rescue.
    c. a trench cave-in.
    d. a confined space rescue.

70. The initial response of the EMS provider to a cave-in should include size-up and:

    a. stabilization of the scene.
    b. establishing a perimeter.
    c. access to the patients.
    d. initiating extrication.

71. The trench rescue team should make access to the cave-in only after:

    a. shoring is in place.
    b. the patient has been located.
    c. all the dirt has been removed.
    d. ropes have been properly placed.

72. What is the greatest hazard when working a highway operation?

    a. Broken glass
    b. Crowds
    c. Fire hazards
    d. Traffic

73. Reduction of the traffic hazards at a highway operation involves a combination of each of the following strategies, *except*:

    a. staging of vehicles.
    b. stopping all flow of traffic.
    c. proper use of emergency lighting.
    d. proper positioning of emergency vehicles.

74. The ambulance and loading area at a highway operation should:

    a. be used as a point to congregate.
    b. not be directly exposed to traffic.
    c. rely on the rear blinking lights to stop cars.
    d. be off the side of the road.

75. When parked at the scene of a highway operation, the ambulance should:

    a. shut off all the lights.
    b. turn on only a minimum of warning lights.
    c. keep on the alternating head lights.
    d. turn on all the emergency lights.

76. When using flares at a highway operation, they should:

    a. direct the flow of traffic away from emergency workers.
    b. only be placed by law enforcement personnel.
    c. be used when the ground is wet.
    d. not be used if there is snow on the road.

77. Non-traffic hazards at a highway operation include:

    a. fuel and fire.
    b. alternate fuel systems.
    c. sharp objects.
    d. all of the above.

78. Why should the paramedic be especially concerned when a vehicle has gone off the road into tall grass?

    a. The potential for a fire hazard is increased.
    b. It will be difficult to find the vehicle.
    c. The potential for an electric hazard is greater.
    d. Patients may wander away from the scene.

79. If the car discussed in question 78 starts a brush fire, this is probably caused by:

    a. spontaneous combustion.
    b. the catalytic converter igniting the grass.
    c. a leaking gasoline tank.
    d. the occupants disposing of cigarettes.

80. Why can an energy-absorbing bumper be a hazard to EMS personnel?

    a. The fluid they leak is highly toxic.
    b. If loaded, they may release when unexpected.
    c. They can hide the true damage to the vehicle.
    d. They have been known to explode.

81. A supplemental restraint system may be a potential hazard to rescue personnel because:

    a. the straps can get in the way.
    b. the straps are difficult to cut.
    c. it can be difficult to remove from the patient.
    d. it can inflate when not expected.

82. If upon arrival at the scene of a car crash, the vehicle is on its side, off the road on an embankment, it will be necessary to rapidly:

    a. gain access.
    b. stabilize the vehicle.
    c. disentangle the patient.
    d. extricate the patient.

83. After assuring that the vehicle's ignition has been turned off, what can the paramedic do to prepare to gain access?

    a. Tell the patient to try to crawl out.
    b. Attempt to climb up on the car and open the door.
    c. Stabilize the vehicle with cribbing and a come-a-long.
    d. Break both the front and rear windows.

84. The part of an auto's anatomy that separates the engine compartment from the occupant compartment is called the:

    a. rocker panel.
    b. firewall.
    c. Nader pin.
    d. "A" post.

85. The reason why the doors do not fly open when a car is involved in a collision is because of the:

    a. firewall.
    b. tempered glass.
    c. Nader pin.
    d. roof support posts.

86. The windshield in vehicles is made of _____ glass.

    a. unbreakable
    b. safety
    c. tempered
    d. plastic

87. Glass which has a plastic laminate layer which limits how it breaks is called _____ glass.

    a. Nader
    b. tempered
    c. safety
    d. UV shield

88. The easiest way to break the _____ glass in the rear window is with a _____ object.

    a. tempered; sharp
    b. safety; sharp
    c. tempered; blunt
    d. safety; blunt

89. Unless the hydraulic spreader is used for accessing a crushed car door, the _____ must be disengaged prior to manually prying the door open.

    a. key
    b. door reinforcement bar
    c. battery cable
    d. Nader pin

90. The first step in accessing a car with a crushed door that has no safety hazards and is stabilized is to:

    a. break the glass in the rear window.
    b. remove the Nader pin.
    c. remove the roof.
    d. try all four doors first.

91. After taking the first step as described in question 90, the paramedic should next consider the need to:

    a. cut off the door at the hinges.
    b. pull the steering wheel through the windshield.
    c. gain access through the window furthest away from the patient.
    d. remove the roof of the vehicle.

92. The area at a collision scene where the rescue takes place is called the:

    a. outer circle.
    b. inner circle.
    c. command post.
    d. hot zone.

93. A steep slope which, in good weather, is capable of being walked up without using your hands is called:

    a. high angle.
    b. low angle.
    c. flat terrain.
    d. limited access terrain.

94. Members of a vertical rescue team should have competency in techniques such as:

    a. rappelling.
    b. belaying.
    c. self-rescue.
    d. all of the above.

95. When transporting a patient over rough terrain, it is recommended that a _____ stretcher be used.

    a. folding
    b. Stokes®
    c. wheeled
    d. limited access

96. The strongest basket stretchers are made of:

    a. wire and tubular metal.
    b. aluminum and plastic.
    c. enduro-plastic.
    d. polycarbonate.

97. Of the following preparations for transporting a patient over rough terrain, which is not necessary?

    a. A harness should be applied to the patient.
    b. A litter should be used to protect the patient's face.
    c. Leg stirrups should be applied to the patient.
    d. The patient should be restrained in a body bag.

98. A team of rescuers to carry out a Stokes® and patient over rough terrain consists of _____ rescuers and _____ teams if the personnel are available.

    a. 4; 4
    b. 6; 3
    c. 4; 3
    d. 6; 2

99. Even though you may not be trained in high angle rescue, there will be a need for helpers at the scene to:

    a. haul on the lines as instructed.
    b. rappel down to the patient.
    c. set up the rigging.
    d. coil the rope.

100. When an aerial ladder is used to remove a Stokes® basket from a building's roof, it is necessary to:

    a. belay the basket with a rope.
    b. use the ladder like a crane.
    c. strap the basket to the end of the ladder.
    d. slide the basket down the top of the ladder.

101. When a helicopter is used to pick up a Stokes® and move it to another nearby location, this is called a:

    a. flying Baker maneuver.
    b. rappel-based rescue.
    c. one skid rescue.
    d. short haul.

102. Paramedics who respond to back country rescues should be trained in all the following, *except*:

    a. long-term hydration management.
    b. termination of CPR.
    c. pain management.
    d. hyperbaric therapy.

103. A patient who has fallen off a cliff, who is still alive and will need a lengthy litter carryout, could benefit from a paramedic being trained to:

    a. cleanse wounds.
    b. reposition dislocations.
    c. manage hyperthermia.
    d. assess a 12-lead ECG.

104. Some of the limitations that may occur in back country rescue include all the following, *except*:

    a. street equipment is not easily transported to the patient.
    b. PPE is not used because it is cumbersome to wear.
    c. access to the patient may be limited.
    d. oxygen needs to be limited to a small aluminum tank.

Test #49 Answer Form

	A	B	C	D			A	B	C	D
1.	❑	❑	❑	❑		27.	❑	❑	❑	❑
2.	❑	❑	❑	❑		28.	❑	❑	❑	❑
3.	❑	❑	❑	❑		29.	❑	❑	❑	❑
4.	❑	❑	❑	❑		30.	❑	❑	❑	❑
5.	❑	❑	❑	❑		31.	❑	❑	❑	❑
6.	❑	❑	❑	❑		32.	❑	❑	❑	❑
7.	❑	❑	❑	❑		33.	❑	❑	❑	❑
8.	❑	❑	❑	❑		34.	❑	❑	❑	❑
9.	❑	❑	❑	❑		35.	❑	❑	❑	❑
10.	❑	❑	❑	❑		36.	❑	❑	❑	❑
11.	❑	❑	❑	❑		37.	❑	❑	❑	❑
12.	❑	❑	❑	❑		38.	❑	❑	❑	❑
13.	❑	❑	❑	❑		39.	❑	❑	❑	❑
14.	❑	❑	❑	❑		40.	❑	❑	❑	❑
15.	❑	❑	❑	❑		41.	❑	❑	❑	❑
16.	❑	❑	❑	❑		42.	❑	❑	❑	❑
17.	❑	❑	❑	❑		43.	❑	❑	❑	❑
18.	❑	❑	❑	❑		44.	❑	❑	❑	❑
19.	❑	❑	❑	❑		45.	❑	❑	❑	❑
20.	❑	❑	❑	❑		46.	❑	❑	❑	❑
21.	❑	❑	❑	❑		47.	❑	❑	❑	❑
22.	❑	❑	❑	❑		48.	❑	❑	❑	❑
23.	❑	❑	❑	❑		49.	❑	❑	❑	❑
24.	❑	❑	❑	❑		50.	❑	❑	❑	❑
25.	❑	❑	❑	❑		51.	❑	❑	❑	❑
26.	❑	❑	❑	❑		52.	❑	❑	❑	❑

	A	B	C	D			A	B	C	D
53.	❏	❏	❏	❏		79.	❏	❏	❏	❏
54.	❏	❏	❏	❏		80.	❏	❏	❏	❏
55.	❏	❏	❏	❏		81.	❏	❏	❏	❏
56.	❏	❏	❏	❏		82.	❏	❏	❏	❏
57.	❏	❏	❏	❏		83.	❏	❏	❏	❏
58.	❏	❏	❏	❏		84.	❏	❏	❏	❏
59.	❏	❏	❏	❏		85.	❏	❏	❏	❏
60.	❏	❏	❏	❏		86.	❏	❏	❏	❏
61.	❏	❏	❏	❏		87.	❏	❏	❏	❏
62.	❏	❏	❏	❏		88.	❏	❏	❏	❏
63.	❏	❏	❏	❏		89.	❏	❏	❏	❏
64.	❏	❏	❏	❏		90.	❏	❏	❏	❏
65.	❏	❏	❏	❏		91.	❏	❏	❏	❏
66.	❏	❏	❏	❏		92.	❏	❏	❏	❏
67.	❏	❏	❏	❏		93.	❏	❏	❏	❏
68.	❏	❏	❏	❏		94.	❏	❏	❏	❏
69.	❏	❏	❏	❏		95.	❏	❏	❏	❏
70.	❏	❏	❏	❏		96.	❏	❏	❏	❏
71.	❏	❏	❏	❏		97.	❏	❏	❏	❏
72.	❏	❏	❏	❏		98.	❏	❏	❏	❏
73.	❏	❏	❏	❏		99.	❏	❏	❏	❏
74.	❏	❏	❏	❏		100.	❏	❏	❏	❏
75.	❏	❏	❏	❏		101.	❏	❏	❏	❏
76.	❏	❏	❏	❏		102.	❏	❏	❏	❏
77.	❏	❏	❏	❏		103.	❏	❏	❏	❏
78.	❏	❏	❏	❏		104.	❏	❏	❏	❏

50

Hazardous Material Awareness and Operations

1. The first standard to guide hazardous material (hazmat) operations specifically for EMS workers was NFPA:

   a. 472
   b. 473
   c. 704
   d. 1500

2. NFPA standard _____ established a system of placarding and labeling fixed facilities for hazardous materials.

   a. 472
   b. 473
   c. 704
   d. 1500

3. _____ is the minimal level of hazmat training at which the responder can perform risk assessment procedures and conduct basic control, containment, and confinement operations.

   a. First responder awareness
   b. First responder operations
   c. Hazardous material technician
   d. Hazardous material specialist

4. Which of the following is not a typical method for identifying hazardous materials?

   a. NFPA 472
   b. Dispatcher obtained information
   c. Material safety data sheets (MSDS)
   d. DOT placards

5. There are _____ levels of hazmat training required by OSHA regulations.

   a. 4
   b. 5
   c. 6
   d. 10

6. The _____ provides written information about the names of substance, UN numbers, placard facsimiles, emergency action guides, and evacuation and isolation information.

   a. *North American Emergency Response Guidebook*
   b. MSDS
   c. CHEMTREC
   d. bill of lading

7. DOT placards classify gasses into all the following categories, *except*:

   a. Poison A
   b. Poison B
   c. Flammable gas
   d. Corrosive gas

8. _____ are used throughout the industry as a means of identifying chemicals and complying with the employee's Right to Know.

   a. Shipping papers
   b. Bills of lading
   c. MSDS
   d. Waybills

9. The stages of metabolism of a poison are the same as with any drug and include all the following, *except*:

   a. absorption.
   b. distribution
   c. elimination.
   d. adaptation.

10. _____ is/are how and what a poison does to the body.

    a. Poison actions
    b. Poison adaptations
    c. Degradation
    d. Absorption

11. Decontamination is the physical or _____ process of removing hazardous material from exposed persons or equipment.

   a. mechanical
   b. chemical
   c. filtration
   d. biodegradable

12. The procedure for the decontamination (decon) of a critical patient is a _____ step process.

   a. 2
   b. 4
   c. 7
   d. 8

13. The decon corridor which consists of _____ stages, is the method used for decontamination of non-critical patients and rescuers.

   a. 5
   b. 6
   c. 7
   d. 8

14. Water is a universal decon solution that dilutes and reduces _____ absorption.

   a. metabolic
   b. topical
   c. enteral
   d. parenteral

15. Which of the following is not a common solution used by EMS providers for decon?

   a. Tincture of green soap
   b. Isopropyl alcohol
   c. Vegetable oil
   d. Milk

16. The properties of potential hazards for chemical substances which are listed on 704 placards and other references include flammability, health hazards, and:

   a. reliability.
   b. toxicity.
   c. relativity.
   d. reactivity.

17. Prior to working at an incident where hazmat is present, _____ is/are established to prevent injury and unnecessary exposure to the substance.

   a. officers
   b. zones
   c. quarters
   d. precedence

18. Examples of emergency actions the paramedic can take at a hazmat include all the following, *except*:

   a. provide first aid by moving victims to fresh air.
   b. keep unnecessary people away.
   c. collect a sample of the material for the ED.
   d. remove and isolate contaminated clothing and shoes at the site.

19. _____ is how much substance it takes to cause a physiologic response.

   a. Dose response
   b. Route of exposure
   c. Synergistic effect
   d. Toxicity

20. Factors that can make field decontamination of a patient difficult include all the following, *except*:

   a. having an MSDS available.
   b. limited level of training.
   c. no single type of PPE is compatible with all chemicals.
   d. critical patient condition.

21. The maximum concentration to which a healthy adult can be exposed to a hazardous material without risk of injury is called the:

   a. ceiling level.
   b. flash point.
   c. permissible exposure limit
   d. threshold limit value.

22. _____ is a time-weighted average concentration that must not be exceeded during any 8-hour work shift or 40-hour work week.

   a. Ceiling level
   b. Short-term exposure limit
   c. Permissible exposure limit
   d. Threshold limit value

23. The reference book *North American Emergency Response Guidebook* gives the paramedic three methods to reference a substance that lead to a guide which provides all the following information, *except*:

   a. potential hazards.
   b. access to MSDS.
   c. first aid treatment.
   d. safety precautions.

24. The Occupational Health and Safety Administration (OSHA) regulations are published in the:

   a. product packaging labels.
   b. Material Safety Data Sheets (MSDS)
   c. *North American Emergency Response Guidebook*
   d. Code of Federal Regulations (CFR)

25. CHEMTREC is an information resource service operated by the _____ and is available by an 800 phone number for detailed information on the chemicals involved and the manufacturer of the chemical.

   a. Centers for Disease Control (CDC)
   b. Federal Regulatory Commission
   c. Department of Transportation (DOT)
   d. Chemical Manufacturers Association

Test #50 Answer Form

	A	B	C	D		A	B	C	D
1.	❏	❏	❏	❏	14.	❏	❏	❏	❏
2.	❏	❏	❏	❏	15.	❏	❏	❏	❏
3.	❏	❏	❏	❏	16.	❏	❏	❏	❏
4.	❏	❏	❏	❏	17.	❏	❏	❏	❏
5.	❏	❏	❏	❏	18.	❏	❏	❏	❏
6.	❏	❏	❏	❏	19.	❏	❏	❏	❏
7.	❏	❏	❏	❏	20.	❏	❏	❏	❏
8.	❏	❏	❏	❏	21.	❏	❏	❏	❏
9.	❏	❏	❏	❏	22.	❏	❏	❏	❏
10.	❏	❏	❏	❏	23.	❏	❏	❏	❏
11.	❏	❏	❏	❏	24.	❏	❏	❏	❏
12.	❏	❏	❏	❏	25.	❏	❏	❏	❏
13.	❏	❏	❏	❏					

51

Crime Scene Awareness

1. Examples of potential exposures for the paramedic in the area of scene violence include which of the following?

   a. Exposure to crowds.
   b. Calls for an assault.
   c. Police on the scene of a call.
   d. Any of the above.

2. As part of the hazard awareness, the paramedic's safety concerns should begin:

   a. in the classroom.
   b. with information obtained from dispatch.
   c. as soon as you enter the neighborhood.
   d. when you arrive at the call address.

3. If while on the scene the paramedic becomes aware of a potential threat, weapons, or any violent or abusive action towards him/her, the paramedic should:

   a. look for a second exit.
   b. retreat right away.
   c. intercede with pepper spray.
   d. wait for police before further intervention.

4. Examples of non-violent dangers that the paramedic should be alert for on the scene include all the following, *except*:

   a. pets.
   b. power lines.
   c. a crowd in front of a residence.
   d. hazardous materials.

5. All the following are reasons that it is not uncommon for a paramedic to be mistaken as a police officer, *except*:

   a. some EMS agencies wear uniforms that resemble the police uniform in their community.
   b. some paramedics wear a badge and holsters with medical equipment in them.
   c. paramedics arrive in vehicles with lights and sirens.
   d. some paramedics have training similar to police training.

6. When dispatched to a known violent scene, the paramedic should stage the vehicle:

   a. at least 50 feet from the scene.
   b. at least 100 feet from the scene.
   c. out of sight of the scene.
   d. directly behind a police vehicle.

7. Safety strategies to practice to avoid injury to yourself and your crew include all the following, *except*:

   a. after you announce your presence or knock on the door, listen for signs of danger.
   b. stand to the side of the door on the doorknob side.
   c. do not backlight yourself by getting between the EMS unit and the residence.
   d. do not broadcast your approach with lights and sirens.

8. When approaching a vehicle that is at the side of the road, clues that typically indicate there may be a dangerous condition include all the following, *except*:

   a. signs of alcohol or drug use.
   b. arguing between the occupants of the vehicle.
   c. any open or unlatched hood or trunks.
   d. all the doors are locked.

9. Before getting out of the ambulance to approach a vehicle on the highway, it is a good idea to notify the dispatcher of the situation and the:

   a. exact location.
   b. color of the vehicle.
   c. number of occupants.
   d. lack of activity where activity is likely.

10. The paramedic should initially approach the vehicle from the passenger side because the:

    a. posts of the vehicle will keep the paramedic safe from a gunshot.
    b. driver would normally expect the police to approach on the driver's side.
    c. paramedic will have a better view of a dangerous situation.
    d. traffic side is usually inaccessible.

11. While approaching a vehicle on the highway, one partner initially remains in the ambulance to watch for hazards, while the other paramedic who is going to approach the vehicle should:

    a. chock the wheels of the vehicle.
    b. copy the license plate number and state.
    c. have a portable radio in hand.
    d. set up a safety zone.

12. In a number of communities the medical personnel wear white shirts and bright colored jackets with retro-reflective stripes and large clear lettering that says "EMS" because:

    a. this is a great public relations tactic.
    b. it keeps them from looking like police officers.
    c. it makes them more visible in traffic.
    d. it is the boss's idea.

13. The Crips, Bloods, Latin Kings, and the Banditos are all names of:

    a. rock bands.
    b. schools.
    c. street gangs.
    d. rap groups.

14. EMS providers may be called to respond to a clandestine drug lab for:

    a. injuries from an explosion.
    b. monitoring suspicious patients.
    c. assisting the DEA with moving chemicals.
    d. assistance in breaking down the cookers.

15. A clandestine drug lab is designed to do chemical:

    a. synthesis and create drugs.
    b. conversion of drugs.
    c. extraction and prepare tablets.
    d. any of the above.

16. It is not uncommon for _____ in or near a clandestine drug lab to warn the criminals of the approach of intruders.

    a. undercover FBI to be
    b. snipers to be staged
    c. booby traps to be set
    d. none of the above

17. The presence of a street gang in a community increases the:

    a. value of the properties.
    b. awareness for graffiti.
    c. potential for street violence.
    d. Good Samaritan effort.

18. Street gangs often have unique clothing they call their _____ , that are an identifier of the group and may represent the member's status within the group.

    a. leathers
    b. rags
    c. colors
    d. stripes

19. If you believe that you have arrived at the scene of a clandestine drug lab, the safest action for you is to:

    a. not move, but call for police.
    b. act as if you do not know that it is a drug lab.
    c. care for the patient but watch out for chemical exposure.
    d. leave immediately and call law enforcement.

20. Who is considered the best personnel to manage an incident at a clandestine drug lab?

    a. The fire department.
    b. The DEA.
    c. A chemical specialist from the nearest college.
    d. The hazmat team.

21. Which of the following types of violence is considered to be domestic violence?

    a. Physical violence by a male cousin.
    b. Sexual violence by an aunt.
    c. Verbal violence from a grandparent.
    d. All of the above.

22. All the following are examples of indications of domestic violence, *except*:

    a. apparent fear of a neighbor.
    b. injuries that do not match the MOI.
    c. one party preventing the other from speaking.
    d. unsanitary living conditions or hygiene.

23. Which of the following actions should the paramedic avoid if he/she suspects domestic violence?

    a. Treat the patient.
    b. Provide a phone number for domestic violence hot line or shelter.
    c. Protect the victim by getting between the victim and the abuser.
    d. Do not be judgmental.

24. All the following rules apply to tactical safety, *except*:

    a. avoidance is always preferable to confrontation.
    b. if you are not sure of a potential danger, call dispatch before entering the scene.
    c. become a keen observer of the warning signs of violence.
    d. always consider staging your unit until law enforcement has secured the scene.

25. If you have to retreat from a dangerous scene be sure to:

    a. document that you did not abandon the patient.
    b. make sure the dispatcher does not send any further EMS units directly into the scene.
    c. bring the patient with you.
    d. bring cover with you.

26. Which of the following is most correct about concealment for the paramedic?

    a. Concealment is positioning the paramedic or crew behind an object that hides them from the view of others.
    b. Concealment offers ballistic protection if the perpetrator begins to fire a weapon.
    c. An example of concealment is hiding behind a brick wall.
    d. None of the above is correct.

27. What can the paramedics do if an aggressor seems to be chasing them?

    a. Strike before the aggressor strikes you.
    b. Do not try to anticipate the moves of the aggressor.
    c. Use pepper spray or mace to slow the aggressor.
    d. Throw the equipment to slow or trip the aggressor.

28. All the following statements about body armor are correct, *except*:

    a. Kevlar® has reduced protection when wet.
    b. body armor does not offer protection against high velocity rifle bullets.
    c. body armor does protect against thin or dull-edged weapons.
    d. one should avoid having a false sense of security when wearing body armor.

29. In some cities a limited number of EMS providers are trained in special tactics to accompany the police on high-risk operations. This program is called:

    a. CONTOMS.
    b. rescue EMS.
    c. tactical EMS.
    d. Superhero EMS.

30. The _____ program started in 1989 was designed to meet the specialized medical training to support law enforcement operations and was funded by the Department of Defense.

    a. CONTOMS
    b. LEA/SWAT team
    c. SWAT–Medic
    d. TEMS

31. When removing clothing from a patient at a crime scene that is stained in blood or body fluids, the paramedic should avoid:

    a. cutting along the seam of the clothing.
    b. cutting through a knife or bullet hole.
    c. having law enforcement assist.
    d. placing items separately.

32. After removing the clothing from a patient at a crime scene, the paramedic should place the clothing in:

    a. a paper bag.
    b. zip lock bag.
    c. a towel.
    d. the patient's bathtub.

33. If a person is found hanging and the paramedic is going to attempt a resuscitation, the paramedic should wear gloves and take the patient down by _____ the knot.

    a. untying
    b. cutting through
    c. getting the police to cut
    d. cutting to avoid

34. Wearing gloves while working at the scene of a crime may prevent the paramedic from leaving finger prints, but does not prevent:

    a. leaving the moisture from his/her skin at the scene.
    b. leaving the oil from his/her skin at the scene.
    c. destroying or "smudging" the perpetrator's prints.
    d. the spread of blood-borne disease.

35. The paramedic can minimize risks when in a suspected dangerous situation by:

    a. not wearing a clip-on tie.
    b. keeping hands in his/her pockets to appear non-threatening.
    c. keeping a safe stance with feet apart, ready to react.
    d. keeping a stethoscope around the neck to look like a doctor.

Test #51 Answer Form

	A	B	C	D			A	B	C	D
1.	❏	❏	❏	❏		19.	❏	❏	❏	❏
2.	❏	❏	❏	❏		20.	❏	❏	❏	❏
3.	❏	❏	❏	❏		21.	❏	❏	❏	❏
4.	❏	❏	❏	❏		22.	❏	❏	❏	❏
5.	❏	❏	❏	❏		23.	❏	❏	❏	❏
6.	❏	❏	❏	❏		24.	❏	❏	❏	❏
7.	❏	❏	❏	❏		25.	❏	❏	❏	❏
8.	❏	❏	❏	❏		26.	❏	❏	❏	❏
9.	❏	❏	❏	❏		27.	❏	❏	❏	❏
10.	❏	❏	❏	❏		28.	❏	❏	❏	❏
11.	❏	❏	❏	❏		29.	❏	❏	❏	❏
12.	❏	❏	❏	❏		30.	❏	❏	❏	❏
13.	❏	❏	❏	❏		31.	❏	❏	❏	❏
14.	❏	❏	❏	❏		32.	❏	❏	❏	❏
15.	❏	❏	❏	❏		33.	❏	❏	❏	❏
16.	❏	❏	❏	❏		34.	❏	❏	❏	❏
17.	❏	❏	❏	❏		35.	❏	❏	❏	❏
18.	❏	❏	❏	❏						

52
Advanced Cardiac Life Support

1. The principles of _____ medicine classifies interventions into one of five categories.

    a. diagnostic
    b. evidence based
    c. homeopathic
    d. osteopathic

2. Class _____ guidelines are supported by very good evidence of effectiveness and safety in humans.

    a. I
    b. IIa
    c. Indeterminate
    d. III

3. Class _____ interventions or actions are proposed guidelines with insufficient evidence to support a final recommendation for clinical use at this time.

    a. IIa
    b. IIb
    c. Indeterminate
    d. III

4. In ACLS, the new unifying approach to assessment and management involves the combination of a Primary ABCD and a Secondary ABCD survey. The ABC remains as airway, breathing, and circulation and the D represents _____ and _____, respectively.

    a. defibrillation; differential diagnosis
    b. defibrillation; disability
    c. disability; defibrillation
    d. disability; differential diagnosis

5. The Guidelines 2000 require the training in the use of a _____ by all health care providers.

    a. BVM
    b. LMA
    c. Combitube®
    d. ET tube

6. All the following are primary techniques for confirmation of endotracheal tube placement, *except:*

    a. direct visualization of the tube going through the cords.
    b. physical examination of the tube placement.
    c. the use of the esophageal detector device (EDD).
    d. five point auscultation.

7. Which of the following is a secondary technique for confirmation of endotracheal tube placement?

    a. Tube condensation.
    b. End tidal CO_2 monitoring.
    c. Bilateral chest expansion.
    d. Physical examination of the tube placement.

8. Which of the following devices provides a continuous visual display of the level of expired CO_2?

    a. Capnometer
    b. Capnograph
    c. Colorimetric device
    d. All of the above

9. Which of the following is incorrect about the Combitube® airway device?

    a. The Combitube® is an advanced airway.
    b. This device is inserted blindly.
    c. It is placed orally and inserted past the hypopharyngeal space.
    d. This device requires extensive training to use.

10. All the following are correct about the LMA airway device, *except:*

    a. This device does not require extensive training to use.
    b. This device is inserted blindly.
    c. This device prevents aspiration of stomach contents into the lungs.
    d. The LMA is an advanced airway device.

11. The primary emphasis of the Guidelines 2000 in the area of ALS for pediatrics includes all the following, *except:*

    a. acute coronary syndromes.
    b. respiratory failure.
    c. shock.
    d. prevention of cardiac arrest.

12. The PALS course has been enriched with new knowledge in the area of managing all the following, *except:*

    a. common poisoning.
    b. toxicologic problems.
    c. electrolyte abnormalities.
    d. trauma.

13. Pediatric post-resuscitation interventions that may improve the neurologic outcome include:

    a. avoiding hyperventilation.
    b. maintaining normal blood sugar levels.
    c. treating hyperthermia and allowing a mild hypothermia to exist.
    d. all of the above.

14. The use of high dose epinephrine in pediatric cardiac arrest has been deemphasized for all the following reasons, *except* it:

    a. is very difficult to accurately dose to the weight.
    b. can increase myocardial oxygen demand.
    c. can cause tachycardia and hypertension.
    d. can cause myocardial necrosis.

15. _____ has been added to the management of potentially fatal pediatric dysrhythmias.

    a. Verapamil
    b. Amiodarone
    c. Cardizem
    d. Vasopressin

16. All the following are recommendations for the care of the neonate in the Guidelines 2000, except:

    a. meconium staining in the newly born who is active and vigorous should not be suctioned.
    b. the two thumb and encircling fingers methods are the preferred methods for two rescuer infant CPR.
    c. the fluid of choice for volume expansion is an albumin-containing solution.
    d. the LMA can be used, by properly trained providers, in newborns where BVM ventilation is ineffective or there is a failed ET.

17. Special circumstances where initiation of CPR in the newborn may not be appropriate include all the following, *except:*

    a. confirmed gestation < 23 weeks.
    b. birth weight < 400 grams.
    c. anencephaly.
    d. confirmed Down syndrome.

18. _____ is the first line antiarrhythmic for shock refractory VF or pulseless VT.

    a. Bretilium
    b. Amiodarone
    c. Vassopressin
    d. Magnesium sulfate

19. _____ has been shown to be effective for VF or pulseless VT, torsades de pointes, and dysrhythmias with known hypomagnesemia.

    a. Sodium bicarbonate
    b. Amiodarone
    c. Vassopressin
    d. Magnesium sulfate

20. _____ is an agent that appears to be as effective as epinephrine in cardiac arrest and lasts between 10 and 20 minutes, so only one dose is recommended.

    a. Lidocaine
    b. Amiodarone
    c. Vassopressin
    d. Procainamide

21. The key changes in the management of asystole include all the following, *except:*

    a. more emphasis on determination of the presence of a DNAR.
    b. the need for improved protocols for stopping CPR.
    c. directing the focus of care toward supporting and comforting the family.
    d. having the ambulance transport the body directly to a funeral home.

22. All the following are key changes in the management of tachycardia, *except:*

    a. the use of more than one antiarrhythmic is no longer recommended.
    b. the patient known to have impaired myocardial function will often do better with antiarrhythmics.
    c. electrical cardioversion should be the intervention of choice or the second antiarrhythmic.
    d. antiarrhythmics are now known to also have proarrhythmic effects.

23. AMI and unstable angina are now recognized as part of a spectrum of disease known as:

    a. acute coronary syndromes.
    b. advanced coronary syndromes.
    c. ACLS disorders.
    d. acute cardiac disorders.

24. Cardiac patients who are not eligible for fibrinolytic therapy because of exclusionary criteria should be considered for transport or transfer to a hospital with _____ facilities.

    a. outpatient placement
    b. hyperbaric oxygen therapy
    c. primary angioplasty and intra-aortic balloon placement.
    d. primary beta-blocking central line

25. IV fibrinolytics have been shown to improve neurologic outcome in stroke patients who meet the criteria, provided they are administered within:

    a. the first 72 hours after symptoms start to resolve.
    b. 2 hours after the symptoms start to resolve.
    c. 3 hours of the onset of the symptoms.
    d. 3 to 6 hours of the onset of the symptoms.

26. Overdose of tricyclic antidepressants has been shown to cause hypotension or:

    a. ventricular dysrhythmias.
    b. TIA or stroke.
    c. hypomagnesium.
    d. hypothermia.

27. The treatment of choice for an overdose of tricyclic antidepressant is the induction of:

    a. systemic alkalosis with a pH of 7.50 to 7.55.
    b. an antiarrhythmic agent like lidocaine.
    c. procainamide.
    d. all of the above.

28. Cocaine overdose has been shown to be associated with serious:

    a. ventricular dysrhythmias.
    b. atrial dysrhythmias.
    c. hypomagnesium.
    d. hypothermia.

29. The Guidelines 2000 recommend all the following for cocaine overdose, *except:*

    a. nitrates as a first line therapy.
    b. benzodiazepines as a first line therapy.
    c. alpha-adrenergic blocking agents as a second line therapy when the first line treatment fails.
    d. beta-blocking agents as a second line therapy when the first line treatment fails.

30. Recommended prehospital medications for all patients with AMI include _____ in the absence of contraindications.

    a. aspirin
    b. nitroglycerin
    c. beta-blockers
    d. none of the above.

Test #52 Answer Form

	A	B	C	D			A	B	C	D
1.	❏	❏	❏	❏		16.	❏	❏	❏	❏
2.	❏	❏	❏	❏		17.	❏	❏	❏	❏
3.	❏	❏	❏	❏		18.	❏	❏	❏	❏
4.	❏	❏	❏	❏		19.	❏	❏	❏	❏
5.	❏	❏	❏	❏		20.	❏	❏	❏	❏
6.	❏	❏	❏	❏		21.	❏	❏	❏	❏
7.	❏	❏	❏	❏		22.	❏	❏	❏	❏
8.	❏	❏	❏	❏		23.	❏	❏	❏	❏
9.	❏	❏	❏	❏		24.	❏	❏	❏	❏
10.	❏	❏	❏	❏		25.	❏	❏	❏	❏
11.	❏	❏	❏	❏		26.	❏	❏	❏	❏
12.	❏	❏	❏	❏		27.	❏	❏	❏	❏
13.	❏	❏	❏	❏		28.	❏	❏	❏	❏
14.	❏	❏	❏	❏		29.	❏	❏	❏	❏
15.	❏	❏	❏	❏		30.	❏	❏	❏	❏

Appendix:
Answer Keys

Chapter 1 Answer Key

1.	A	14.	D	27.	B	40.	A	53.	B
2.	C	15.	B	28.	C	41.	D	54.	B
3.	D	16.	A	29.	B	42.	D	55.	D
4.	D	17.	C	30.	A	43.	A	56.	A
5.	B	18.	D	31.	B	44.	D	57.	B
6.	A	19.	B	32.	B	45.	B	58.	C
7.	C	20.	A	33.	C	46.	D	59.	B
8.	A	21.	B	34.	B	47.	D	60.	D
9.	C	22.	B	35.	A	48.	C	61.	B
10.	B	23.	A	36.	D	49.	B	62.	B
11.	A	24.	D	37.	A	50.	C		
12.	C	25.	B	38.	D	51.	A		
13.	C	26.	D	39.	B	52.	B		

Chapter 2 Answer Key

1.	B	16.	D	31.	B	46.	A	61.	B
2.	A	17.	C	32.	B	47.	C	62.	B
3.	A	18.	C	33.	D	48.	A	63.	D
4.	D	19.	A	34.	D	49.	B	64.	D
5.	B	20.	A	35.	B	50.	A	65.	C
6.	D	21.	D	36.	B	51.	D	66.	A
7.	C	22.	B	37.	A	52.	D	67.	B
8.	A	23.	C	38.	C	53.	B	68.	B
9.	C	24.	A	39.	C	54.	B	69.	B
10.	C	25.	D	40.	A	55.	A	70.	C
11.	B	26.	A	41.	B	56.	D	71.	A
12.	A	27.	B	42.	D	57.	C	72.	C
13.	C	28.	D	43.	D	58.	B	73.	B
14.	A	29.	C	44.	B	59.	D	74.	D
15.	D	30.	A	45.	C	60.	A	75.	C

Chapter 3 Answer Key

1. D	8. A	15. D	22. D	29. D
2. A	9. B	16. C	23. A	30. A
3. A	10. B	17. B	24. D	31. D
4. C	11. C	18. A	25. C	32. A
5. B	12. C	19. A	26. B	33. A
6. A	13. A	20. A	27. D	34. B
7. D	14. D	21. B	28. D	35. C

Chapter 4 Answer Key

1. D	16. A	31. C	46. B	61. D
2. A	17. D	32. A	47. B	62. C
3. C	18. A	33. C	48. B	63. D
4. B	19. B	34. B	49. B	64. D
5. C	20. D	35. C	50. D	65. A
6. B	21. B	36. A	51. B	66. D
7. C	22. C	37. D	52. D	67. B
8. D	23. A	38. B	53. A	68. C
9. B	24. B	39. D	54. B	69. B
10. B	25. A	40. B	55. C	70. A
11. D	26. C	41. D	56. A	71. D
12. C	27. C	42. C	57. D	72. B
13. B	28. D	43. C	58. B	73. D
14. C	29. B	44. A	59. A	74. C
15. B	30. B	45. B	60. C	75. D

Chapter 5 Answer Key

1. B	6. A	11. A	16. B	21. C
2. A	7. B	12. B	17. A	22. C
3. D	8. D	13. D	18. C	23. D
4. D	9. D	14. D	19. D	24. B
5. A	10. D	15. A	20. B	25. D

Chapter 6 Answer Key

1. D	27. C	53. D	79. B	105. C
2. B	28. C	54. C	80. B	106. B
3. C	29. B	55. B	81. A	107. C
4. B	30. B	56. A	82. C	108. C
5. C	31. B	57. C	83. D	109. B
6. A	32. A	58. C	84. A	110. A
7. B	33. B	59. A	85. B	111. C
8. C	34. D	60. C	86. D	112. C
9. D	35. C	61. D	87. B	113. B
10. A	36. A	62. A	88. C	114. D
11. A	37. A	63. C	89. C	115. B
12. D	38. D	64. A	90. D	116. A
13. C	39. B	65. B	91. C	117. C
14. B	40. B	66. A	92. C	118. C
15. C	41. C	67. B	93. B	119. C
16. D	42. A	68. D	94. B	120. C
17. C	43. C	69. A	95. D	121. C
18. A	44. D	70. C	96. C	122. D
19. B	45. B	71. A	97. C	123. B
20. D	46. C	72. B	98. D	124. A
21. C	47. B	73. C	99. B	125. B
22. B	48. C	74. B	100. B	126. B
23. B	49. A	75. B	101. C	127. C
24. A	50. D	76. A	102. D	128. C
25. B	51. B	77. C	103. C	129. B
26. D	52. C	78. C	104. A	130. B
				131. C

Chapter 7 Answer Key

1. B	11. D	21. A	31. B	41. D
2. A	12. C	22. D	32. A	42. A
3. A	13. A	23. D	33. D	43. B
4. D	14. D	24. B	34. C	44. B
5. D	15. A	25. A	35. A	45. D
6. A	16. D	26. D	36. D	46. B
7. A	17. A	27. A	37. A	47. B
8. B	18. B	28. D	38. B	48. C
9. D	19. A	29. A	39. A	49. A
10. A	20. B	30. C	40. C	50. A

Chapter 8 Answer Key

1. B	11. C	21. B	31. A	41. A
2. A	12. B	22. B	32. C	42. D
3. C	13. C	23. B	33. B	43. D
4. D	14. A	24. B	34. D	44. C
5. D	15. D	25. C	35. B	45. B
6. A	16. B	26. C	36. A	46. D
7. C	17. B	27. C	37. A	47. D
8. A	18. A	28. A	38. B	48. B
9. A	19. D	29. B	39. C	49. B
10. C	20. D	30. D	40. A	

Chapter 9 Answer Key

1. C	11. C	21. A	31. D	41. B
2. D	12. B	22. C	32. B	42. D
3. B	13. B	23. B	33. B	43. C
4. C	14. C	24. B	34. D	44. B
5. B	15. D	25. C	35. A	45. A
6. A	16. D	26. C	36. B	46. D
7. C	17. C	27. C	37. D	47. A
8. B	18. B	28. A	38. D	48. C
9. C	19. C	29. C	39. B	49. B
10. D	20. D	30. B	40. A	50. D

Chapter 10 Answer Key

1. B	11. B	21. A	31. D	41. C
2. B	12. C	22. A	32. D	42. A
3. C	13. B	23. A	33. B	43. C
4. A	14. A	24. D	34. A	44. B
5. A	15. A	25. B	35. C	45. B
6. D	16. B	26. B	36. B	46. D
7. A	17. B	27. B	37. B	47. C
8. C	18. D	28. A	38. C	48. D
9. C	19. D	29. B	39. D	49. C
10. B	20. C	30. C	40. A	50. A

Chapter 11 Answer Key

1. A	21. D	41. B	61. D	81. A
2. C	22. C	42. A	62. D	82. D
3. B	23. B	43. A	63. C	83. B
4. D	24. D	44. B	64. A	84. A
5. D	25. A	45. A	65. B	85. C
6. A	26. B	46. A	66. C	86. A
7. C	27. C	47. A	67. C	87. B
8. A	28. D	48. D	68. D	88. C
9. C	29. C	49. B	69. D	89. A
10. B	30. B	50. B	70. D	90. D
11. A	31. A	51. A	71. A	91. C
12. B	32. D	52. C	72. D	92. C
13. A	33. B	53. B	73. D	93. C
14. D	34. C	54. D	74. B	94. A
15. C	35. A	55. C	75. A	95. B
16. A	36. B	56. C	76. C	96. C
17. B	37. C	57. A	77. C	97. D
18. C	38. B	58. C	78. D	98. D
19. B	39. D	59. B	79. A	99. B
20. D	40. C	60. C	80. B	100. B

Chapter 12 Answer Key

1. B	9. D	17. C	25. A	33. C
2. D	10. C	18. D	26. B	34. C
3. C	11. A	19. A	27. C	35. D
4. A	12. B	20. B	28. A	36. B
5. B	13. B	21. B	29. D	37. B
6. D	14. D	22. A	30. A	38. C
7. D	15. C	23. C	31. C	39. A
8. A	16. B	24. D	32. D	40. D

Chapter 13 Answer Key

1. B	11. B	21. B	31. D	41. D
2. A	12. A	22. D	32. A	42. A
3. B	13. C	23. D	33. D	43. D
4. B	14. B	24. A	34. B	44. C
5. D	15. D	25. B	35. A	45. D
6. A	16. A	26. C	36. A	46. B
7. B	17. C	27. A	37. C	47. C
8. A	18. B	28. B	38. C	48. C
9. B	19. D	29. A	39. B	49. B
10. D	20. A	30. B	40. D	50. C

Chapter 14 Answer Key

1. C	6. A	11. B	16. B	21. A
2. D	7. C	12. C	17. C	22. B
3. B	8. C	13. C	18. D	23. B
4. A	9. D	14. D	19. D	24. C
5. C	10. B	15. A	20. B	25. A

CHAPTER 15 Answer Key

1. B	11. C	21. A	31. B	41. C
2. A	12. A	22. A	32. C	42. B
3. D	13. B	23. D	33. A	43. A
4. A	14. B	24. B	34. B	44. B
5. A	15. D	25. B	35. B	45. B
6. A	16. C	26. B	36. B	46. A
7. C	17. A	27. A	37. D	47. C
8. B	18. C	28. C	38. D	48. A
9. D	19. B	29. A	39. D	49. B
10. A	20. C	30. D	40. A	50. C

Chapter 16 Answer Key

1. B	11. A	21. B	31. D	41. D
2. C	12. C	22. A	32. A	42. A
3. A	13. C	23. A	33. B	43. B
4. A	14. B	24. C	34. A	44. A
5. C	15. C	25. B	35. B	45. C
6. B	16. D	26. B	36. D	46. D
7. D	17. C	27. A	37. A	47. A
8. D	18. A	28. A	38. C	48. D
9. B	19. C	29. B	39. B	49. B
10. C	20. D	30. B	40. A	50. A

Chapter 17 Answer Key

1. C	10. C	19. C	28. C	37. A
2. B	11. B	20. D	29. B	38. C
3. A	12. D	21. B	30. A	39. C
4. D	13. A	22. A	31. D	40. B
5. B	14. D	23. B	32. C	41. C
6. B	15. B	24. B	33. D	42. A
7. A	16. B	25. C	34. C	43. D
8. D	17. A	26. A	35. A	44. B
9. B	18. A	27. B	36. B	45. B

Chapter 18 Answer Key

1. B	7. A	13. C	19. A	25. B
2. C	8. C	14. A	20. B	26. B
3. B	9. B	15. B	21. D	27. C
4. D	10. A	16. D	22. D	28. A
5. A	11. C	17. B	23. C	29. D
6. A	12. D	18. C	24. A	30. C

Chapter 19 Answer Key

1. C	8. A	15. B	22. B	29. C
2. B	9. D	16. A	23. D	30. A
3. C	10. C	17. C	24. A	31. A
4. D	11. D	18. D	25. C	32. D
5. D	12. B	19. A	26. B	33. B
6. A	13. C	20. C	27. A	34. D
7. B	14. C	21. D	28. D	35. A

Chapter 20 Answer Key

1. A	8. B	15. D	22. B	29. D
2. C	9. A	16. B	23. B	30. B
3. B	10. B	17. B	24. C	31. A
4. D	11. B	18. A	25. C	32. D
5. C	12. A	19. B	26. A	33. D
6. C	13. B	20. D	27. D	34. B
7. D	14. B	21. D	28. C	35. B

Chapter 21 Answer Key

1. B	11. A	21. C	31. A	41. D
2. C	12. B	22. A	32. B	42. B
3. A	13. D	23. C	33. C	43. C
4. C	14. C	24. C	34. B	44. A
5. A	15. C	25. C	35. C	45. D
6. D	16. B	26. B	36. C	46. D
7. D	17. A	27. B	37. A	47. A
8. B	18. A	28. D	38. A	48. D
9. A	19. C	29. D	39. C	49. A
10. B	20. D	30. D	40. C	50. A

Chapter 22 Answer Key

1. D	22. C	43. D	64. D	85. D
2. A	23. C	44. B	65. A	86. D
3. C	24. A	45. A	66. A	87. A
4. B	25. D	46. B	67. A	88. A
5. A	26. D	47. C	68. B	89. D
6. C	27. B	48. B	69. C	90. B
7. D	28. C	49. D	70. D	91. A
8. A	29. A	50. A	71. C	92. D
9. D	30. A	51. B	72. C	93. C
10. B	31. A	52. D	73. C	94. C
11. C	32. A	53. B	74. A	95. D
12. A	33. C	54. A	75. D	96. B
13. D	34. B	55. C	76. B	97. A
14. B	35. A	56. A	77. D	98. C
15. C	36. B	57. C	78. C	99. B
16. D	37. C	58. A	79. A	100. A
17. A	38. B	59. B	80. C	101. A
18. A	39. A	60. D	81. D	102. C
19. B	40. C	61. B	82. A	103. D
20. D	41. B	62. B	83. B	104. A
21. A	42. B	63. B	84. B	

Chapter 23 Answer Key

1. A	21. D	41. A	61. C	81. C
2. A	22. A	42. A	62. C	82. B
3. B	23. C	43. C	63. A	83. B
4. C	24. D	44. D	64. B	84. A
5. A	25. A	45. A	65. D	85. D
6. C	26. A	46. A	66. B	86. A
7. D	27. B	47. C	67. A	87. B
8. B	28. B	48. B	68. A	88. D
9. C	29. C	49. B	69. C	89. A
10. B	30. A	50. D	70. B	90. B
11. C	31. C	51. C	71. C	91. B
12. B	32. B	52. A	72. A	92. B
13. D	33. A	53. B	73. D	93. D
14. B	34. B	54. D	74. B	94. C
15. C	35. D	55. D	75. A	95. D
16. A	36. A	56. B	76. B	96. A
17. C	37. C	57. D	77. A	97. B
18. B	38. B	58. A	78. B	98. C
19. B	39. B	59. A	79. D	99. D
20. A	40. B	60. D	80. C	

Chapter 24 Answer Key

1. A	21. A	41. D	61. B	81. B
2. B	22. B	42. C	62. A	82. A
3. B	23. B	43. B	63. A	83. B
4. C	24. A	44. C	64. B	84. D
5. C	25. C	45. B	65. D	85. B
6. A	26. D	46. A	66. C	86. D
7. A	27. B	47. C	67. D	87. B
8. C	28. C	48. D	68. A	88. A
9. D	29. A	49. A	69. D	89. C
10. D	30. D	50. A	70. B	90. D
11. B	31. C	51. B	71. A	91. A
12. B	32. B	52. C	72. D	92. C
13. C	33. C	53. C	73. C	93. C
14. A	34. B	54. D	74. A	94. C
15. B	35. B	55. B	75. B	95. D
16. D	36. A	56. A	76. D	96. B
17. C	37. C	57. B	77. C	97. A
18. A	38. A	58. D	78. A	98. B
19. D	39. A	59. A	79. C	99. D
20. A	40. A	60. C	80. A	100. A

Chapter 25 Answer Key

1. C	14. A	27. B	40. B	53. C
2. A	15. A	28. A	41. A	54. D
3. B	16. A	29. D	42. D	55. B
4. A	17. C	30. D	43. A	56. B
5. D	18. D	31. C	44. A	57. A
6. B	19. C	32. D	45. D	58. A
7. D	20. A	33. B	46. C	59. A
8. A	21. A	34. D	47. B	60. D
9. C	22. D	35. A	48. C	61. A
10. A	23. B	36. A	49. A	62. A
11. C	24. B	37. B	50. A	63. B
12. D	25. C	38. A	51. B	64. C
13. B	26. A	39. C	52. C	65. D

Chapter 26 Answer Key

1. C	7. A	13. B	19. B	25. B
2. C	8. D	14. A	20. D	26. B
3. A	9. B	15. B	21. A	27. B
4. B	10. B	16. A	22. C	28. A
5. D	11. D	17. C	23. D	29. D
6. C	12. C	18. D	24. A	30. C

Chapter 27 Answer Key

1. C	11. A	21. C	31. A	41. A
2. A	12. B	22. D	32. B	42. A
3. B	13. B	23. A	33. B	43. A
4. B	14. D	24. C	34. A	44. B
5. A	15. B	25. D	35. A	45. D
6. C	16. D	26. B	36. A	46. B
7. C	17. B	27. B	37. C	47. B
8. B	18. A	28. D	38. B	48. C
9. A	19. A	29. C	39. B	49. D
10. B	20. C	30. C	40. D	50. B

Chapter 28 Answer Key

1. A	11. D	21. A	31. A	41. A
2. C	12. C	22. C	32. B	42. C
3. B	13. B	23. C	33. C	43. D
4. C	14. C	24. C	34. B	44. B
5. B	15. A	25. A	35. C	45. B
6. C	16. C	26. C	36. C	46. A
7. B	17. B	27. A	37. B	47. A
8. C	18. A	28. D	38. C	48. C
9. A	19. C	29. C	39. B	49. D
10. B	20. C	30. C	40. C	50. B

Chapter 29 Answer Key

1. A	17. A	33. D	49. C	65. B
2. C	18. B	34. A	50. C	66. D
3. C	19. A	35. B	51. D	67. B
4. D	20. C	36. A	52. A	68. C
5. A	21. A	37. B	53. A	69. A
6. B	22. D	38. D	54. C	70. A
7. D	23. A	39. C	55. B	71. D
8. C	24. B	40. D	56. A	72. A
9. C	25. A	41. C	57. B	73. C
10. A	26. D	42. A	58. D	74. C
11. A	27. D	43. B	59. A	75. A
12. B	28. B	44. B	60. C	76. C
13. D	29. B	45. C	61. D	77. B
14. A	30. B	46. B	62. D	78. B
15. B	31. D	47. A	63. A	79. A
16. B	32. A	48. B	64. A	80. A

Chapter 30 Answer Key

1. B	11. B	21. C	31. C	41. B
2. A	12. C	22. A	32. C	42. C
3. B	13. A	23. B	33. D	43. B
4. D	14. A	24. B	34. B	44. C
5. D	15. A	25. A	35. B	45. B
6. D	16. D	26. D	36. A	46. C
7. C	17. D	27. D	37. B	47. B
8. B	18. C	28. B	38. A	48. C
9. B	19. C	29. A	39. D	49. A
10. D	20. C	30. A	40. C	50. B

Chapter 31 Answer Key

1. B	11. B	21. D	31. C	41. B
2. B	12. A	22. B	32. D	42. C
3. A	13. C	23. A	33. C	43. A
4. C	14. D	24. B	34. C	44. B
5. C	15. C	25. B	35. C	45. C
6. A	16. B	26. D	36. B	46. D
7. B	17. C	27. C	37. D	47. B
8. D	18. D	28. A	38. C	48. A
9. C	19. A	29. B	39. C	49. D
10. A	20. A	30. A	40. D	50. B

Chapter 32 Answer Key

1. C	8. C	15. B	22. D	29. D
2. B	9. A	16. C	23. C	30. A
3. D	10. C	17. B	24. B	31. A
4. C	11. D	18. A	25. C	32. B
5. B	12. A	19. A	26. D	33. C
6. D	13. C	20. B	27. B	34. B
7. B	14. B	21. C	28. C	35. A

Chapter 33 Answer Key

1. B	13. A	25. B	37. C	49. B
2. A	14. C	26. A	38. A	50. C
3. B	15. D	27. A	39. D	51. B
4. A	16. D	28. C	40. C	52. C
5. B	17. D	29. B	41. D	53. A
6. D	18. B	30. D	42. B	54. C
7. D	19. B	31. B	43. C	55. B
8. A	20. B	32. A	44. B	56. D
9. C	21. B	33. A	45. A	57. B
10. D	22. C	34. C	46. B	58. A
11. A	23. D	35. B	47. A	59. D
12. B	24. C	36. C	48. D	60. B

Chapter 34 Answer Key

1. C	11. B	21. B	31. D	41. B
2. A	12. A	22. A	32. B	42. A
3. D	13. C	23. C	33. D	43. A
4. A	14. B	24. A	34. A	44. C
5. B	15. D	25. D	35. B	45. B
6. B	16. A	26. D	36. C	46. B
7. A	17. D	27. D	37. C	47. D
8. D	18. C	28. C	38. D	48. C
9. C	19. A	29. B	39. A	49. C
10. D	20. C	30. A	40. D	50. A

Chapter 35 Answer Key

1. C	9. C	17. C	25. B	33. A
2. B	10. B	18. B	26. A	34. A
3. B	11. C	19. B	27. D	35. B
4. C	12. C	20. C	28. A	36. C
5. C	13. D	21. A	29. B	37. B
6. D	14. C	22. D	30. B	38. D
7. B	15. D	23. B	31. C	39. C
8. C	16. B	24. A	32. C	40. A

Chapter 36 Answer Key

1. D	13. C	25. C	37. A	49. B
2. A	14. C	26. B	38. B	50. A
3. B	15. D	27. D	39. B	51. C
4. C	16. A	28. A	40. C	52. D
5. B	17. B	29. B	41. A	53. C
6. A	18. A	30. B	42. A	54. A
7. D	19. C	31. D	43. D	55. B
8. A	20. A	32. D	44. C	56. C
9. D	21. C	33. A	45. B	57. A
10. B	22. D	34. C	46. A	58. B
11. A	23. A	35. C	47. A	59. B
12. C	24. B	36. D	48. D	60. A

Chapter 37 Answer Key

1. A	13. C	25. C	37. B	49. A
2. B	14. D	26. D	38. C	50. A
3. D	15. B	27. C	39. B	51. C
4. C	16. B	28. C	40. D	52. B
5. A	17. C	29. B	41. A	53. D
6. D	18. C	30. C	42. C	54. A
7. B	19. A	31. A	43. D	55. D
8. B	20. D	32. A	44. A	56. C
9. C	21. A	33. B	45. C	57. D
10. A	22. B	34. D	46. C	58. B
11. D	23. A	35. B	47. B	59. C
12. B	24. B	36. B	48. D	60. C

Chapter 38 Answer Key

1. C	13. D	25. C	37. B	49. C
2. B	14. D	26. B	38. C	50. D
3. A	15. B	27. C	39. C	51. B
4. D	16. B	28. C	40. A	52. A
5. D	17. A	29. D	41. C	53. D
6. C	18. A	30. A	42. A	54. B
7. A	19. B	31. C	43. D	55. B
8. A	20. C	32. C	44. B	56. A
9. C	21. C	33. D	45. A	57. C
10. D	22. B	34. A	46. B	58. A
11. C	23. A	35. B	47. D	59. B
12. B	24. D	36. D	48. A	60. A

Chapter 39 Answer Key

1. B	13. B	25. B	37. D	49. C
2. C	14. D	26. C	38. A	50. B
3. D	15. C	27. C	39. A	51. A
4. B	16. B	28. A	40. B	52. C
5. C	17. A	29. D	41. D	53. C
6. C	18. B	30. D	42. D	54. B
7. D	19. C	31. B	43. C	55. C
8. C	20. A	32. C	44. D	56. D
9. B	21. C	33. C	45. B	57. A
10. D	22. B	34. B	46. A	58. B
11. B	23. C	35. C	47. C	59. A
12. B	24. B	36. A	48. B	60. B

Chapter 40 Answer Key

1.	B	13.	A	25.	C	37.	C	49.	C
2.	A	14.	D	26.	D	38.	D	50.	B
3.	A	15.	C	27.	A	39.	C	51.	D
4.	B	16.	B	28.	D	40.	C	52.	C
5.	C	17.	A	29.	C	41.	C	53.	B
6.	D	18.	B	30.	B	42.	D	54.	A
7.	B	19.	D	31.	D	43.	A	55.	C
8.	A	20.	D	32.	A	44.	B	56.	A
9.	B	21.	A	33.	D	45.	B	57.	C
10.	D	22.	B	34.	B	46.	C	58.	D
11.	A	23.	B	35.	D	47.	A	59.	C
12.	D	24.	C	36.	A	48.	D	60.	A

Chapter 41 Answer Key

1.	A	7.	C	13.	B	19.	A	25.	D
2.	B	8.	B	14.	A	20.	B	26.	C
3.	D	9.	A	15.	C	21.	A	27.	A
4.	C	10.	C	16.	B	22.	D	28.	B
5.	C	11.	A	17.	C	23.	C	29.	C
6.	B	12.	D	18.	A	24.	B	30.	D

Chapter 42 Answer Key

1.	D	11.	A	21.	C	31.	C	41.	A
2.	A	12.	C	22.	B	32.	D	42.	C
3.	D	13.	D	23.	D	33.	B	43.	D
4.	A	14.	B	24.	A	34.	A	44.	A
5.	D	15.	A	25.	B	35.	A	45.	A
6.	B	16.	D	26.	C	36.	B	46.	B
7.	C	17.	D	27.	A	37.	D	47.	A
8.	A	18.	C	28.	B	38.	B	48.	D
9.	C	19.	A	29.	C	39.	C	49.	C
10.	D	20.	B	30.	D	40.	B	50.	C

Chapter 43 Answer Key

1. D	11. B	21. B	31. D	41. B
2. C	12. D	22. A	32. B	42. D
3. A	13. A	23. A	33. A	43. B
4. A	14. A	24. C	34. A	44. A
5. C	15. B	25. C	35. B	45. B
6. D	16. A	26. A	36. D	46. C
7. B	17. C	27. B	37. C	47. B
8. B	18. A	28. B	38. C	48. C
9. A	19. B	29. D	39. A	49. C
10. D	20. D	30. A	40. D	50. B

Chapter 44 Answer Key

1. C	13. A	25. C	37. A	49. B
2. C	14. D	26. A	38. D	50. D
3. D	15. D	27. D	39. C	51. D
4. D	16. A	28. B	40. B	52. C
5. B	17. B	29. B	41. A	53. B
6. A	18. B	30. B	42. B	54. A
7. B	19. B	31. C	43. C	55. A
8. A	20. D	32. A	44. D	56. B
9. D	21. A	33. C	45. A	57. C
10. A	22. D	34. D	46. A	58. B
11. C	23. A	35. C	47. D	59. B
12. B	24. C	36. D	48. C	

Chapter 45 Answer Key

1. D	11. D	21. C	31. A	41. C
2. B	12. C	22. B	32. D	42. B
3. B	13. A	23. D	33. D	43. A
4. A	14. D	24. A	34. D	44. A
5. B	15. B	25. B	35. C	45. B
6. D	16. C	26. C	36. B	46. D
7. A	17. C	27. A	37. B	47. C
8. B	18. D	28. B	38. C	48. D
9. C	19. A	29. D	39. D	49. B
10. B	20. D	30. B	40. D	50. C

Chapter 46 Answer Key

1. C	11. B	21. D	31. D	41. B
2. A	12. C	22. B	32. C	42. C
3. B	13. B	23. A	33. A	43. A
4. C	14. A	24. A	34. B	44. A
5. A	15. C	25. A	35. D	45. C
6. D	16. D	26. B	36. A	46. B
7. A	17. D	27. C	37. D	47. D
8. B	18. A	28. B	38. B	48. D
9. D	19. B	29. A	39. A	49. B
10. A	20. A	30. B	40. A	50. B

Chapter 47 Answer Key

1. A	11. D	21. A	31. B	41. A
2. B	12. B	22. A	32. D	42. C
3. D	13. C	23. A	33. A	43. D
4. D	14. D	24. C	34. B	44. C
5. D	15. D	25. B	35. B	45. C
6. A	16. A	26. D	36. B	46. D
7. B	17. B	27. A	37. D	47. B
8. A	18. C	28. A	38. A	48. A
9. C	19. C	29. A	39. C	49. C
10. A	20. C	30. D	40. B	50. A

Chapter 48 Answer Key

1. B	11. A	21. D	31. C	41. A
2. D	12. D	22. B	32. D	42. A
3. D	13. D	23. B	33. B	43. B
4. C	14. C	24. D	34. D	44. C
5. A	15. B	25. D	35. D	45. A
6. C	16. C	26. C	36. A	46. B
7. B	17. C	27. A	37. C	47. C
8. B	18. C	28. B	38. D	48. C
9. D	19. A	29. C	39. B	49. D
10. B	20. A	30. A	40. D	50. A

Chapter 49 Answer Key

1.	C	22.	B	43.	D	64.	D	85.	C
2.	C	23.	B	44.	B	65.	A	86.	B
3.	A	24.	D	45.	C	66.	D	87.	C
4.	C	25.	C	46.	B	67.	C	88.	A
5.	D	26.	A	47.	B	68.	D	89.	D
6.	B	27.	B	48.	B	69.	C	90.	D
7.	A	28.	C	49.	D	70.	B	91.	C
8.	B	29.	D	50.	D	71.	A	92.	B
9.	D	30.	A	51.	A	72.	D	93.	B
10.	A	31.	D	52.	A	73.	B	94.	D
11.	D	32.	C	53.	D	74.	B	95.	B
12.	C	33.	C	54.	B	75.	B	96.	A
13.	D	34.	C	55.	D	76.	A	97.	D
14.	B	35.	C	56.	B	77.	D	98.	B
15.	C	36.	B	57.	A	78.	A	99.	A
16.	B	37.	C	58.	A	79.	B	100.	A
17.	D	38.	B	59.	D	80.	B	101.	D
18.	D	39.	B	60.	C	81.	D	102.	D
19.	C	40.	D	61.	C	82.	B	103.	B
20.	D	41.	D	62.	D	83.	C	104.	B
21.	D	42.	D	63.	D	84.	B		

Chapter 50 Answer Key

1.	B	6.	A	11.	B	16.	D	21.	A
2.	C	7.	B	12.	A	17.	B	22.	C
3.	B	8.	C	13.	D	18.	C	23.	B
4.	A	9.	D	14.	B	19.	A	24.	D
5.	B	10.	A	15.	D	20.	A	25.	D

Chapter 51 Answer Key

1.	D	8.	D	15.	D	22.	A	29.	C
2.	B	9.	A	16.	C	23.	C	30.	A
3.	B	10.	B	17.	C	24.	B	31.	B
4.	C	11.	C	18.	C	25.	B	32.	A
5.	D	12.	B	19.	D	26.	A	33.	D
6.	C	13.	C	20.	B	27.	D	34.	C
7.	A	14.	A	21.	D	28.	C	35.	C

Chapter 52 Answer Key

1. B	7. B	13. D	19. D	25. C
2. B	8. B	14. A	20. C	26. A
3. C	9. D	15. B	21. D	27. A
4. A	10. C	16. C	22. B	28. A
5. A	11. A	17. D	23. A	29. D
6. C	12. D	18. B	24. C	30. A

Set-Up Instructions for
Elling/*The Paramedic Review*

Instructions:

1. Insert disk into CD ROM player
2. From the Start Menu, choose *RUN*
3. In the Open text box, enter *d: setup.exe* then click the OK
   button.(Substitute the letter of your CD ROM drive for d:)
4. Follow the installation prompts from there.

System Requirements:

• Microsoft®Windows 95® or better • 486 Mhz CPU (Pentium recommended) • 16 MB or more of RAM
• Double-spin CD-ROM drive • 10 MB or more of free hard drive space • 256 color display or better

Microsoft® is a registered trademark and Windows™ and
NT™ are trademarks of Microsoft Corporation.
